Next-Gen Blood Purification

Silvia De Rosa • Sergio Lassola
Editors

Next-Gen Blood Purification

Advancing Technologies and Emerging Trends in Hemofiltration and Dialysis

Springer

Editors
Silvia De Rosa
Anesthesiology and Intensive Care Medicine
CisMed University of Trento
Trento, Italy

Sergio Lassola
Anesthesia and Intensive Care
Ospedale Santa Chiara
Trento, Italy

ISBN 978-3-032-27032-0 ISBN 978-3-032-27033-7 (eBook)
https://doi.org/10.1007/978-3-032-27033-7

This Springer imprint is published by the registered company Springer Nature Switzerland AG
The registered company address is: Gewerbestrasse 11, 6330 Cham, Switzerland

To our parents, whose love, sacrifices, and constant encouragement have been the foundation of everything we have achieved.

Foreword

Advances in extracorporeal blood purification technologies have significantly transformed the landscape of critical care and nephrology over the past decades. What began primarily as renal replacement therapy for patients with acute or chronic kidney failure has progressively evolved into a broader platform capable of supporting multiple organ systems and modulating complex pathophysiological processes.

In recent years, the increasing understanding of systemic inflammation, immune dysregulation, and multi-organ failure has driven the development of innovative extracorporeal approaches aimed at removing inflammatory mediators, toxins, and other harmful circulating factors. These emerging strategies are opening new therapeutic perspectives in conditions such as sepsis, acute respiratory distress syndrome, and multi-organ dysfunction.

The volume *Next-Gen Blood Purification: Advancing Technologies and Emerging Trends in Hemofiltration and Dialysis* provides a timely and comprehensive overview of the current state of the art in this rapidly evolving field. The editors and contributing authors bring together a wide range of expertise, spanning nephrology, intensive care medicine, bioengineering, and translational research. This multidisciplinary approach reflects the complexity of modern extracorporeal therapies and the collaborative efforts required to further advance patient care.

The chapters included in this book explore both the scientific foundations and the clinical applications of blood purification technologies, while also addressing emerging innovations such as artificial intelligence, nanotechnology, and personalized extracorporeal therapies. Such perspectives are particularly relevant in an era where precision medicine and technological integration are becoming increasingly important in critical care.

As President of the Italian Society of Anesthesia, Analgesia, Resuscitation and Intensive Care (SIAARTI), I strongly welcome initiatives that foster scientific exchange and contribute to the dissemination of knowledge in fields that have a direct impact on the management of critically ill patients.

This book represents an important contribution to the ongoing dialogue between clinicians, researchers, and engineers working to improve extracorporeal therapies and patient outcomes.

I hope that this volume will serve as a valuable reference for clinicians, investigators, and trainees interested in the future of blood purification technologies and their role in modern critical care medicine.

Professor of Anesthesiology and Intensive Care, University of Parma
Parma, Italy
President, Italian Society of Anesthesia, Analgesia, Resuscitation and Intensive Care (SIAARTI)
Rome, Italy

Elena Bignami

Preface

Extracorporeal blood purification has undergone remarkable development over the past decades, evolving far beyond its original role as a therapy for renal replacement. Advances in membrane technologies, adsorption systems, and integrated extracorporeal support platforms have progressively expanded the clinical applications of these therapies in critical care medicine.

Today, extracorporeal blood purification represents an important therapeutic strategy not only for acute and chronic kidney failure but also for complex conditions such as sepsis, cytokine storm syndromes, and multi-organ dysfunction. The growing understanding of systemic inflammation and immune dysregulation has stimulated the development of innovative extracorporeal approaches aimed at removing harmful mediators, modulating the host response, and supporting organ function.

This volume, *Next-Gen Blood Purification: Advancing Technologies and Emerging Trends in Hemofiltration and Dialysis*, aims to provide a comprehensive overview of the current state of the art and emerging perspectives in this rapidly evolving field. The book brings together contributions from international experts with different backgrounds, including intensive care medicine, nephrology, biomedical engineering, and translational research.

The chapters address fundamental principles of blood purification, innovative adsorption technologies, extracorporeal CO_2 removal, multi-organ support systems, and emerging applications involving artificial intelligence and advanced bioengineering. Particular attention is also devoted to clinical applications in infectious diseases, organ failure, and critical illness, as well as to the regulatory and ethical aspects surrounding the development of next-generation extracorporeal devices.

The multidisciplinary nature of this book reflects the complexity of modern extracorporeal therapies, which require close collaboration among clinicians, engineers, and researchers. By bringing together these different perspectives, the aim of this volume is to contribute to the advancement of knowledge and to support the development of innovative therapeutic strategies for critically ill patients.

We would like to sincerely thank all the authors who contributed their expertise and dedication to this project, as well as the editorial team at Springer Nature for their support throughout the development of this volume.

We hope that this book will serve as a useful resource for clinicians, researchers, and trainees interested in extracorporeal therapies and their expanding role in modern critical care medicine.

Trento, Italy Silvia De Rosa
Trento, Italy Sergio Lassola

Acknowledgments

The editors would like to express their sincere gratitude to all the authors who contributed to this volume. Their expertise, dedication, and scientific insight made it possible to develop a comprehensive overview of current advances and emerging perspectives in extracorporeal blood purification.

We are also grateful to the many colleagues and collaborators who have contributed, directly or indirectly, to the development of the ideas and research presented in this book. Their work continues to advance knowledge and innovation in the field of critical care and extracorporeal therapies.

Special thanks are extended to the editorial and production team at Springer Nature for their support and guidance throughout the preparation of this volume.

Finally, we would like to acknowledge the commitment of clinicians, researchers, and healthcare professionals who work every day to improve the care of critically ill patients. Their dedication remains the true driving force behind the progress of modern medicine.

Contents

Introduction: The Evolution and Future of Blood Purification Technologies

1

Sergio Lassola and Silvia De Rosa

1.1 Introduction

For decades, Professors Claudio Ronco and Rinaldo Bellomo have been at the forefront of this discipline, not only using and refining these techniques at the bedside but also meticulously documenting their historical evolution [1]. Their work has traced the journey from Willem Kolff's pioneering rotating drum kidney in the 1940s, through the shift from cellulose sheets to high-performance synthetic membranes, to the development of sorbent-based systems and hybrid extracorporeal platforms [2]. At the same time, they have championed the exploration of new technologies, multi-layer asymmetric membranes, biocompatible polymer blends, nanostructured sorbents, and, more recently, wearable and portable blood purification devices. Their research bridges engineering innovation and clinical application, always aiming to improve safety, efficiency, and patient outcomes [3]. The goal of this chapter is to connect that historical knowledge with the technological advances shaping the present and future of extracorporeal therapy. By understanding where we started, and how innovators like Ronco and Bellomo have steered the field, we can better appreciate the current state of the art and imagine the next generation of solutions for life-saving blood purification.

S. Lassola (✉)
Anesthesia and Intensive Care, Santa Chiara Hospital, Azienda Provinciale per i Servizi Sanitari di Trento, Trento, Italy
e-mail: sergio.lassola@apss.tn.it

S. De Rosa
Anesthesia and Intensive Care, Santa Chiara Hospital, Azienda Provinciale per i Servizi Sanitari di Trento, Trento, Italy

Centre for Medical Sciences, University of Trento, Trento, Italy
e-mail: silvia.derosa@unitn.it

S. De Rosa, S. Lassola (eds.), *Next-Gen Blood Purification*,
https://doi.org/10.1007/978-3-032-27033-7_1

1.2 Principles of Solute Removal

In clinical settings, blood purification techniques achieve molecular solute separation primarily through membrane-based processes, such as diffusion, convection, or a combination of both, and through adsorptive mechanisms [3]. The term dialysis refers to the exchange process that occurs between two compartments: the blood and the dialysis fluid, separated by a semipermeable membrane. This exchange can take place via a concentration gradient (diffusion), as seen in standard hemodialysis (HD); through hydrostatic pressure (convection), as in hemofiltration (HF); or by combining both mechanisms, as in hemodiafiltration (HDF) [4].

The membrane plays a key role in removing toxic solutes (TS) and excess water during this process. Its properties, including material composition, structure, biophysical characteristics, pore size, permeability, and biocompatibility, are critical in determining the effectiveness and safety of dialysis. Therefore, membrane geometry is essential for optimizing solute mass transfer [5].

In contrast, adsorption is a separation process based on the interaction between a solid agent (sorbent) and the solutes. It involves the binding of the adsorbate (the molecule being removed) onto the surface of the adsorbent (the material facilitating adsorption) [6]. This mechanism differs fundamentally from transport processes across a membrane barrier and can overcome the limitations imposed by dialysis membranes, allowing the removal of a broader spectrum of solutes [7]. The evolution of hemodialysis membranes from the first cellophane membranes used in rotating drum kidneys to the widespread adoption of hollow-fiber, high-flux membranes in modern practice has been remarkable [8].

Today's hollow-fiber synthetic membranes are commonly made from polymers such as polysulfone (PS), polyethersulfone, polyacrylonitrile (including sulfonated polyacrylonitrile, AN69), and polymethyl methacrylate (PMMA). Over time, the wall thickness of these membranes has been significantly reduced; modern membranes typically range from 20 to 50 μm in thickness and offer high permeability, which facilitates both diffusive and convective transport. This makes them suitable for high-flux HD and HDF.

1.3 Historical Evolution of Dialysis Membranes

Over the past 80 years, dialysis membranes have undergone a remarkable transformation, from simple cellulose sheets to highly engineered synthetic hollow fibers designed for maximum permeability, precise selectivity, and better patient safety [9].

1.3.1 Early Cellulose Membranes (1943–1960s)

The story begins in *1943*, when Willem Kolff's rotating-drum kidney used regenerated cellulose tubing as its filter [2]. These membranes were *symmetric*, meaning the pore size and density were uniform across the entire wall. In a symmetric membrane, a molecule traveling from one side to the other encounters the same structure all the way through [10]. They typically had wall thicknesses of 5–15 μm, were hydrophilic and inexpensive, and could remove small waste molecules effectively through diffusion. However, their uniform density created higher resistance to water and solute transport, leading to low water permeability, poor clearance of larger "middle" molecules, and immune activation that reduced biocompatibility. In practice, they could only support *low-flux diffusive hemodialysis* [11].

1.3.2 Modified Cellulose (1970s–1980s)

In the *1970s*, chemists tried to improve cellulose by modifying it into cellulose acetate (CA) and cellulose triacetate (CTA) [12]. These changes reduced immune reactions and improved blood compatibility. Most of these membranes remained symmetric, although some CTA versions were made *asymmetric*. In an asymmetric membrane, the structure changes across the wall, with a very thin, dense "skin" layer for filtration, and a thicker, more porous support layer to reduce flow resistance. The improvements were helpful but modest, and these membranes were still mainly low flux [13].

1.3.3 Synthetic Membranes (Late 1970s–1990s)

A major leap came in the *late 1970s* with synthetic materials like PS, PES, polyacrylonitrile (PAN), sulfonated PAN (AN69), and PMMA. These could be made with *asymmetric structures*, which allowed much greater water and solute movement without losing selectivity [14].

- *PS/PES*: Strong, durable, and either hydrophobic or modified to be more hydrophilic; ideal for high-flux dialysis and hemodiafiltration.
- *PMMA*: Symmetric but able to adsorb certain toxins.
- *AN69*: Hydrophilic, reducing protein fouling, and improving compatibility.

1.3.4 Hollow-Fiber Technology (Late 1970s–Present)

Also in the *late 1970s*, switching from flat sheets to thousands of fine hollow fibers was another revolution. This design packed more surface area into a smaller space, reduced the amount of blood needed to fill the dialyzer, and allowed precise control over pore size and wall structure. It's still the basis for most dialyzers today [15].

1.3.5 High-Flux, High Cut-Off, and Medium Cut-Off Membranes (1980s–Present)

In the *1980s*, high-flux membranes boosted clearance of middle molecules like β_2-microglobulin, helping prevent dialysis-related amyloidosis. High cut-off (HCO) membranes went even further, but their high albumin loss meant they were used mainly for special cases like removing myeloma light chains. Medium cut-off

(MCO) membranes, introduced in the *2010s*, were designed as the best of both worlds—strong middle-molecule clearance with minimal albumin leakage—making them the new standard in many settings [16].

1.3.6 Modern Multi-Layer Designs (2010s–Present)

Today's cutting-edge membranes often have three distinct layers: a selective inner skin, a supportive porous core, and an outer protective layer. The *Polyflux* family is a good example, using a blend of polyamide, PES, and PVP to balance hydrophilic and hydrophobic properties. Advances in nanotechnology now allow engineers to fine-tune pore size and shape for the best possible clearance without sacrificing vital proteins [17].

Table 1.1 pulls together the key milestones—from the first cellulose membranes to modern multi-layer designs—showing how materials, structure, and performance have evolved over time, with Polyflux highlighted as a prime example of the latest generation.

Table 1.1 Evolution of dialysis membranes: materials, structure, performance, and clinical use

Historical period	Main material/ examples	Structure	Wall thickness (μm)	Hydraulic permeability (KUF, mL/ m^2·h·mmHg)	Typical clinical application
1940s–1960s	Regenerated cellulose (Cuprophan)	Symmetric	5–15	10–20 (low-flux)	Low-permeability diffusive hemodialysis
1970s–1980s	Modified cellulose (CA, CTA)	Symmetric (CTA sometimes asymmetric)	6–15	10–20 (low-flux)	Improved diffusive HD
1970s–1990s	Synthetic (PS, PES, PAN, AN69, PMMA)	Asymmetric (PMMA symmetric)	20–50	200–400 (high-flux)	High-flux HD, HDF, convective therapies
2000s	Hydrophilized PS/PES, high cut-off membranes	Asymmetric	30–100	600–1100	HDF, β_2-microglobulin removal, light-chain removal
2010s–present	Medium cut-off (MCO, PAES/ PVP), *Polyflux* family	Multi-layer asymmetric	30–50	600–850	HD and HDF with high middle-molecule removal and minimal albumin loss

Abbreviations: *CA* cellulose acetate, *CTA* cellulose triacetate, *PS* polysulfone, *PES* polyethersulfone, *PAN* polyacrylonitrile, *PMMA* polymethyl methacrylate, *PAES* polyarylethersulfone, *PVP* polyvinylpyrrolidone, *HD* hemodialysis, *HDF* hemodiafiltration, *MCO* medium cut-off, *KUF* ultrafiltration coefficient.

1.4 The Polyflux Membrane

The Polyflux membrane family represents a modern generation of high-performance hemodialysis membranes, designed to combine efficient solute removal with excellent biocompatibility. These membranes employ a three-layer asymmetric structure that integrates a selective inner layer, a supportive intermediate matrix (stroma), and an outer protective skin [18]. The inner selective layer serves as the primary filtration barrier, engineered to allow passage of water, electrolytes, and uremic toxins up to middle-molecule size, while minimizing albumin loss [18].

The supportive stroma provides mechanical stability and maintains structural integrity under transmembrane pressure, ensuring consistent pore geometry. The outer skin acts as a protective envelope, reducing shear stress and safeguarding the membrane against handling damage during manufacturing and clinical use. Polyflux membranes are manufactured using a polymer blend of polyamide (PA), polyethersulfone (PES), and polyvinylpyrrolidone (PVP) [18]. This combination balances hydrophilic and hydrophobic properties: PES and PA offer strength, chemical resistance, and durability, while PVP enhances surface hydrophilicity, reducing protein adsorption and platelet activation. The incorporation of PVP throughout the membrane matrix, rather than as a surface coating, contributes to the long-term stability of the hydrophilic character, even after repeated sterilization cycles. Nanotechnology plays a role in the manufacturing process, enabling precise control of pore size distribution within the inner layer [19]. This allows for a high degree of selectivity, maximizing removal of middle molecules such as β_2-microglobulin (11.8 kDa) while retaining essential proteins like albumin (~66 kDa). The optimized pore structure also promotes high ultrafiltration coefficients (KUF) without compromising selectivity, making these membranes suitable for both high-flux hemodialysis and online hemodiafiltration (HDF) [20].

Clinically, the Polyflux family has demonstrated excellent clearance of small and middle molecules while maintaining minimal albumin leakage. High permeability enables enhanced convective transport in HDF, which has been associated with improved patient outcomes, including reduced inflammation and better nutritional status [8]. The balanced hydrophilic—hydrophobic interface reduces complement activation, leukocyte adhesion, and cytokine release, contributing to a favorable biocompatibility profile. The membranes are also designed to maintain performance across a range of treatment modalities, including standard HD, high-flux HD, and HDF. Their mechanical robustness minimizes fiber breakage and maintains stable performance over the treatment session, which is particularly important in high-efficiency convective therapies [21].

The Polyflux membrane family exemplifies the latest stage in the evolution of dialysis membranes, integrating multi-layer asymmetric architecture, polymer blend chemistry, and nanoprecision pore engineering [18]. This combination delivers a balance of high solute clearance, low albumin loss, and superior hemocompatibility, making Polyflux a versatile and clinically reliable choice for contemporary dialysis practice [22].

1.5 Sorbent-Based Blood Purification

Sorbent-based blood purification removes solutes through *adsorption*, in contrast to membrane-based separation, which relies on size exclusion. Adsorption occurs when molecules bind to the sorbent surface via weak ionic bonds, van der Waals forces, or hydrophobic interactions.

Common sorbent materials include *activated carbon*, *synthetic porous resins* (e.g., polystyrene-divinylbenzene), and advanced *nanostructured adsorbents*. These can be natural or synthetic, shaped as beads, granules, flakes, fibers, or cylinders (50 μm–1.2 cm) [1]. High surface-to-mass ratios (300–1200 m^2/g) enhance binding capacity. Pore size defines sorbent classes: *macroporous* (>500 Å), *mesoporous* (20–500 Å), and *microporous* (<20 Å), influencing target solute range [1].

When blood flows through a sorbent, it can interact in three main ways: between particles (interparticle flow), over the external surface (interphase flow), or deep inside the pores (intraphase flow). Adsorption occurs in stages: the solute is transported to the sorbent surface (external mass transfer), diffuses into the internal pore structure (internal mass transfer), moves along the pore surfaces, and finally binds firmly to them [23]. Different forces drive this binding: van der Waals forces are relatively weak and reversible, ionic bonds arise from electrostatic attraction and are typical of ion-exchange resins, while hydrophobic bonds are stronger, relying on the affinity between hydrophobic surfaces [1, 24].

Clinically, sorbents are used in direct hemoperfusion (HP), where blood passes through a sorbent cartridge to remove protein-bound uremic toxins, inflammatory mediators, and poisons. In hybrid systems (HP-HD or HP-CRRT), adsorption is combined with diffusion and convection, expanding the range of toxins removed while maintaining fluid balance [1].

The concept is not new: it began in the mid-1800s with natural zeolites for ion exchange. By the 1930s, synthetic polymeric ion-exchange resins had been developed. Since the 1970s–1980s, coated activated charcoal and polymer resins have been widely used in toxicology, liver failure, sepsis, and autoimmune diseases (see Table 1.2) [1].

Table 1.2 The story of sorbents in extracorporeal therapies

Period	What happened	Why it mattered
1850	Scientists discovered that inorganic aluminosilicates (zeolites) could swap ammonium (NH_4^+) and calcium (Ca^{2+}) ions	First glimpse of how minerals could be used to purify fluids
1910	Zeolites began to be used in water softeners, but they proved unstable in acidic conditions	Highlighted the limits of early sorbent materials
1935	Adams and Holmes created the first organic polymer ion exchange resin	Marked the birth of synthetic sorbents
1948	First published case of hemoperfusion using ionic resin to treat uremia in dogs	Proof-of-concept that sorbents could work inside extracorporeal circuits

(continued)

Table 1.2 (continued)

Period	What happened	Why it mattered
1950s	Synthetic porous polymers like Amberlyte, Duolite, and Dowex entered experimental blood purification	Expanded the toolbox for removing toxins from blood
1958	Ion exchange resin used clinically to treat barbiturate poisoning	Showed sorbents could save lives in acute poisoning cases
1960s	Hemoperfusion with ion exchange resins used to clear salicylate and phenobarbital in dogs	Extended applications beyond uremia
1970s	Coated charcoal and resin therapies became widespread for poisoning treatment	Mainstream adoption in toxicology
1980s	These coated materials applied to broader diseases like liver failure, vasculitis, and autoimmune disorders	Sorbents became a versatile extracorporeal therapy tool

1.6 Wearable and Miniaturized Blood Purification Systems

The wearable artificial kidney (WAK) is an innovative device designed to enable prolonged and frequent dialysis for patients with end-stage renal disease (ESRD). It offers a potential solution to the limitations of conventional dialysis by improving accessibility, mobility, and patient quality of life [25]. Over the years, several WAK prototypes have been developed, each exploring different engineering methods and treatment approaches. An optimal WAK design may emerge from combining the best features of these existing models.

ESRD remains a growing global health concern, with rising incidence and prevalence contributing to significant healthcare costs. Studies show that daily and prolonged dialysis can enhance the quality of life and survival of patients [26]. However, implementing such frequent treatments with traditional dialysis machines is impractical. In this context, wearable hemodialysis offers a promising alternative, allowing patients to undergo treatment with minimal disruption to their daily lives [27].

The current most advanced WAK prototype is the belt-type device developed by Gura and colleagues. It operates by drawing blood through a double-lumen catheter, circulating it via micro-pumps through a dialyzer, and cleansing it using a sorbent-based dialysate regeneration system. This process mimics natural kidney function while maintaining portability [25].

Despite progress, several technical and clinical challenges remain before a fully wearable, practical artificial kidney can become widely available. These challenges include ensuring device safety, miniaturization, battery efficiency, clot prevention, and low toxicity, while also delivering high filtration performance and maintaining electrolyte and acid-base balance [28].

An ideal WAK should be lightweight, biocompatible, ergonomically designed, and easy to use without expert supervision. It must function independently of external power sources, which requires the development of compact, efficient batteries and pumps. Additionally, the device should enable continuous use, allowing patients to sleep, walk, and perform daily activities comfortably [29].

Looking ahead, the future of dialysis aligns with the broader trend toward personalized medicine. The WAK fits into this vision by offering patient-specific, daily treatments. However, its continued development depends not only on overcoming engineering hurdles but also on addressing social, ethical, economic, and legal considerations. Multidisciplinary collaboration is essential, involving engineers, clinicians, biologists, economists, and social scientists working together to meet the complex demands of wearable renal replacement therapy [30].

In summary, while WAK technology has advanced significantly and entered a phase of reliability testing, achieving widespread clinical adoption requires further innovation and cooperation across various fields to deliver a safe, effective, and truly wearable dialysis solution.

1.7 Conclusions

Over the past decades, blood purification has evolved from rudimentary cellulose membranes to sophisticated multi-layer, nanostructured systems and advanced sorbent technologies. These innovations have expanded therapeutic possibilities, improved toxin clearance, and enhanced patient safety. The next generation, driven by Artificial Intelligence, biohybrid designs, implantable devices, and portable platforms, promises to extend treatment beyond traditional renal indications, delivering precision, autonomy, and multi-organ support. Achieving this vision will require close collaboration between engineers, clinicians, material scientists, and industry partners. By uniting technological innovation with clinical insight, the future of blood purification can transform outcomes for patients with kidney failure and beyond.

References

1. Ronco C, Bellomo R. Hemoperfusion: technical aspects and state of the art. Crit Care. 2022;26:135. https://doi.org/10.1186/s13054-022-04009-w.
2. Sharma N, Khav E, Elahmadi A, Ong J, Parag S. Dr. Willem Kolff: the father of the artificial kidney. Cureus. 2024;16:e69098. https://doi.org/10.7759/cureus.69098.
3. Clark WR, Ferrari F, La Manna G, Ronco C. Extracorporeal sorbent technologies: basic concepts and clinical application. In: La Manna G, Ronco C, editors. Contributions to nephrology, vol. 190. S. Karger AG; 2017. p. 43–57. https://doi.org/10.1159/000468911.
4. Erdélyi L, Trásy D. CRRT is more than just continuous renal replacement therapy. Pharmaceuticals. 2024;17:1571. https://doi.org/10.3390/ph17121571.
5. Clark WR, Hamburger RJ, Lysaght MJ. Effect of membrane composition and structure on solute removal and biocompatibility in hemodialysis. Kidney Int. 1999;56:2005–15. https://doi.org/10.1046/j.1523-1755.1999.00784.x.
6. Mahdavi P, Siol A, Thöming J. Adsorption-based removal of pharmaceutical from water: a critical review on adsorbent performance. J Environ Chem Eng. 2025;13:117520. https://doi.org/10.1016/j.jece.2025.117520.
7. Clark WR, Gao D, Neri M, Ronco C. Solute transport in hemodialysis: advances and limitations of current membrane technology. In: Ronco C, editor. Contributions to nephrology, vol. 191. S. Karger AG; 2017. p. 84–99. https://doi.org/10.1159/000479258.

8. Canaud B. Recent advances in dialysis membranes. Curr Opin Nephrol Hypertens. 2021;30:613–22. https://doi.org/10.1097/MNH.0000000000000744.
9. Macleod AM, Campbell M, Cody JD, Daly C, Donaldson C, Grant A, et al. Cellulose, modified cellulose and synthetic membranes in the haemodialysis of patients with end-stage renal disease. Cochrane Database Syst Rev. 2005;2005:CD003234. https://doi.org/10.1002/14651858.CD003234.pub2.
10. Chang X, Zhang C, He Y, Dong X, Jin W, Xu N. A comparative study of the performance of symmetric and asymmetric mixed-conducting membranes. Chin J Chem Eng. 2009;17:562–70. https://doi.org/10.1016/S1004-9541(08)60245-1.
11. García-Rollán M, Sanz-Santos E, Belver C, Bedia J. Key adsorbents and influencing factors in the adsorption of micro- and nanoplastics: a review. J Environ Manag. 2025;383:125394. https://doi.org/10.1016/j.jenvman.2025.125394.
12. Raza A, Farrukh S, Hussain A, Khan I, Othman MHD, Ahsan M. Performance analysis of blended membranes of cellulose acetate with variable degree of acetylation for CO2/CH4 separation. Membranes. 2021;11:245. https://doi.org/10.3390/membranes11040245.
13. Akizawa T, Kinugasa E, Sato Y, Kohjiro S, Naitoh H, Azuma M, et al. Development of a new cellulose triacetate membrane with a microgradient porous structure for hemodialysis. ASAIO J. 1998;44:M584–6. https://doi.org/10.1097/00002480-199809000-00055.
14. Su B, Shi Y, Fu P, Tao Y, Nie S, Zhao C. Clinical evaluation of polyethersulfone high-flux hemodialysis membrane compared to other membranes. J Appl Polym Sci. 2012;124:E91–8. https://doi.org/10.1002/app.35589.
15. Davenport A. The changing face of dialyzer membranes and dialyzers. Semin Dial. 2025;38:25–34. https://doi.org/10.1111/sdi.13161.
16. Zweigart C, Boschetti-de-Fierro A, Hulko M, Nilsson L-G, Beck W, Storr M, et al. Medium cut-off membranes – closer to the natural kidney removal function. Int J Artif Organs. 2017;40:328–34. https://doi.org/10.5301/ijao.5000603.
17. Setiawan L, Wang R, Tan S, Shi L, Fane AG. Fabrication of poly(amide-imide)-polyethersulfone dual layer hollow fiber membranes applied in forward osmosis by combined polyelectrolyte cross-linking and depositions. Desalination. 2013;312:99–106. https://doi.org/10.1016/j.desal.2012.10.032.
18. Ronco C. Evolution of synthetic membranes for blood purification: the case of the Polyflux family. Nephrol Dial Transplant. 2003;18:10vii–20. https://doi.org/10.1093/ndt/gfg1073.
19. Liu M, Yu F, Niu L, Chi H. Advances in nanofiltration membrane pore size adjustment techniques: a review. Environ Funct Mater. 2025:S2773058125000109. https://doi.org/10.1016/j.efmat.2025.02.002.
20. Sakurai K. Biomarkers for evaluation of clinical outcomes of hemodiafiltration. Blood Purif. 2013;35:64–8. https://doi.org/10.1159/000346364.
21. Siagian UWR, Khoiruddin K, Wardani AK, Aryanti PTP, Widiasa IN, Qiu G, et al. High-performance ultrafiltration membrane: recent progress and its application for wastewater treatment. Curr Pollut Rep. 2021;7:448–62. https://doi.org/10.1007/s40726-021-00204-5.
22. Battaglia Y, Shroff R, Meijers B, Nistor I, Alfano G, Franssen C, et al. Haemodiafiltration versus high-flux haemodialysis-a consensus statement from the EuDial Working Group of the ERA. Nephrol Dial Transplant. 2025;40:1590–614. https://doi.org/10.1093/ndt/gfaf024.
23. Alaqarbeh M. Adsorption phenomena: definition, mechanisms, and adsorption types: short review. RHAZES Green Appl Chem. 2021:43–51. https://doi.org/10.48419/IMIST.PRSM/RHAZES-V13.28283.
24. Ricci Z, Romagnoli S, Reis T, Bellomo R, Ronco C. Hemoperfusion in the intensive care unit. Intensive Care Med. 2022;48:1397–408. https://doi.org/10.1007/s00134-022-06810-1.
25. Gura V, Rivara MB, Bieber S, Munshi R, Smith NC, Linke L, et al. A wearable artificial kidney for patients with end-stage renal disease. JCI Insight. 2016;1:e86397. https://doi.org/10.1172/jci.insight.86397.
26. Hu Y-H, Liu Y-L, Meng L-F, Zhang Y-X, Cui W-P. Selection of dialysis methods for end-stage kidney disease patients with diabetes. World J Diabetes. 2024;15:1862–73. https://doi.org/10.4239/wjd.v15.i9.1862.

27. Armignacco P, Lorenzin A, Neri M, Nalesso F, Garzotto F, Ronco C. Wearable devices for blood purification: principles, miniaturization, and technical challenges. Semin Dial. 2015;28:125–30. https://doi.org/10.1111/sdi.12346.
28. Hueso M, Navarro E, Sandoval D, Cruzado JM. Progress in the development and challenges for the use of artificial kidneys and wearable dialysis devices. Kidney Dis. 2019;5:3–10. https://doi.org/10.1159/000492932.
29. Kim JC, Garzotto F, Nalesso F, Cruz D, Kim JH, Kang E, et al. A wearable artificial kidney: technical requirements and potential solutions. Expert Rev Med Devices. 2011;8:567–79. https://doi.org/10.1586/erd.11.33.
30. Chan MM, Sadeghi-Alavijeh O, Evans RD, Davenport A, Nitsch D. The future of nephrology in 2050. Future Healthc J. 2025;12:100236. https://doi.org/10.1016/j.fhj.2025.100236.

Core Principles of Blood Purification: Filtration, Adsorption, and Bioengineering

2

Niamh Corcoran, David Keane, and Bairbre McNicholas

2.1 Introduction

Extracorporeal therapies such as continuous renal replacement therapy (CRRT) are used to support patients with organ failure, inflammatory conditions, or toxidromes. A core component of these therapies is the removal of substances from the blood via transport across a semipermeable membrane, either based on concentration gradient (as in hemodialysis) or pressure gradient (as in hemofiltration). The performance of these therapies depends on characteristics of the membrane, defining their effectiveness in either clearing an injurious state or altering the trajectory of an illness. Clinically suitable membranes must deliver consistent ultrafiltration and withstand transmembrane pressure gradients while maintaining efficient diffusive mass transfer [1].

N. Corcoran
Department of Nephrology, School of Medicine, University of Galway, Galway, Ireland
e-mail: niamh.corcoran2@hse.ie

D. Keane
Department of Nephrology, School of Medicine, University of Galway, Galway, Ireland

CÚRAM Research Ireland Centre for Medical Devices, University of Galway, Galway, Ireland
e-mail: keanedd@universityofgalway.ie

B. McNicholas (✉)
Department of Nephrology, School of Medicine, University of Galway, Galway, Ireland

Department of Anaesthesia and Intensive Care Medicine, School of Medicine, University of Galway, Galway, Ireland
e-mail: bmcnicholas@universityofgalway.ie

S. De Rosa, S. Lassola (eds.), *Next-Gen Blood Purification*,
https://doi.org/10.1007/978-3-032-27033-7_2

Membrane design has evolved considerably since the early use of cellulose filters, progressing to high-flux, high cut-off (HCO), and medium cut-off (MCO) systems to better meet clinical needs. Key material and surface properties, including hydrophobicity, surface charge, and incorporation of functional groups, influence membrane performance and biological interactions [2]. In this chapter, we link the engineering physics of solute and fluid transport with their clinical translation and highlight emerging bioengineered membranes that integrate filtration and adsorption. It is organized into three parts. The first addresses the physical principles and technological evolution of dialysis and filtration, the second explores adsorption as both a surface phenomenon and therapeutic mechanism, and the third describes contemporary bioengineering strategies that unify these processes into advanced, biocompatible blood-purification systems.

2.2 Historical Development

Understanding how these principles evolved from early cellulosic dialyzers to bioengineered systems is essential to appreciate current design priorities. The concept of blood purification through selective filtration originated with early cellulosic dialyzers in the 1940s. Cellulose, a naturally derived polymer of β-D-glucose, offered mechanical stability but was highly reactive with complement and leukocytes, causing febrile reactions and membrane fouling. The advent of *modified cellulose* in the 1970s, acetylated or substituted acetylation, etherification, or carbamate substitution, improved biocompatibility by masking hydroxyl moieties and reducing complement activation [3].

The next major advance was the introduction of *synthetic and semisynthetic membranes* such as polyacrylonitrile (PAN), polysulfone (PS), polyethersulfone (PES), polyamide, and cellulose triacetate (CTA). Synthetic membranes offered superior hemocompatibility, reduced inflammatory mediator release, and enabled high-flux dialysis modalities, which were not achievable with cellulosic materials [4]. These materials provided high mechanical strength, consistent pore formation, and tolerance to steam sterilization properties essential for the high fluid-exchange rates used in CRRT. Synthetic polymers also enabled precise control of porosity and thickness, allowing fine-tuning of the ultrafiltration coefficient and solute selectivity. The dry/wet spinning technique evolved in the 1960s and 1970s, and the adoption of phase inversion for asymmetric membrane types [5, 6] and the introduction of an air gap allowed for precise tuning of pore size, wall thickness, and permeability by adjusting parameters such as polymer concentration, air gap distance, extrusion rate, and bath composition [6]. This made it ideal for bioengineered dialysis membranes, where both diffusion (for small solutes like urea) and adsorption (for protein-bound toxins) must be optimized.

The shift from intermittent hemodialysis to continuous modalities transformed design priorities. CRRT membranes must sustain 24-hour operation with minimal transmembrane-pressure drift, maintain thermal and chemical stability in citrate or bicarbonate solutions, and demonstrate high endotoxin retention. Polysulfone and polyethersulfone, often blended with polyvinylpyrrolidone (PVP) to enhance hydrophilicity, became dominant materials because they combined excellent mechanical resilience with low protein adsorption [7].

The 1990s and early 2000s saw the development of *high-flux* membranes with larger pore radii, increasing permeability for molecules up to 20–30 kDa, followed by *high-cut-off* (HCO) membranes with nominal cut-offs of 60–100 kDa, approximating the molecular weight of albumin [8–10]. HCO membranes enabled clearance of myoglobin, cytokines, and free light chains but risked albumin loss [11]. *Medium-cut-off* (MCO) membranes subsequently bridged this gap, offering more uniform pore distributions (35–45 kDa) that enhance middle-molecule removal while retaining albumin [12].

With historical context in mind, we will next explore two major defining characteristics of membranes, that is, filtration and adsorption. We will outline a number of alterations and engineering adjustments that can be made in order to optimize the CRRT process.

2.3 Membrane Characteristics: Filtration

The first key process in CRRT is filtration. Purely from an engineering perspective, a semipermeable membrane is designed to allow selective transport of different molecules between two compartments. In the case of filtration, we are interested in the transport of harmful molecules from the blood compartment into the dialysate compartment, the retention of beneficial molecules in the blood compartment, and the transport of certain molecules from the dialysate compartment into the blood.

How is this achieved? The key design features of the membrane are pore size, thickness and distribution, membrane material, and membrane size. Further, it is important to consider the drivers of the selective transport (diffusion and convection) and the ability of the membranes to minimize fouling (e.g., clotting) [1].

Solute transport mechanisms The primary drivers of solute transport in dialysis are diffusion, convection, and backfiltration. Diffusion is driven by a solute concentration gradient and is effective at the removal of small solutes such as urea or potassium, which can build up in patients indicated for CRRT, and for the movement of molecules, such as bicarbonate and citrate from the dialysate into the blood. Convective clearance refers to the removal of molecules in fluid that is pulled across the dialysis membrane (ultrafiltration) and is more effective than diffusion at removing middle molecular weight toxins. Convection is maximized in filtration modalities, such as hemofiltration or hemodiafiltration, compared to hemodialysis. However, convective clearance can also occur through internal pressure gradients in a dialyzer, a process known as backfiltration. This is where fluid moves from the dialyzer compartment back into the blood (a form of internal substitution), which is caused by differential pressure gradients and is offset by balanced movement of fluid in the opposite direction, causing a convective clearance. The rate of backfiltration is linked to ultrafiltration, blood and dialysate flow rates, dialyzer flow patterns, and sieving coefficients.

Membrane pores The membrane pores are effectively channels that connect the blood compartment to the dialysate compartment. The physical dimensions of the pores define transport characteristics: smaller pores retain more larger molecules (e.g., essential proteins) and favor removal of smaller molecules (e.g., urea), with larger pores improving clearance of some middle molecular weight uremic toxins while risking loss of beneficial molecules. In reality, membranes have a distribution of pore sizes that is designed to optimize this balance. The density of the pores influences hydraulic permeability, or the ultrafiltration coefficient, as well as diffusive permeability. Manufacturing techniques from air- to water-drying influence the size of pores [13, 14]. The thickness of a membrane defines the path length a molecule needs to travel to cross the membrane, where diffusion rates decrease with increasing thickness, and this has an increased impact as molecular size increases. As well as reducing loss of middle molecules, thicker membranes are structurally more robust and less likely to rupture. Pore radius, density, and tortuosity determine both selectivity and hydraulic resistance. Thicker membranes reduce diffusive transport but provide mechanical robustness; thinner ones maximize permeability at the expense of structural stability. Real membranes exhibit a distribution of pore sizes rather than a single cut-off, producing a smooth transition in sieving behavior. The effective "cut-off" therefore corresponds to the smallest molecular weight that is 90–95% retained.

MCO membranes achieve their performance by narrowing the pore-size distribution and optimizing wall thickness, thereby sustaining albumin retention while permitting cytokine passage. Symmetric triacetate designs further control pore orientation to balance flow resistance and biocompatibility [15].

Membrane material The material of a dialysis membrane can impact therapy in several ways. One of the most significant advances in renal replacement therapy has been the improvements in biocompatibility of dialyzer membrane materials in the transition from naturally occurring, cellulosic membranes to a variety of synthetic membranes. However, other advances include the potential for adsorption onto the membrane, which can help remove molecules that may have limited diffusive clearance, such as cytokines, and developments in surface charge to try to minimize unwanted protein binding to the membrane and activation of clotting factors. Finally, the addition of specific materials onto the dialyzer material has been trialed, including heparin (reducing anticoagulation requirements), vitamin E, and polyethyleneimine (PEI) grafting, which neutralizes negative surface charge and enables electrostatic binding of endotoxin (as in AN69ST and oXiris) [16].

Blood flow characterization The dialyzer header refers to the polyurethane potting in which the hollow fibers are fixed and distributed. Blood entering the header tends to preferentially flow through the inner fibers; therefore, fiber packing density and header geometry are engineered to promote uniform flow distribution across all fibers, which maximizes clearance. Subtle fiber undulation also helps minimize flow mismatch between blood and dialysate and reduces boundary layer effects on the dialysate side. Within a hollow-fiber dialyzer, blood flows through thousands of micro-capillary fibers arranged in counter-current to the dialysate. Achieving uniform flow prevents channeling and maintains consistent transmembrane pressures along the fiber bundle. Fiber inner diameters (typically 180–200 μm) and packing densities are selected to balance shear forces, high enough to avoid stagnation and clotting, yet low enough to prevent hemolysis. Computational fluid-dynamic (CFD) studies show that longitudinal pressure gradients establish regions of internal filtration and backfiltration, underscoring the importance of precise header design in achieving optimal solute exchange and ultrafiltration performance. Each dialyzer will contain 10–17 K individual hollow fibers and fiber spiral arrangement, and diameter is optimized to reduce shear, improving dialysis over differing blood flow levels. Internal filtration increases with membrane permeability and smaller fiber inner diameter, which facilitates backfiltration.

2.4 Fouling and Performance Stability

Protein deposition and microthrombus formation progressively reduce effective pore area, increasing transmembrane pressure and shortening filter life. This *fouling* arises from electrostatic and hydrophobic interactions between plasma proteins and polymer surfaces [17–19]. Strategies to mitigate fouling include hydrophilic coatings, dynamic flow modulation, and surface charge neutralization. Maintaining high shear rates and adequate anticoagulation further prolongs performance stability, critical in continuous therapies [2].

2.5 Membrane Characteristics: Adsorption

Adsorption is the second core process of CRRT. It refers to the physical or chemical binding of solutes from a fluid phase onto the surface of a solid material. In the context of CRRT, this process occurs when plasma constituents adhere to the membrane or to sorbent particles incorporated within it. Unlike absorption, which implies penetration into a bulk matrix, adsorption is a surface phenomenon governed by the physicochemical interactions between solute molecules and the solid interface. Adsorption is an additional method of toxin clearance which acts as an important barrier against endotoxin transfer. An ideal membrane has maximal adsorptive capacity to aid in endotoxin removal while also not impeding solute clearance. Adsorption capacity is determined by the surface properties of the membrane.

Two main types of adsorption are recognized. Physisorption relies on weak van der Waals forces, hydrogen bonding, and hydrophobic interactions; it is reversible and nonspecific. Chemisorption involves stronger ionic or covalent bonding based on electrostatic attraction or chemical affinity, leading to more selective and often irreversible binding.

The overall adsorption capacity of a membrane depends on its available surface area, pore structure, surface charge, and hydrophobic–hydrophilic balance [1]. An ideal adsorptive membrane must maximize beneficial binding (e.g., cytokines, endotoxins, uremic toxins) while minimizing unwanted loss of essential proteins or drugs. The design challenge lies in tuning surface chemistry to achieve this selectivity without compromising permeability or biocompatibility.

In hemodialysis and CRRT, adsorption serves dual purposes. It contributes to solute removal, particularly of middle and protein-bound molecules that diffuse poorly, and acts as a protective barrier against back-transfer of endotoxins or bacterial products from the dialysate. The membrane is therefore the final safeguard before blood returns to the patient [5, 20]. Quantifying adsorption is complex because it involves both instantaneous surface binding and dynamic equilibrium with the plasma phase. Operational factors such as blood flow rate, contact time, and competing solutes strongly influence these parameters. In CRRT, continuous exposure and low shear favor sustained adsorption but also accelerate fouling; thus, balancing duration and efficiency is key.

2.6 Mechanism and Determinants of Adsorption

How is effective adsorption achieved? When blood contacts an artificial surface, an ultrathin layer of adsorbed proteins forms within milliseconds. This "conditioning film" dictates subsequent interactions, including platelet activation and complement cascades. Engineering the initial adsorptive event rather than eliminating it has become a central design strategy for hemocompatibility [21].

The extent and selectivity of adsorption are determined by several interrelated factors, including surface area and porosity, surface charge, hydrophobicity or hydrophilicity, functional groups and specific affinity, and conditioning film formation. Larger surface areas achieved through microporous or nanoporous structures offer more binding sites. For example, polymethylmethacrylate (PMMA) membranes possess a sponge-like morphology with interconnected pores that enable high cytokine uptake [22].

Surface charge plays a key role in the selective binding of charged solutes. Cationic membranes, such as PEI-functionalized cryogels, efficiently adsorb negatively charged endotoxin via strong electrostatic interactions. However, this same mechanism can increase nonspecific protein deposition, accelerating fouling unless balanced by hydrophilic surface engineering molecules [23], and nonspecific protein adsorption, leading to fouling and reduced hemocompatibility [24].

Hydrophobic surfaces readily bind lipophilic toxins but also tend to attract plasma proteins and promote platelet adhesion. Increasing hydrophilicity commonly through the incorporation or grafting of hydrophilic polymers such as polyvinylpyrrolidone (PVP) or polyethylene glycol (PEG) reduces nonspecific protein adsorption and improves hemocompatibility [25]. Many modern membranes incorporate these hydrophilic additives to reduce nonspecific binding [26]. Increased protein deposition is a recognized risk unless hydrophilicity is adequately engineered into the surface [27].

In addition to modulating surface energy, functional ligand modification can provide targeted bioactivity. For example, chemical modification with ligands (e.g., heparin) provides targeted binding through coordination or ionic exchange mechanisms. Heparin is immobilized onto membrane surfaces via covalent bonding, layer-by-layer assembly, or polyelectrolyte blending. This provides a negatively charged, anticoagulant surface that interacts with blood components through ionic exchange, reducing protein adsorption, platelet adhesion, and clot formation [28]. Heparinized membranes show improved hemocompatibility and prolonged clotting times, with various immobilization strategies enhancing stability and performance [29].

Understanding the complexity of these membranes and their numerous modifiable variables is key to appreciating the differences between individual membrane subtypes. The next section comprises an outline of a number of membranes commonly used in modern practice.

2.7 Examples of Membranes

The most widely used membrane materials in continuous renal replacement therapy (CRRT) today are synthetic polymers such as polyethersulfone (PES), polysulfone (PS), polyacrylonitrile (PAN), and polyamide [30]. These polymers offer excellent chemical stability and tensile strength but vary in hydrophilicity, charge, and surface roughness [31]. Blending or co-polymerizing these materials allows fine control over porosity and surface energy [32]. Commonly used membrane types, their base materials, key functional properties, and representative commercial examples are summarized in Table 2.1.

Table 2.1 Overview of commonly used dialysis and CRRT membranes, summarizing base material composition, key physicochemical properties, and representative commercial examples relevant to filtration and adsorption performance

Membrane type	Base material/ modification	Key features/notes	Examples
Polyacrylonitrile (AN69)	Acrylonitrile + sodium methallyl sulfonate copolymer	High permeability; negatively charged surface enhances biocompatibility; moderate cytokine adsorption	AN69 (Baxter/ Gambro)
Polysulfone (PS)	Synthetic polymer (sulfonated polyether)	Highly biocompatible; strong mechanical stability; minimal adsorption; used widely in ICU CRRT	Ultraflux, FX (Fresenius)

(continued)

Table 2.1 (continued)

Membrane type	Base material/ modification	Key features/notes	Examples
Polyethersulfone (PES)	Synthetic polymer related to PS	Similar to polysulfone; high hydraulic permeability and good solute clearance	Prismaflex ST150/ST100 (Baxter), Multifiltrate (Fresenius)
Polyamide	Synthetic polymer	High flux; used for diffusive and convective clearance	Hemofilter PAN (Asahi)
AN69ST	Polyethyleneimine (PEI) surface treatment of AN69	Neutralizes negative surface charge → allows use with heparin or citrate anticoagulation; reduces bradykinin generation	AN69ST (Baxter)
oXiris	AN69 base + PEI treatment + immobilized heparin + enhanced adsorption capacity	Combines RRT with adsorption of cytokines and endotoxin; intended for septic shock, COVID-19, and hyperinflammation	oXiris (Baxter)
PMMA (Polymethylmethacrylate)	Intrinsically adsorptive polymer	Strong cytokine and middle-molecule adsorption; limited solute clearance	Hemofeel (Toray)
EMiC2	Polysulfone with high cutoff	Designed for middle molecule clearance (β2-microglobulin, myoglobin)	EMiC2 (Fresenius)
High cutoff (HCO)	Cutoff ~60–100 kDa	Enhanced removal of myoglobin, cytokines, light chains; may lead to albumin loss	HCO1100 (Baxter), SepteX (Gambro)
Medium cutoff (MCO)	Cutoff ~40–50 kDa	Better middle molecule clearance with limited albumin loss; more physiological pore distribution	Theranova

2.8 Polyacrylonitrile-Based Membranes

Polyacrylonitrile-based membranes, exemplified by AN69 and its derivatives, continue to evolve through surface treatments that modify charge and adsorption properties. The AN69 membrane, composed of acrylonitrile and sodium methallyl sulfonate copolymer, carries negatively charged sulfonate groups that attract positively charged cytokines and basic proteins. These innovations demonstrate how relatively minor chemical modifications, such as introducing amino or sulfonate groups, can radically alter the biological interactions of a membrane. Its high hydrophilicity promotes moderate endotoxin binding and favorable hemocompatibility. The AN69 membrane promotes contact activation of the kallikrein-kinin system, leading to bradykinin generation. In patients treated with ACE inhibitors who have impaired bradykinin degradation, this may cause hypotension or angioedema at dialysis initiation. Additionally, in vitro drug adsorption of antifungals such as caspofungin has been noted, leading to concern about inconsistent bioavailability from sequestration [33], although other factors may be at play. The surface-treated derivative AN69ST neutralizes the charge by grafting PEI, reducing bradykinin generation, and enhancing adsorption of negatively charged molecules such as endotoxin, without an associated increased absorption of caspofungin.

2.9 Polyethersulfone (PES)–Polyvinylpyrrolidone (PVP)

Polyvinylpyrrolidone (PVP) is commonly added to polysulfone or PES formulations to enhance hydrophilicity, reduce protein adsorption, and improve resistance to fouling. The PES–PVP composite remains the benchmark for high-performance CRRT filters [34]. Recent work by Oprea et al. [35] introduced *crown-ether functionalized* PES membranes capable of selectively binding calcium to reduce clotting at the filter membranes through host–guest chemistry. Such functionalization exemplifies the trend toward membranes that not only separate solutes by size but also recognize them chemically; however, the effect of fouling on longer use has not been reported. The EMiC2 polysulfone filter (cut-off 45 kDa) exemplifies MCO design. In vitro studies demonstrate higher clearance of IL-6 (26 kDa) and IL-10 (17 kDa) compared with standard low-cut-off membranes [36]. Clinical trials [37] show efficient cytokine removal without excessive albumin loss, although plasma concentrations often decline similarly between groups, suggesting endogenous metabolism outweighs extracorporeal clearance. While biochemical and hemodynamic benefits are consistently demonstrated [38], mortality improvements remain inconsistent across trials, underscoring the need for targeted use based on inflammatory phenotype [37].

2.10 Polymethylmethacrylate (PMMA)

Polymethyl methacrylate (PMMA) possesses an intrinsic three-dimensional microporous structure that promotes the adsorption of β_2-microglobulin, pro-inflammatory cytokines, and complement fragments via hydrophobic interactions. PMMA has been widely used in chronic dialysis and is increasingly applied in inflammatory states such as sepsis, supporting the concept of extracorporeal immunomodulation [39].

2.11 PEPA Membranes

Polyester Polymer Alloy (PEPA) membrane was developed as an advanced synthetic polymer membrane that combines the benefits of multiple polymer components, and was first marketed by Nikkiso as FLX. Specifically, it is composed of two key polymers: polyethersulfone (PES) and polyacrylate (PAR). PEPA membranes consist of a three-layer architecture: an inner hydrophobic polyester for mechanical strength, a middle microporous layer providing adsorption sites, and an outer hydrophilic polymer ensuring blood compatibility. They demonstrate enhanced clearance of middle molecules and endotoxin retention but can adsorb essential plasma proteins, limiting routine use [40].

2.12 Mixed-Matrix Membranes

Mixed-matrix membranes (MMMs) embed adsorptive particles (activated carbon, zeolites, porous organic polymers) within a polymer matrix, combining the hemocompatibility of polymers with the high sorption capacity of porous solids [41, 42]. These membranes expand clearance to protein-bound and hydrophobic uremic toxins while preserving albumin. Molecularly imprinted zeolite–PES–PVP hollow-fiber MMMs have demonstrated up to 40% increased p-cresol removal compared with conventional PES filters [43]. When activated carbon is incorporated, endotoxin removal from dialysate increases tenfold, preventing pyrogen transfer when water purity is suboptimal [44, 45].

2.13 Nanostructured Membrane

Nanostructured membranes combine a conventional polymer matrix with embedded adsorptive particles such as activated carbon or imprinted zeolites. Carbon-based nanomaterials, including *multiwalled carbon nanotubes (MWCNTs),* increase surface area and electrical conductivity, although biocompatibility remains a concern. Added particles capture water-soluble uremic toxins (WSUTs) and protein-bound uremic toxins (PBUTs), while the surrounding polymer maintains structural integrity and selective permeability. Dual-layer structures further minimize albumin loss by restricting adsorbent exposure to the plasma phase [43]. Irfan et al. [46] reported a composite membrane of polyethersulfone blended with PVP-k25 and carboxylated MWCNTs that exhibited improved uremic toxin clearance, enhanced permeability, and intrinsic anticoagulant activity. The carboxyl functional groups reduced platelet adhesion while preserving diffusive transport. Similarly, Raharjo et al. [43] incorporated molecularly imprinted zeolites into a mixed-matrix membrane to target *p-cresol* and *indoxyl sulfate*. The imprinted cavities enhanced selectivity by recognizing the three-dimensional structure of the toxin molecule, achieving higher binding efficiency than conventional adsorbents. These examples illustrate the potential of nanostructured materials to achieve precise molecular targeting.

As stated in the previous section, mixed matrix membranes incorporating activated carbon improve endotoxin removal and prevent pyrogen transfer even when water purity is suboptimal [42]. The high surface area of nano-sized carbon particles (20–40 μm) enhances adsorption kinetics, and their uniform dispersion within the polymer prevents channel formation [45].

These composites maintain selective permeability, minimizing albumin loss while increasing clearance of protein-bound toxins such as *p-cresol* and *indoxyl sulfate,* two key uremic toxins implicated in cardiovascular morbidity. The dual-layer configuration of some systems ensures that blood contacts a biocompatible outer surface, while adsorption occurs in an internal sorbent layer protected from direct cell interaction [47, 48].

2.14 Clinical Scenarios

With improved understanding of the variety of membranes available, it is imperative to understand when and where to use each membrane to its maximal potential, and to translate that knowledge into clinical practice. We discuss three common indications for CRRT and the specific role a membrane can play therein.

2.15 Sepsis and Systemic Inflammatory Response

Adsorptive membranes and cartridges can attenuate cytokine storm and endotoxin load. Although biochemical markers frequently improve, large trials have not demonstrated a consistent mortality benefit [49]. The optimal timing, duration, and patient selection remain active areas of investigation.

Sepsis is defined as a dysregulated host immune response to infection. This response involves a complex interplay of numerous cells and plasma components, triggering both pro- and anti-inflammatory responses. An imbalance between these mediators of inflammation leads to deleterious clinical outcomes, including organ failure and death. Conventional hemodialysis clears small solutes but removes cytokines inefficiently because of their larger molecular weights (8–60 kDa). Alternate methods of extracorporeal blood purification (ECBP), such as CVVH, hemoadsorption, and plasma exchange, may instead be utilized. The goal of ECBP is to remove cytokines and bacterial toxins, thus attenuating the systemic inflammatory response in sepsis. This is done via both convective removal and adsorption. The membranes we use can be engineered to optimize both processes. Pathogens, endotoxins, and cytokines are just three plasma components implicated in the pathogenesis of sepsis. Clearance of these mediators and thus restoration of the pro- and anti-inflammatory equilibrium is a potential therapeutic target in sepsis. Unfortunately, these small molecules are poorly removed by hemodialysis. Advanced adsorptive membranes (e.g., AN69 ST, Oxiris, polymethyl methacrylate) may be used to enhance cytokine and endotoxin removal [50], although robust outcome data are still emerging. High cut-off membranes have larger pore sizes and thus improved clearance of large middle molecules. This includes most inflammatory cytokines such as IL-8, IL-6, and TNF-α. In addition to altering pore size, membranes can be engineered to better adsorb endotoxins and inflammatory cytokines.

High-flux and HCO membranes broaden the spectrum of removal. Early studies by Morgera and colleagues [51–53] demonstrated enhanced IL-6 and IL-1ra clearance and reduced vasopressor dependence with 60 kDa polyamide filters, albeit with measurable protein loss. Subsequent trials, including Chelazzi et al. [54] and Atan et al. [55], reported improved hemodynamics but no mortality difference. The *HICOSS* multicenter trial confirmed biochemical improvements without outcome benefit, highlighting the need for patient-phenotype targeting [56].

The oXiris® filter evolved from the AN69 platform, a copolymer of acrylonitrile and sodium methallyl sulfonate whose negatively charged sulfonate groups enable cytokine adsorption. Surface treatment with PEI converts the charge to positive, facilitating endotoxin binding and allowing covalent heparin grafting that enhances hemocompatibility [57]. The resulting design integrates convective and diffusive clearance with selective adsorption of endotoxin and cytokines.

Multiple observational studies and small RCTs have examined oXiris in septic AKI and, more recently, COVID-19–related hyperinflammation. Meta-analyses indicate reductions in IL-6 levels, lactate, and vasopressor dose, with trends toward improved 28-day survival [58].

2.16 Acute Liver Failure

Albumin-coated charcoal or resin sorbents are employed within molecular adsorbent recirculating systems (MARS) to remove bilirubin and bile acids. These platforms paved the way for incorporating selective adsorption into renal replacement therapy. High-flux synthetic membranes (typically polysulfone or polyacrylonitrile) are used, but these are specifically adapted to allow the passage of albumin-bound toxins from blood into an albumin-containing dialysate, while retaining albumin itself [59]. The membrane is often impregnated or coated with albumin, or used in conjunction with an albumin-rich dialysate circuit, to maximize the transfer of protein-bound toxins. Experimental approaches have also included albumin-fixed membranes, such as polysulfone membranes covalently bonded to albumin, which enhance the removal of protein-bound toxins like bilirubin [60].

2.17 Drug and Toxin Intoxications

Adsorptive systems extend clearance to hydrophobic and protein-bound xenobiotics that are poorly removed by conventional dialysis, including tricyclic antidepressants, digoxin, and carbamazepine. This can be achieved through the incorporation of adsorptive components such as mixed-matrix membranes, activated carbon, or composite polymers like PEPA. Membrane engineering strategies that adjust surface charge, hydrophilicity, and pore architecture can further enhance binding and removal of highly protein-bound drugs. However, these approaches also carry the risk of nonselective adsorption, potentially depleting essential plasma proteins and nutrients. Consequently, most clinical experience with drug removal to date derives from sorbent-based systems rather than routine dialysis membranes.

2.18 Conclusion

The evolution of dialysis membranes from early cellulosic filters to advanced bioengineered platforms reflects sustained innovation in polymer chemistry, pore architecture, and surface functionalization. These advances have expanded the scope of extracorporeal therapy from simple solute removal to targeted modulation of inflammation and toxin clearance. Yet, real clinical benefit depends not only on engineering ingenuity, but on rigorous translational evaluation. Future progress will require close collaboration between biomaterial scientists, nephrologists, and intensivists to ensure that promising physicochemical improvements translate into meaningful patient outcomes.

Next-generation membranes will more closely mimic the clearance capacity of the kidney. Artificial intelligence and machine-learning models will be utilized to predict blood-membrane and solute-membrane interactions and further advance our understanding of each individual membrane. As these novel bioengineering strategies continue to refine the balance between filtration, adsorption, and biocompatibility, there is significant potential for next-generation membranes to deliver more personalized and effective extracorporeal support across acute and chronic diseases.

References

1. Ronco C, Clark WR. Haemodialysis membranes. Nat Rev Nephrol. 2018;14(6):394–410.
2. Zawada AM, Lang T, Ottillinger B, Kircelli F, Stauss-Grabo M, Kennedy JP. Impact of hydrophilic modification of synthetic dialysis membranes on hemocompatibility and performance. Membranes (Basel). 2022;12(10):932.
3. Woffindin C, Hoenich NA, Matthews JNS. Cellulose-based haemodialysis membranes: biocompatibility and functional performance compared. Nephrol Dial Transplant. 1992;7(4):340–5.
4. Hoenich NA, Woffindin C, Stamp S, Roberts SJ, Turnbull J. Synthetically modified cellulose: an alternative to synthetic membranes for use in haemodialysis? Biomaterials. 1997;18(19):1299–303.
5. Clark WR, Gao D, Ronco C. Membranes for dialysis. Composition, structure and function. Contrib Nephrol. 2002;(137):70–7.
6. Strathmann H, Kock K, Amar P, Baker RW. The formation mechanism of asymmetric membranes. Desalination. 1975;16(2):179–203.
7. Malard B, Hulko M, Koch J, Speidel R, Pouchoulin D, Echeverri J, et al. Comparison of different membranes for continuous renal replacement therapies: an in vitro study. ASAIO J. 2025;71(6):510–8.
8. Clark WR, Hamburger RJ, Lysaght MJ. Effect of membrane composition and structure on solute removal and biocompatibility in hemodialysis. Kidney Int. 1999;56(6):2005–15.

9. Ronco C, Marchionna N, Brendolan A, Neri M, Lorenzin A, Martínez Rueda AJ. Expanded haemodialysis: from operational mechanism to clinical results. Nephrol Dial Transplant. 2018;33(suppl_3):iii41–i7.
10. Fiorentino M, La Fergola F, De Rosa S. Medium cut-off dialyzer for middle molecular uremic toxins in AKI and chronic dialysis. J Nephrol. 2024;37(1):23–37.
11. Boschetti-de-Fierro A, Voigt M, Storr M, Krause B. Extended characterization of a new class of membranes for blood purification: the high cut-off membranes. Int J Artif Organs. 2013;36(7):455–63.
12. Atan R, Peck L, Visvanathan K, Skinner N, Eastwood G, Bellomo R, et al. High cut-off hemofiltration versus standard hemofiltration: effect on plasma cytokines. Int J Artif Organs. 2016;39(9):479–86.
13. Barzin J, Feng C, Khulbe K, Matsuura T, Madaeni SS. Characterization of polyethersulfone hemodialysis membrane by ultrafiltration and atomic force microscopy. J Membr Sci. 2004;237:77–85.
14. Miyata M, Konishi S, Shimamoto Y, Kamada A, Umimoto K. Influence of sterilization and storage period on elution of polyvinylpyrrolidone from wet-type polysulfone membrane dialyzers. ASAIO J. 2015;61(4):468–73.
15. Albalate Ramón M, Martínez Miguel P, Bohorquez L, de Sequera P, Bouarich H, Pérez-García R, et al. El triacetato de celulosa asimétrico es una alternativa segura y eficaz para la hemodiafiltración en línea. Nefrologia. 2018;38(3):315–20.
16. Cruz DN, De Cal M, Garzotto F, Brendolan A, Nalesso D, Corradi V, et al. Effect of vitamin E-coated dialysis membranes on anemia in patients with chronic kidney disease: an Italian multicenter study. Int J Artif Organs. 2008;31(6):545–52.
17. Huang Z, Gao D, Letteri JJ, Clark WR. Blood-membrane interactions during dialysis. Semin Dial. 2009;22(6):623–8.
18. Langsdorf LJ, Zydney AL. Effect of blood contact on the transport properties of hemodialysis membranes: a two-layer membrane model. Blood Purif. 1994;12(6):292–307.
19. Morti SM, Zydney AL. Protein-membrane interactions during hemodialysis: effects on solute transport. ASAIO J. 1998;44(4):319–26.
20. Florens N, Guebre-Egziabher F, Juillard L. Reconsidering adsorption in hemodialysis: is it just an epiphenomenon? A narrative review. J Nephrol. 2022;35(1):33–41.
21. Westphalen H, Saadati S, Eduok U, Abdelrasoul A, Shoker A, Choi P, et al. Case studies of clinical hemodialysis membranes: influences of membrane morphology and biocompatibility on uremic blood-membrane interactions and inflammatory biomarkers. Sci Rep. 2020;10(1):14808.
22. Phasuk A, Putthabucha N, Winuprasith T, Srisawat N, Khomein P. Hemoperfusion adsorbents from porous PMMA microspheres: synthesis approaches and their cytokine removal efficiency. J Mater Chem B. 2025;13(39):12614–23.
23. Akın A, Akgönüllü S, Çimen D, Denizli A, Yavuz H. Supermacroporous cryogel membranes via polyethyleneimine-assisted decoration for efficient removal of bacterial endotoxin. J Chromatogr B. 2025;1261:124636.
24. Kiguchi T, Ito H, Yamashita AC. Effect of membrane surface area on solute removal performance of dialyzers with fouling. Membranes (Basel). 2022;12(7):684.
25. Higuchi A, Shirano K, Harashima M, Yoon BO, Hara M, Hattori M, et al. Chemically modified polysulfone hollow fibers with vinylpyrrolidone having improved blood compatibility. Biomaterials. 2002;23(13):2659–66.
26. Bernhard C, Roeters SJ, Franz J, Weidner T, Bonn M, Gonella G. Repelling and ordering: the influence of poly(ethylene glycol) on protein adsorption. Phys Chem Chem Phys. 2017;19(41):28182–8.
27. Bergstrand A, Rahmani-Monfared G, Ostlund A, Nydén M, Holmberg K. Comparison of PEI-PEG and PLL-PEG copolymer coatings on the prevention of protein fouling. J Biomed Mater Res A. 2009;88(3):608–15.

28. Tangvoraphonkchai K, Riddell A, Davenport A. Platelet activation and clotting cascade activation by dialyzers designed for high volume online hemodiafiltration. Hemodial Int. 2018;22(2):192–200.
29. Aryanti PTP, Nugroho FA, Kusmala YY. Heparin and heparin-like modifications in hemodialysis membranes: current innovations and future directions. Biotechnol Adv. 2025;80:108527.
30. Mandolfo S, Malberti F, Imbasciati E, Cogliati P, Gauly A. Impact of blood and dialysate flow and surface on performance of new polysulfone hemodialysis dialyzers. Int J Artif Organs. 2003;26(2):113–20.
31. Hoenich NA, Katopodis KP. Clinical characterization of a new polymeric membrane for use in renal replacement therapy. Biomaterials. 2002;23(18):3853–8.
32. Oshihara W, Ueno Y, Fujieda H. A new polysulfone membrane dialyzer, NV, with low-fouling and antithrombotic properties. Contrib Nephrol. 2017;189:222–9.
33. Baud FJ, Jullien V, Desnos-Ollivier M, Lamhaut L, Lortholary O. Caspofungin sequestration in a polyacrylonitrile-derived filter: increasing the dose does not mitigate sequestration. Int J Antimicrob Agents. 2023;62(6):107007.
34. Su BH, Fu P, Li Q, Tao Y, Li Z, Zao HS, et al. Evaluation of polyethersulfone highflux hemodialysis membrane in vitro and in vivo. J Mater Sci Mater Med. 2008;19(2):745–51.
35. Oprea M, Pandele AM, Enachescu CI, Antoniac IV, Voicu SI, Fratila AM. Crown ether-functionalized polyethersulfone membranes with potential applications in hemodialysis. Polym Int. 2025;17(16):2184.
36. Eichhorn T, Hartmann J, Harm S, Linsberger I, König F, Valicek G, et al. Clearance of selected plasma cytokines with continuous veno-venous hemodialysis using Ultraflux EMiC2 versus Ultraflux AV1000S. Blood Purif. 2017;44(4):260–6.
37. Lumlertgul N, Hall A, Camporota L, Crichton S, Ostermann M. Clearance of inflammatory cytokines in patients with septic acute kidney injury during renal replacement therapy using the EMiC2 filter (Clic-AKI study). Crit Care (Lond, Engl) [Internet]. 2021;25(1):39. Available from: http://europepmc.org/abstract/MED/33509215; https://doi.org/10.1186/s13054-021-03476-x; https://europepmc.org/articles/PMC7845048; https://europepmc.org/articles/PMC7845048?pdf=render.
38. Díaz-Tejeiro R, Regidor D, Morales J, Padrón M, Cueto L, Muñoz MA, et al. Acute renal failure due to rhabdomyolysis. Renal replacement therapy with intermediate cut-off membranes (EMIC2). Nefrologia (Engl Ed). 2018;38(6):664–5.
39. Kishikawa T, Fujieda H, Sakaguchi H. Comprehensive analysis of cytokine adsorption properties of polymethyl methacrylate (PMMA) membrane material. J Artif Organs. 2022;25(4):343–9.
40. Nakatani T, Tsuchida K, Sugimura K, Yoshimura R, Takemoto Y. Investigation of endotoxin adsorption with polyether polymer alloy dialysis membranes. Int J Mol Med. 2003;11(2):195–7.
41. Geremia I, Pavlenko D, Maksymow K, Rüth M, Lemke HD, Stamatialis D. Ex vivo evaluation of the blood compatibility of mixed matrix haemodialysis membranes. Acta Biomater. 2020;111:118–28.
42. Geremia I, Bansal R, Stamatialis D. In vitro assessment of mixed matrix hemodialysis membrane for achieving endotoxin-free dialysate combined with high removal of uremic toxins from human plasma. Acta Biomater. 2019;90:100–11.
43. Raharjo Y, Ismail AF, Dzarfan Othman MH, Fahmi MZ, Saiful, Santoso D, et al. Selectively mixed matrix hemodialysis membrane for adequate clearance of p-cresol by the incorporation of imprinted zeolite. RSC Adv. 2023;13(5):2972–83.
44. Cheng Y, Ying Y, Japip S, Jiang SD, Chung TS, Zhang S, et al. Advanced porous materials in mixed matrix membranes. Adv Mater. 2018;30(47):e1802401.
45. Pavlenko D, van Geffen E, van Steenbergen MJ, Glorieux G, Vanholder R, Gerritsen KG, et al. New low-flux mixed matrix membranes that offer superior removal of protein-bound toxins from human plasma. Sci Rep. 2016;6:34429.
46. Irfan M, Irfan M, Shah SM, Baig N, Saleh TA, Ahmed M, et al. Hemodialysis performance and anticoagulant activities of PVP-k25 and carboxylic-multiwall nanotube composite blended Polyethersulfone membrane. Mater Sci Eng C. 2019;103:109769.

47. ter Beek OEM, van Gelder MK, Lokhorst C, Hazenbrink DHM, Lentferink BH, Gerritsen KGF, et al. In vitro study of dual layer mixed matrix hollow fiber membranes for outside-in filtration of human blood plasma. Acta Biomater. 2021;123:244–53.
48. Chow CM, Persad AH, Karnik R. Effect of membrane permeance and system parameters on the removal of protein-bound uremic toxins in hemodialysis. Ann Biomed Eng. 2024;52(3):526–41.
49. Honore PM, Blackman S, Perriens E, Oueslati I, Haddad C, Al-Sammour C, et al. Adsorptive therapies in sepsis and inflammation: description of the various adsorptive techniques and their failure to improve outcomes. Rev Investig Clin. 2023;75(6):359–76.
50. Chanard J, Lavaud S, Paris B, Toure F, Rieu P, Renaux JL, et al. Assessment of heparin binding to the AN69 ST hemodialysis membrane: I. Preclinical studies. ASAIO J. 2005;51(4):342–7.
51. Morgera S, Haase M, Rocktäschel J, Böhler T, Vargas-Hein O, Melzer C, et al. Intermittent high-permeability hemofiltration modulates inflammatory response in septic patients with multiorgan failure. Nephron Clin Pract. 2003;94(3):c75–80.
52. Morgera S, Slowinski T, Melzer C, Sobottke V, Vargas-Hein O, Volk T, et al. Renal replacement therapy with high-cutoff hemofilters: impact of convection and diffusion on cytokine clearances and protein status. Am J Kidney Dis. 2004;43(3):444–53.
53. Morgera S, Haase M, Kuss T, Vargas-Hein O, Zuckermann-Becker H, Melzer C, et al. Pilot study on the effects of high cutoff hemofiltration on the need for norepinephrine in septic patients with acute renal failure. Crit Care Med. 2006;34(8):2099–104.
54. Chelazzi C, Villa G, D'Alfonso MG, Mancinelli P, Consales G, Berardi M, et al. Hemodialysis with high cut-off hemodialyzers in patients with multi-drug resistant gram-negative sepsis and acute kidney injury: a retrospective, case-control study. Blood Purif. 2016;42(3):186–93.
55. Atan R, Peck L, Prowle J, Licari E, Eastwood GM, Storr M, et al. A double-blind randomized controlled trial of high cutoff versus standard hemofiltration in critically ill patients with acute kidney injury. Crit Care Med. 2018;46(10):e988.
56. Honore P, Clark W, editors. Novel therapeutical concepts for extracorporeal treatment of hyperinflammation and sepsis: immunomodulation. Approach with a novel high Cut-OFF membrane: the SepteX membrane. In: Proceedings of 10th congress of World Federation of CCU (WFSICCM). Florence, Italy; 2009.
57. Broman ME, Hansson F, Vincent JL, Bodelsson M. Endotoxin and cytokine reducing properties of the oXiris membrane in patients with septic shock: a randomized crossover double-blind study. PLoS One. 2019;14(8):e0220444.
58. Wang G, He Y, Guo Q, Zhao Y, He J, Chen Y, et al. Continuous renal replacement therapy with the adsorptive oXiris filter may be associated with the lower 28-day mortality in sepsis: a systematic review and meta-analysis. Crit Care. 2023;27(1):275.
59. Mitzner SR, Stange J, Klammt S, Peszynski P, Schmidt R. Albumin dialysis using the molecular adsorbent recirculating system. Curr Opin Nephrol Hypertens. 2001;10(6):777–83.
60. Ge D, Wu D, Shi W, Ma Y, Tian X, Liang P, et al. An albumin-fixed membrane for the removal of protein-bound toxins. Biomed Mater. 2006;1(3):170–4.

Artificial Intelligence and Personalized Blood Purification

3

Salvatore Lucio Cutuli

3.1 Introduction

Extracorporeal therapies have become a central component of organ support in the contemporary management of critically ill patients [1]. Extracorporeal blood purification therapies (EBPTs) [2], that includes continuous renal replacement therapy (CRRT), adsorptive membranes, and cartridges within multiorgan support platforms, are now widely available in many intensive care units (ICUs). However, the way these technologies are applied remains relatively protocolized and far from a personalized approach. This stands in stark contrast to the biological complexity of critical ill patients who receive these therapies.

Sepsis and septic shock are leading causes of disability and mortality worldwide [3] that frequently demand the application of extracorporeal blood purification as complementary therapy. However, these conditions are acknowledged as heterogeneous syndromes with distinct inflammatory, metabolic, and immunological endotypes, rather than homogeneous entities [4–6]. For these reasons, the evidence supporting the role of EBPTs in the management of these conditions is controversial, and a standardized EBPT prescription cannot reasonably be expected to serve all of patients affected by these syndromes equally well. Artificial intelligence (AI) may offer a framework for resolving this mismatch. Machine learning, deep learning, and reinforcement learning can integrate high-frequency physiological data, biomarker trajectories, multiomics, microbiology, pharmacokinetics, and device-generated signals into predictive and prescriptive models that operate in real time [7]. In this setting, artificial intelligence (AI) may drive the clinician to identify

S. L. Cutuli (✉)
Università Cattolica del Sacro Cuore, Dipartimento di Scienze Biotecnologiche di Base, Cliniche Intensivologiche e Perioperatorie, Rome, Italy

Fondazione Policlinico Universitairo Agostino Gemelli IRCCS, Dipartimento di Scienze dell'Emergenza, Anestesiologiche e della Rianimazione, Rome, Italy

S. De Rosa, S. Lassola (eds.), *Next-Gen Blood Purification*,
https://doi.org/10.1007/978-3-032-27033-7_3

patients who are most likely to benefit from extracorporeal treatments. Specifically, AI may help to determine timing, modality, intensity, and duration of a specific EBPT, as well as to anticipate technical failures and to individualize antimicrobial dosing, while it is running in place.

This chapter provides a detailed and extensive exploration of the intersection between AI and EBPTs in critical care practice. It first reviews the biological heterogeneity of sepsis and the conventional evidence surrounding CRRT, adsorptive membrane, and cartridges. Then, it examines the methodological foundations of AI in critical care and describes how AI may be potentially applied across the entire life cycle of EBPT to orient the management of critically ill patients requiring these therapies.

3.2 Biological Heterogeneity and the Rationale for Personalized Blood Purification

3.2.1 Sepsis as a Spectrum of Endotypes

The modern definition of sepsis moves away from a purely infection-based framework and emphasizes the "dysregulated host response" as the key pathogenic challenge [4]. This conceptual shift has been supported by large-scale transcriptomic, proteomic, and clinical clustering studies [5, 8]. Rather than a single disease, sepsis comprises multiple, biologically distinct endotypes [6] that are not visible in routine laboratory tests or conventional scores. Specifically, Seymour et al. [5] derived four reproducible clinical sepsis phenotypes (α, β, γ, δ) in an analysis of more than 20,000 patients, who met Sepsis-3 criteria [4] within 6 hours of hospital presentation at 12 Pennsylvania hospitals (2010–2012). In this study, exploratory analyses also suggested differential treatment responses, with certain phenotypes exhibiting greater benefit or harm from specific interventions. These findings may suggest the physiological rationale for a personalized approach to specific therapy, like the EBPT. Techniques such as cytokine adsorption or endotoxin removal are biologically plausible only in patients who actually exhibit cytokine storm or endotoxemia, while they appear harmful in those with negligible levels of these mediators. The implications of this hypothesis are straightforward: blood purification must be targeted to the right biological state to allow for immunomodulation and adequate organ support.

3.2.2 Temporal Dynamics of Inflammation and Endotoxin

Sepsis is not only heterogeneous between patients but also evolves dynamically within a single patient over time [9]. For this reason, the effectiveness of EBPT was acknowledged to be maximal during periods of high mediator flux, like early in the course of acute diseases [10]. In daily clinical practice, mediator kinetic curves are rarely measured, and the progression of mediator concentration remains unknown in most of the patients. In these regards, AI models designed for time-series data (e.g., recurrent neural networks or temporal convolutional networks) may help to infer the underlying trajectory of mediators concentration from sparse measurements and physiological data, estimate peaks and inflection points, and even forecast future values.

The potential of unraveling the "hidden kinetics" of mediators' concentration makes it possible to time blood purification to biologically meaningful windows rather than administratively convenient slots.

3.2.3 Organ Crosstalk and the Inflammatory Load

Conventional scoring systems, such as SOFA and SOFA-2 scores [11, 12], play a pivotal role in the evaluation of organ dysfunction, although they are not designed to evaluate the burden of inflammatory response altering organ interplay, as well as to predict the progression of organ function. AI models can be trained to use full trajectories of organ function biomarkers, and, potentially, estimate a composite "inflammatory and organ-dysfunction burden" in real time. Such a metric, although latent, could inform both the decision to initiate a specific EBPT and set its intensity and duration.

3.3 Conventional Evidence on CRRT and Hemoadsorption: The Case for AI-Driven Selection

Sepsis is implicated in the pathophysiology of AKI and is acknowledged as a major determinant of this syndrome [13]. Moreover, several investigations have demonstrated that AKI is a heterogeneous clinical condition [14], whose trajectories are unpredictable and may lead to RRT requirement in a nonnegligible proportion of these patients [15]. In this context, many aspects of RRT remain a matter of controversy due to conflicting evidence, for which AI application may offer the possibility to optimize patient selection, in order to orient the physician to provide the best personalized patient care.

3.3.1 Timing of CRRT

The question of "early" versus "delayed" initiation of RRT has generated conflicting evidence over the past decades [16–20]. The rationale for early RRT initiation—aimed at preventing metabolic derangements—has driven the design of several pivotal trials, which overall failed to demonstrate a clinical benefit of this approach [16, 18, 19] with the exception of postsurgical critically ill patients with refractory fluid overload [17]. Conversely, further postponement of RRT initiation did not confer additional benefit and was associated with potential harm [20].

Importantly, post hoc analyses of these trials identified patient subgroups that might derive differential benefit from one strategy over another [21–24]. These findings suggest that, rather than pursuing a single universal RRT initiation strategy, a personalized approach, guided by the identification of specific patient subgroups, may improve clinical outcomes. However, distinguishing such subgroups based solely on baseline serum creatinine or urine output is implausible. In this context, AI models integrating demographic, clinical, and biomarker data may help estimate an individual patient's probability of requiring RRT, as well as identify the most appropriate timing for RRT initiation. Although Tomasev et al. [7] reported the potential role of deep learning systems to predict AKI up to 48 hours before clinical recognition, there is currently no evidence supporting the use of AI to guide RRT initiation strategies within a personalized management framework. The generation of such evidence is therefore strongly warranted.

3.3.2 Dose and Intensity of CRRT

High-intensity CRRT, defined as effluent doses above 35 mL/kg/h, was initially hypothesized to confer survival benefit by more aggressively removing inflammatory mediators and toxins. The VA/NIH ATN trial and the RENAL study [25, 26] both disproved this hypothesis, and current KDIGO guidelines recommend standard doses of 25–30 mL/kg/h [27]. Nonetheless, even this standard dose is crude, as it does not account for biological heterogeneity. Apart from the heterogeneous degree of organ dysfunction, solute generation rates vary between patients, with non-standardizable requirements and tolerance to fixed effluent rates. For these reasons, the potential of AI-based dosing systems to predict solute kinetics and multiorgan function in real time, estimating the volume of effluent rate safely. As an example, AI-based dosing systems may increase dose temporarily during periods of high catabolic stress and reduce it when metabolic demands lessen, potentially sparing resources and lowering the risk of excessive nutrient and drug clearance.

3.3.3 Evidence on Adsorptive Therapies

Clinical evidence supporting the role of extracorporeal immunomodulation by specific membranes [28, 29] and cartridges [30–33] is heterogeneous and remains a matter of controversy. When looking at pragmatic trials enrolling heterogeneous patients, no evidence supports the benefit of nonselective cytokine removal via acrylonitrile-sodium methallyl sulfonate/polyethylenimine membrane [28], as well as selective endotoxin removal via Polymyxin-B Hemoperfusion [33]. However, the early use of acrylonitrile-sodium methallyl sulfonate/polyethylenimine membrane during cardiopulmonary bypass in cardiac surgical patients was demonstrated to be effective in preventing the occurrence of postoperative AKI [29]. Likewise, endotoxin removal via Polymyxin-B hemoperfusion in septic patients with endotoxin activity (EA) [34] between 0.6 and 0.89 was reported to be effective in reducing the 28-day mortality [35]. In line with what has already been discussed in the previous sections, the implementation of AI-modeling appears to be of interest for potentially identifying clinical phenotypes of patients at risk of immune dysregulation, or with life-threatening endotoxemia, to early identify subgroup responders that may benefit from these therapies..

3.3.4 Variability in Pharmacokinetics During Extracorporeal Therapies

CRRT, adsorptive membranes, and cartridges may also significantly alter the pharmacokinetics and pharmacodynamics of drugs and nutrients (e.g., antimicrobials and vitamins) [36]. Variability in drug clearance—driven by membrane characteristics, effluent dose, and patient factors—makes standard dosing protocols suboptimal [37]. With respect to antimicrobials, Roberts et al. [38] demonstrated that β-lactam underexposure is common in critically ill patients, particularly in those undergoing extracorporeal therapies. In this setting, AI-driven precision dosing systems informed by therapeutic drug monitoring and integrating clinical and EBPT characteristics may help to maintain therapeutic drug levels by reducing the occurrence of both drug underexposure and toxicity.

3.4 AI for Technical Performance: Circuit Monitoring, Clotting, and Safety

Extracorporeal circuits are mechanically complex systems with numerous failure modes: filter clotting, access recirculation, catheter dysfunction, pump malfunctions, leaks, and sensor errors. AI may function as an always-on, high-resolution monitor for these technical variables. Pressure transducers along the circuit generate continuous streams of data; under normal circumstances, these follow stable patterns. Before a filter clots, subtle changes in transmembrane pressure, prefilter and postfilter pressure gradients, and blood flow–resistance relationships appear, often well before alarm thresholds are reached. Machine learning models trained on labeled data, like clotting episodes, may potentially detect these patterns and issue early warnings.

In units using regional citrate anticoagulation, AI-modeling may track the relationship between citrate dose, ionized calcium, total calcium, and acid–base balance, identifying patients at risk of citrate accumulation or insufficient anticoagulation. Also, AI-modeling may suggest titrations that maintain filter patency while minimizing metabolic disturbances.

3.5 Foundations of Artificial Intelligence in Extracorporeal Therapy

3.5.1 Machine Learning and Deep Learning for Prediction

Machine learning techniques have demonstrated superior performance compared with traditional scoring systems in a variety of ICU prediction tasks. From the EBPT perspective, these predictive capabilities can be redirected to estimate when a patient is about to cross a threshold where these therapies become beneficial. Rather than regarding CRRT, adsorptive membranes, and cartridges as binary present/absent interventions, AI may allow them to be viewed as timed responses within a continuous trajectory.

3.5.2 Reinforcement Learning for Treatment Strategies

Reinforcement learning differs fundamentally from supervised prediction: instead of forecasting an outcome given a set of features, RL learns a policy for selecting actions in a dynamic environment. The same paradigm should be applied to extracorporeal therapy. An RL agent can be trained to adjust CRRT dose, blood flow, anticoagulation, and membrane choice in response to evolving physiological and biochemical states, with a reward signal defined in terms of short-term stability and long-term outcomes. In simulation environments constructed from historical data, the agent can explore a wide range of strategies without risk to patients, converging on policies that outperform static protocols. Then, these policies may be embedded as decision-support tools rather than fully autonomous controllers.

3.5.3 AI, Multiomics, and Digital Twins in Blood Purification

The future of personalized blood purification lies not only in better use of existing clinical data but also in integrating multiomics. Transcriptomics, proteomics, metabolomics, and even single-cell analyses are increasingly feasible, at least in research settings, and they provide a granular view of the host response.

AI methods are essential for making sense of such high-dimensional data. Unsupervised clustering algorithms may be useful to identify novel inflammatory endotypes based on multiomic signatures. Then, supervised models may be trained to recognize these endotypes from a small subset of clinically accessible biomarkers and physiological signals, potentially enabling their use in routine practice. In this setting, the concept of a "digital twin" is particularly relevant. A digital twin consists of a computational model that emulates an individual patient's physiology, updated continuously with real-time data. In the context of EBPTs, a digital twin may simulate how different extracorporeal strategies (e.g., CRRT dose profiles, membrane types, adsorption intensities) would affect solute kinetics, cytokine levels, hemodynamics, and drug concentrations in a specific patient. AI models would serve both as the engine of the twin and as the inference mechanism that updates it as new data arrive. Such digital twins could be used to perform virtual trials of extracorporeal strategies before applying them in vivo, effectively conducting a kind of $N = 1$ randomized trial in silico. While still largely experimental, this approach aligns well with the broader movement toward model-informed precision dosing and personalized organ support.

3.6 Future Directions and Research Agenda

The integration of AI and blood purification invites a rich research agenda. Prospective interventional studies are urgently needed to test whether AI modeling may play a role in the management of EBPTs. In light of this view, collaborative registries that link detailed extracorporeal device logs, physiological monitoring, laboratory data, omics, and outcome measures are necessary for training robust models. Accordingly, federated learning frameworks appear to be of interest to allow multiple institutions to contribute to model development without sharing raw patient data, thus preserving privacy while improving generalizability. In order to make it possible, there is also a need for standards that include: standards for representing extracorporeal device data in interoperable formats; standards for reporting AI models in critical care; and standards for evaluating AI-guided interventions in clinical trials. For these reasons, multinational collaborative initiatives and consensus are strongly advocated.

3.7 Conclusion

Blood purification in critically ill patients has historically been delivered according to simple, largely uniform protocols that fail to account for the biological and temporal heterogeneity of sepsis and organ failure. At the same time, extracorporeal technologies have become increasingly sophisticated, capable of nuanced modulation of solutes, cytokines, endotoxin, and volume status. Artificial intelligence is the missing integrative layer that can reconcile these two trajectories. By leveraging predictive models, reinforcement learning, multiomics integration, and explainable decision-support, AI may help patient identification, EBPT choice, and online management. Moreover, AI may potentially help to re-interpret the equivocal evidence of traditional trials by analyzing raw data and uncovering the responsive subgroups hidden within heterogeneous populations.

If these challenges are met, AI-enabled personalized blood purification has the potential to transform extracorporeal therapy from a blunt instrument into a precise, adaptive, biologically informed intervention that may play a pivotal role in improving patient-related outcomes.

References

1. Husain-Syed F, Ricci Z, Brodie D, Vincent J-L, Ranieri VM, Slutsky AS, Taccone FS, Gattinoni L, Ronco C. Extracorporeal organ support (ECOS) in critical illness and acute kidney injury: from native to artificial organ crosstalk. Intensive Care Med. 2018;44:1447–59. https://doi.org/10.1007/s00134-018-5329-z.
2. De Rosa S, Cutuli SL, Lorenzin A, Zanella M. Sequential extracorporeal therapy in sepsis. In: Bellomo R, Ronco C, editors. Contributions to nephrology. S. Karger AG; 2023. p. 149–59.
3. Rudd KE, Johnson SC, Agesa KM, Shackelford KA, Tsoi D, Kievlan DR, Colombara DV, Ikuta KS, Kissoon N, Finfer S, Fleischmann-Struzek C, Machado FR, Reinhart KK, Rowan K, Seymour CW, Watson RS, West TE, Marinho F, Hay SI, Lozano R, Lopez AD, Angus DC, Murray CJL, Naghavi M. Global, regional, and national sepsis incidence and mortality, 1990–2017: analysis for the Global Burden of Disease Study. Lancet. 2020;395:200–11. https://doi.org/10.1016/S0140-6736(19)32989-7.
4. Singer M, Deutschman CS, Seymour CW, Shankar-Hari M, Annane D, Bauer M, Bellomo R, Bernard GR, Chiche J-D, Coopersmith CM, Hotchkiss RS, Levy MM, Marshall JC, Martin GS, Opal SM, Rubenfeld GD, van der Poll T, Vincent J-L, Angus DC. The third international consensus definitions for sepsis and septic shock (Sepsis-3). JAMA. 2016;315:801–10. https://doi.org/10.1001/jama.2016.0287.
5. Seymour CW, Kennedy JN, Wang S, Chang C-CH, Elliott CF, Xu Z, Berry S, Clermont G, Cooper G, Gomez H, Huang DT, Kellum JA, Mi Q, Opal SM, Talisa V, Van Der Poll T, Visweswaran S, Vodovotz Y, Weiss JC, Yealy DM, Yende S, Angus DC. Derivation, validation, and potential treatment implications of novel clinical phenotypes for sepsis. JAMA. 2019;321:2003. https://doi.org/10.1001/jama.2019.5791.
6. Scicluna BP, Van Vught LA, Zwinderman AH, Wiewel MA, Davenport EE, Burnham KL, Nürnberg P, Schultz MJ, Horn J, Cremer OL, Bonten MJ, Hinds CJ, Wong HR, Knight JC, Van Der Poll T, De Beer FM, Bos LDJ, Frencken JF, Koster-Brouwer ME, Van De Groep K, Verboom DM, Glas GJ, Van Hooijdonk RTM, Hoogendijk AJ, Huson MA, Klouwenberg PMK, Ong DSY, Schouten LRA, Straat M, Witteveen E, Wieske L. Classification of patients with sepsis according to blood genomic endotype: a prospective cohort study. Lancet Respir Med. 2017;5:816–26. https://doi.org/10.1016/S2213-2600(17)30294-1.
7. Tomašev N, Glorot X, Rae JW, Zielinski M, Askham H, Saraiva A, Mottram A, Meyer C, Ravuri S, Protsyuk I, Connell A, Hughes CO, Karthikesalingam A, Cornebise J, Montgomery H, Rees G, Laing C, Baker CR, Peterson K, Reeves R, Hassabis D, King D, Suleyman M, Back T, Nielson C, Ledsam JR, Mohamed S. A clinically applicable approach to continuous prediction of future acute kidney injury. Nature. 2019;572:116–9. https://doi.org/10.1038/s41586-019-1390-1.
8. Evans L, Rhodes A, Alhazzani W, Antonelli M, Coopersmith CM, French C, Machado FR, Mcintyre L, Ostermann M, Prescott HC, Schorr C, Simpson S, Wiersinga WJ, Alshamsi F, Angus DC, Arabi Y, Azevedo L, Beale R, Beilman G, Belley-Cote E, Burry L, Cecconi M, Centofanti J, Coz Yataco A, De Waele J, Dellinger RP, Doi K, Du B, Estenssoro E, Ferrer R, Gomersall C, Hodgson C, Møller MH, Iwashyna T, Jacob S, Kleinpell R, Klompas M, Koh Y, Kumar A, Kwizera A, Lobo S, Masur H, McGloughlin S, Mehta S, Mehta Y, Mer M, Nunnally M, Oczkowski S, Osborn T, Papathanassoglou E, Perner A, Puskarich M, Roberts J, Schweickert W, Seckel M, Sevransky J, Sprung CL, Welte T, Zimmerman J, Levy M. Surviving sepsis campaign: international guidelines for management of sepsis and septic shock 2021. Intensive Care Med. 2021;47:1181–247. https://doi.org/10.1007/s00134-021-06506-y.
9. Hotchkiss RS, Moldawer LL, Opal SM, Reinhart K, Turnbull IR, Vincent J-L. Sepsis and septic shock. Nat Rev Dis Primers. 2016;2:16045. https://doi.org/10.1038/nrdp.2016.45.
10. Rimmel T, Kellum JA. Clinical review: blood purification for sepsis. Crit Care. 2011;15:205. https://doi.org/10.1186/cc9411.
11. Vincent J-L, Moreno R, Takala J, Willatts S, De Mendonça A, Bruining H, Reinhart CK, Suter PM, Thijs LG. The SOFA (Sepsis-related Organ Failure Assessment) score to describe organ dysfunction/failure: on behalf of the Working Group on Sepsis-Related Problems of the

European Society of Intensive Care Medicine (see contributors to the project in the appendix). Intensive Care Med. 1996;22:707–10. https://doi.org/10.1007/BF01709751.
12. Ranzani OT, Singer M, Salluh JIF, Shankar-Hari M, Pilcher D, Berger-Estilita J, Coopersmith CM, Juffermans NP, Laffey J, Reinikainen M, Neto AS, Tavares M, Timsit J-F, Arias Lopez MDP, Arulkumaran N, Aryal D, Azoulay E, Celi LA, Chaudhuri D, De Lange D, De Waele J, Dos Santos CC, Du B, Einav S, Engelbrecht T, Fazla F, Ferrer R, Finazzi S, Fujii T, Gershengorn HB, Greene JD, Haniffa R, Hao S, Hasan MS, Hollenberg S, Ippolito M, Jung C, Kirov M, Kobari S, Lakbar I, Lipman J, Liu V, Liu X, Lobo SM, Magatti D, Martin GS, Metnitz B, Metnitz P, Myatra SN, Oczkowski S, Paiva J-A, Paruk F, Pekkarinen PT, Piquilloud L, Pölkki A, Prescott HC, Blaser AR, Rezende E, Robba C, Rochwerg B, Ruckly S, Samei R, Schenck EJ, Secombe P, Sendagire C, Siaw-Frimpong M, Simpkin AJ, Soares M, Summers C, Szczeklik W, Takala J, Tanaka S, Tricella G, Vincent J-L, Wendon J, Zampieri FG, Rhodes A, Moreno R. Development and validation of the sequential organ failure assessment (SOFA)-2 score. JAMA. 2025;334:2090–103. https://doi.org/10.1001/jama.2025.20516.
13. Hoste EAJ, Bagshaw SM, Bellomo R, Cely CM, Colman R, Cruz DN, Edipidis K, Forni LG, Gomersall CD, Govil D, Honoré PM, Joannes-Boyau O, Joannidis M, Korhonen A-M, Lavrentieva A, Mehta RL, Palevsky P, Roessler E, Ronco C, Uchino S, Vazquez JA, Vidal Andrade E, Webb S, Kellum JA. Epidemiology of acute kidney injury in critically ill patients: the multinational AKI-EPI study. Intensive Care Med. 2015;41:1411–23. https://doi.org/10.1007/s00134-015-3934-7.
14. Vaara ST, Bhatraju PK, Stanski NL, McMahon BA, Liu K, Joannidis M, Bagshaw SM. Subphenotypes in acute kidney injury: a narrative review. Crit Care. 2022;26:251. https://doi.org/10.1186/s13054-022-04121-x.
15. White KC, Serpa-Neto A, Hurford R, Clement P, Laupland KB, See E, McCullough J, White H, Shekar K, Tabah A, Ramanan M, Garrett P, Attokaran AG, Luke S, Senthuran S, McIlroy P, Bellomo R, the Queensland Critical Care Research Network (QCCRN), Ramanan M, Marella P, Young P, McIlroy P, Nash B, McCullough J, Tallott M, Marshall A, Moore D, White H, Sane S, Morrison L, Dipplesman P, Luke S, Paasilahti A, Asimus R, Taylor J, White K, Cook D, Kruger P, Meyer J, Hurford R, Plumpton K, Barlow A, Tabah A, Pollock H, Young P, Attokaran AG, Poggenpoel J, Reoch J, Laupland KB, Edwards F, Dhanani J, Kirrane M, Clement P, Karamujic N, Lister P, Masurkar V, Murray L, Brailsford J, Erbacher T, Shekar K, Lavana J, Cornell G, Senthuran S, Whebell S, Henson G, Gatton M, Tyack Z, Andrews R, Ter Hofstede A, Wynn M, Laupland KB, Edwards F. Sepsis-associated acute kidney injury in the intensive care unit: incidence, patient characteristics, timing, trajectory, treatment, and associated outcomes. A multicenter, observational study. Intensive Care Med. 2023;49:1079–89. https://doi.org/10.1007/s00134-023-07138-0.
16. Gaudry S, Hajage D, Schortgen F, Martin-Lefevre L, Pons B, Boulet E, Boyer A, Chevrel G, Lerolle N, Carpentier D, De Prost N, Lautrette A, Bretagnol A, Mayaux J, Nseir S, Megarbane B, Thirion M, Forel J-M, Maizel J, Yonis H, Markowicz P, Thiery G, Tubach F, Ricard J-D, Dreyfuss D. Initiation strategies for renal-replacement therapy in the intensive care unit. N Engl J Med. 2016;375:122–33. https://doi.org/10.1056/NEJMoa1603017.
17. Zarbock A, Kellum JA, Schmidt C, Van Aken H, Wempe C, Pavenstädt H, Boanta A, Gerß J, Meersch M. Effect of early vs delayed initiation of renal replacement therapy on mortality in critically ill patients with acute kidney injury: the ELAIN randomized clinical trial. JAMA. 2016;315:2190. https://doi.org/10.1001/jama.2016.5828.
18. Barbar SD, Clere-Jehl R, Bourredjem A, Hernu R, Montini F, Bruyère R, Lebert C, Bohé J, Badie J, Eraldi J-P, Rigaud J-P, Levy B, Siami S, Louis G, Bouadma L, Constantin J-M, Mercier E, Klouche K, Du Cheyron D, Piton G, Annane D, Jaber S, Van Der Linden T, Blasco G, Mira J-P, Schwebel C, Chimot L, Guiot P, Nay M-A, Meziani F, Helms J, Roger C, Louart B, Trusson R, Dargent A, Binquet C, Quenot J-P. Timing of renal-replacement therapy in patients with acute kidney injury and sepsis. N Engl J Med. 2018;379:1431–42. https://doi.org/10.1056/NEJMoa1803213.
19. The STARRT-AKI Investigators. Timing of initiation of renal-replacement therapy in acute kidney injury. N Engl J Med. 2020;383:240–51. https://doi.org/10.1056/NEJMoa2000741.

20. Gaudry S, Hajage D, Martin-Lefevre L, Lebbah S, Louis G, Moschietto S, Titeca-Beauport D, Combe BL, Pons B, De Prost N, Besset S, Combes A, Robine A, Beuzelin M, Badie J, Chevrel G, Bohé J, Coupez E, Chudeau N, Barbar S, Vinsonneau C, Forel J-M, Thevenin D, Boulet E, Lakhal K, Aissaoui N, Grange S, Leone M, Lacave G, Nseir S, Poirson F, Mayaux J, Asehnoune K, Geri G, Klouche K, Thiery G, Argaud L, Rozec B, Cadoz C, Andreu P, Reignier J, Ricard J-D, Quenot J-P, Dreyfuss D. Comparison of two delayed strategies for renal replacement therapy initiation for severe acute kidney injury (AKIKI 2): a multicentre, open-label, randomised, controlled trial. Lancet. 2021;397:1293–300. https://doi.org/10.1016/S0140-6736(21)00350-0.
21. Gaudry S, Verney C, Hajage D, Ricard JD, Dreyfuss D. Hypothesis: early renal replacement therapy increases mortality in critically ill patients with acute on chronic renal failure. A post hoc analysis of the AKIKI trial. Intensive Care Med. 2018;44:1360–1. https://doi.org/10.1007/s00134-018-5210-0.
22. Gaudry S, Hajage D, Schortgen F, Martin-Lefevre L, Verney C, Pons B, Boulet E, Boyer A, Chevrel G, Lerolle N, Carpentier D, De Prost N, Lautrette A, Bretagnol A, Mayaux J, Nseir S, Megarbane B, Thirion M, Forel J-M, Maizel J, Yonis H, Markowicz P, Thiery G, Tubach F, Ricard J-D, Dreyfuss D. Timing of renal support and outcome of septic shock and acute respiratory distress syndrome. A post hoc analysis of the AKIKI randomized clinical trial. Am J Respir Crit Care Med. 2018;198:58–66. https://doi.org/10.1164/rccm.201706-1255OC.
23. Zampieri FG, Serpa-Neto A, Wald R, Bellomo R, Bagshaw SM. Hierarchical endpoints in critical care: a post-hoc exploratory analysis of the standard versus accelerated initiation of renal-replacement therapy in acute kidney injury and the intensity of continuous renal-replacement therapy in critically ill patients trials. J Crit Care. 2024;82:154767. https://doi.org/10.1016/j.jcrc.2024.154767.
24. Barbar SD, Bourredjem A, Trusson R, Dargent A, Binquet C, Quenot J-P, IDEAL-ICU Study, Clere-Jehl R, Hernu R, Montini F, Bruyère R, Lebert C, Bohé J, Badie J, Eraldi J-P, Rigaud J-P, Levy B, Siami S, Louis G, Bouadma L, Constantin J-M, Mercier E, Klouche K, Du Cheyron D, Piton G, Annane D, Jaber S, Van Der Linden T, Blasco G, Mira J-P, Schwebel C, Chimot L, Guiot P, Nay M-A, Meziani F, Helms J, Roger C, Louart B. Differential effect on mortality of the timing of initiation of renal replacement therapy according to the criteria used to diagnose acute kidney injury: an IDEAL-ICU substudy. Crit Care. 2023;27:316. https://doi.org/10.1186/s13054-023-04602-7.
25. VA/NIH Acute Renal Failure Trial Network. Intensity of renal support in critically ill patients with acute kidney injury. N Engl J Med. 2008;359:7–20. https://doi.org/10.1056/NEJMoa0802639.
26. RENAL Replacement Therapy Study Investigators. Intensity of continuous renal-replacement therapy in critically ill patients. N Engl J Med. 2009;361:1627–38. https://doi.org/10.1056/NEJMoa0902413.
27. Kellum JA, Lameire N, for the KDIGO AKI Guideline Work Group. Diagnosis, evaluation, and management of acute kidney injury: a KDIGO summary (Part 1). Crit Care. 2013;17:204. https://doi.org/10.1186/cc11454.
28. Broman ME, Hansson F, Vincent J-L, Bodelsson M. Endotoxin and cytokine reducing properties of the oXiris membrane in patients with septic shock: a randomized crossover double-blind study. PLoS One. 2019;14:e0220444. https://doi.org/10.1371/journal.pone.0220444.
29. Pérez-Fernández X, Ulsamer A, Cámara-Rosell M, Sbraga F, Boza-Hernández E, Moret-Ruíz E, Plata-Menchaca E, Santiago-Bautista D, Boronat-García P, Gumucio-Sanguino V, Peñafiel-Muñoz J, Camacho-Pérez M, Betbesé-Roig A, Forni L, Campos-Gómez A, Sabater-Riera J, SIRAKI02 Study Group, Ballus Noguera J, Huguet Briba M, Máñez Mendiluce R, Esteve Urbano F, Santafosta Gómez E, Alanez Saavedra BH, Alonso Juste V, Anguela Calvet L, Ávila Espinoza RS, Cárdenas Campos P, Carrió Cardona ML, Casanovas Lorenzo T, Corral Ansa L, Corral VF, Farrero Bayarri E, Fuset Cabanes MP, Granada Vicente R, López Delgado JC, López Suñe N, Maisterra Santos K, Moreno GJ, Oliver Juan E, Pons Serra M, Periche Pedra E, Sastre Pérez P, Soley Corderas R, Rodríguez Castro D, Torrado Santos HR, Belda Ley M-D, Di Paolo FA, Lores AC, Luna Solis S-M, Ochagavía Calvo AR, Serra Paya P, Garcia Zaloña A, Via Clavero G, Boza Hernández E, Gil Dorado A, Bonet Burguera A, Mendez Arias E, Garcia Ballester S, Leon Moreno A, Herrera RS, Sanz Iturbe M, Toscano Fernández J, Sbraga

F, Potocnik Potocnik M, Osorio Higa K, Miralles Cassina A, Ortiz Berbel D, Toral Sepúlveda D, Blasco Lucas A, Dantas A, Cevallos B, Tejero J, Martinez Sepena L, Iglesias Gordillo F, Bautista Correa MJ, Gutiérrez Y, Modrego Montiel E, Albendea Perell C, Castillo J, Bruguera E, Oliveras M, Badia Gamarra S, Berastegui Garcia E, Torres Aparicio O, Finestres Martin M, Buys S, Escudero Teixidó A, Massó Lago E, Ródenas Gómez F, Rodríguez Núñez M, Sariñena Fernandez MT, Ayala Gallardo M, Charlotte Philibert VJ, Sánchez Satorra M, Tomasa Irriguible T, Valls Estrada EA, Hueso M, Montero N, Estruch M, Ordoñez Llanos J, Hernandez Platero L, Rigo Bonnin R, Mora V, Arnaiz Francos A, Moreno Durán A, Farigola Munuera ME, Julià Valls C, Gonzalez Pujol A, Romera Peregrina I, Lerma Brianso C, Vera Martinez A, Prieto Palomino S, Carretero Aguilà J, Querol Parra, Torà Navarro L, Gonzalez Romero M, Gonzalez Barrera L, Puente Mora E, Briones Roc M, Pérez Sanchez J, Sanz Mellado C, Garcia-Morron Gallego A, Campoy A, Clavería O, Martinez Ocon S, Vazquez Guillamet B, Costa Capela L, Torreguitart I, Duran Colacios M, Puig Aragon A, Martinez Orellana M, Perez Soria D, Peribañez Biedma C, Gonzalez Del Hoyo S, Montoya Perez A, Sanchez Escudero M, Mendoza Jimenez C, Mesa Carrizosa C, Ibern Navarro L, Lopez Gonzalez O, Burgos Naranjo MA, Moreno Duran AM, Rodriguez Contreras P, Mora Muñiz V, Cabezas Garrido S, CarrionSanchez A, Ausio Navarro M, Gascon Tomas L, Fuentes Mila V, Chinchilla Perez A, Castaño Camuñez J, Nogales Ibañez R, Gimenez Vila V, Sanjuan Navais M, Rodriguez Gonzalez D, Gracia Martinez A, Ojeda Jimenez V, Hamed Loukili S, Perea Sanchez L, Buendia Flores R, Ramos Puig JM, Piquer Robles C, Marti Massanas L, Gil Ginebra C, Moreno Santoro A, Llamas Ruiz J, Hurtado Hidalgo S, Pujadas Fernandez-Cordeiro M, Barranco Rodriguez A, Olivera Rodriguez T, Cardenete Villarroyo A, Cruz Bardina S, Serrano Jaureguizar S, Del Rio Sanchez A, Llamas Bolta M, Gonzalez Lopez C, Justel Garcia RF, Ruiz De Pablo B, Figuereo Beltre D, Fernandez Gallego C, Julià Amill I, Delgado Ramis L, Romero Ferrer B, Roig Pineda R, Cabaña Benjumea A, Anglada Oliván M, Catalán Eraso B, Farré Estebe A, Ruiz Artola V, Bonet Cruces E, González Martínez E, Fabra Raduà M, Manciño Contreras JM, Martinez Vega S, Raguer Pardo L, Perez González V, Velázquez Torres M, Diago Ferré M, Blasco Torres C, Bielsa Berrocal L, Garces Gimeno B, Rodriguez Pedreira P, Muñoz Del Rio G, Bervel Franco D, Rodriguez Fanjul J, Benveniste Perez E, Chavez Diandreras F, Bauça Socies M, Pons López T, Mota Montané DP, Coluccio Pereira EE. Extracorporeal blood purification and acute kidney injury in cardiac surgery: the SIRAKI02 randomized clinical trial. JAMA. 2024;332:1446. https://doi.org/10.1001/jama.2024.20630.
30. Schädler D, Pausch C, Heise D, Meier-Hellmann A, Brederlau J, Weiler N, Marx G, Putensen C, Spies C, Jörres A, Quintel M, Engel C, Kellum JA, Kuhlmann MK. The effect of a novel extracorporeal cytokine hemoadsorption device on IL-6 elimination in septic patients: a randomized controlled trial. PLoS One. 2017;12:e0187015. https://doi.org/10.1371/journal.pone.0187015.
31. Supady A, Weber E, Rieder M, Lother A, Niklaus T, Zahn T, Frech F, Müller S, Kuhl M, Benk C, Maier S, Trummer G, Flügler A, Krüger K, Sekandarzad A, Stachon P, Zotzmann V, Bode C, Biever PM, Staudacher D, Wengenmayer T, Graf E, Duerschmied D. Cytokine adsorption in patients with severe COVID-19 pneumonia requiring extracorporeal membrane oxygenation (CYCOV): a single centre, open-label, randomised, controlled trial. Lancet Respir Med. 2021;9:755–62. https://doi.org/10.1016/S2213-2600(21)00177-6.
32. Cruz DN, Antonelli M, Fumagalli R, Foltran F, Brienza N, Donati A, Malcangi V, Petrini F, Volta G, Bobbio Pallavicini FM, Rottoli F, Giunta F, Ronco C. Early use of polymyxin B hemoperfusion in abdominal septic shock: the EUPHAS randomized controlled trial. JAMA. 2009;301:2445. https://doi.org/10.1001/jama.2009.856.
33. Dellinger RP, Bagshaw SM, Antonelli M, Foster DM, Klein DJ, Marshall JC, Palevsky PM, Weisberg LS, Schorr CA, Trzeciak S, Walker PM, for the EUPHRATES Trial Investigators. Effect of targeted polymyxin B hemoperfusion on 28-day mortality in patients with septic shock and elevated endotoxin level: the EUPHRATES randomized clinical trial. JAMA. 2018;320:1455. https://doi.org/10.1001/jama.2018.14618.
34. Marshall JC, Foster D, Vincent J, Cook DJ, Cohen J, Dellinger RP, Opal S, Abraham E, Brett SJ, Smith T, Mehta S, Derzko A, Romaschin A. Diagnostic and prognostic implications of

endotoxemia in critical illness: results of the MEDIC study. J Infect Dis. 2004;190:527–34. https://doi.org/10.1086/422254.

35. Klein DJ, Foster D, Walker PM, Bagshaw SM, Mekonnen H, Antonelli M. Polymyxin B hemoperfusion in endotoxemic septic shock patients without extreme endotoxemia: a post hoc analysis of the EUPHRATES trial. Intensive Care Med. 2018;44:2205–12. https://doi.org/10.1007/s00134-018-5463-7.
36. Cutuli SL, Cascarano L, Lazzaro P, Tanzarella ES, Pintaudi G, Grieco DL, De Pascale G, Antonelli M. Antimicrobial exposure in critically ill patients with sepsis-associated multi-organ dysfunction requiring extracorporeal organ support: a narrative review. Microorganisms. 2023;11:473. https://doi.org/10.3390/microorganisms11020473.
37. Roberts JA, Joynt GM, Lee A, Choi G, Bellomo R, Kanji S, Mudaliar MY, Peake SL, Stephens D, Taccone FS, Ulldemolins M, Valkonen MM, Agbeve J, Baptista JP, Bekos V, Boidin C, Brinkmann A, Buizen L, Castro P, Cole CL, Creteur J, De Waele JJ, Deans R, Eastwood GM, Escobar L, Gomersall C, Gresham R, Jamal JA, Kluge S, König C, Koulouras VP, Lassig-Smith M, Laterre P-F, Lei K, Leung P, Lefrant J-Y, Llauradó-Serra M, Martin-Loeches I, Mat Nor MB, Ostermann M, Parker SL, Rello J, Roberts DM, Roberts MS, Richards B, Rodríguez A, Roehr AC, Roger C, Seoane L, Sinnollareddy M, Sousa E, Soy D, Spring A, Starr T, Thomas J, Turnidge J, Wallis SC, Williams T, Wittebole X, Zikou XT, Paul SK, Lipman J, SMARRT Study Collaborators and the ANZICS Clinical Trials Group, Andresen M, Baltazar SF, Barbar S, Costa E, Durand D, Freitas R, Frey OR, Guerra Valero Y, Haughton M, Koeberer A, Kollef M, Klein K, Mehta R, McKenzie C, Muller L, Nair P, Nayyar V, Ordóñez Mejia JL, Panagou G-L, Paxton J, Peck L, Samanta M, Vincent J-L, Wan R, Young H. The effect of renal replacement therapy and antibiotic dose on antibiotic concentrations in critically ill patients: data from the multinational sampling antibiotics in renal replacement therapy study. Clin Infect Dis. 2021;72:1369–78. https://doi.org/10.1093/cid/ciaa224.
38. Roberts JA, Paul SK, Akova M, Bassetti M, De Waele JJ, Dimopoulos G, Kaukonen K-M, Koulenti D, Martin C, Montravers P, Rello J, Rhodes A, Starr T, Wallis SC, Lipman J, DALI Study, Roberts JA, Lipman J, Starr T, Wallis SC, Paul SK, Margarit Ribas A, De Waele JJ, De Crop L, Spapen H, Wauters J, Dugernier T, Jorens P, Dapper I, De Backer D, Taccone FS, Rello J, Ruano L, Afonso E, Alvarez-Lerma F, Gracia-Arnillas MP, Fernandez F, Feijoo N, Bardolet N, Rovira A, Garro P, Colon D, Castillo C, Fernado J, Lopez MJ, Fernandez JL, Arribas AM, Teja JL, Ots E, Carlos Montejo J, Catalan M, Prieto I, Gonzalo G, Galvan B, Blasco MA, Meyer E, Del Nogal F, Vidaur L, Sebastian R, Garde PM, Martin Velasco MDM, Zaragoza Crespo R, Esperatti M, Torres A, Montravers P, Baldesi O, Dupont H, Mahjoub Y, Lasocki S, Constantin JM, Payen JF, Martin C, Albanese J, Malledant Y, Pottecher J, Lefrant J-Y, Jaber S, Joannes-Boyau O, Orban C, Ostermann M, McKenzie C, Berry W, Smith J, Lei K, Rubulotta F, Gordon A, Brett S, Stotz M, Templeton M, Rhodes A, Ebm C, Moran C, Kaukonen K-M, Pettila V, Dimopoulos G, Koulenti D, Xristodoulou A, Theodorou V, Kouliatsis G, Sertaridou E, Anthopoulos G, Choutas G, Rantis T, Karatzas S, Balla M, Papanikolaou M, Myrianthefs P, Gavala A, Fildisis G, Koutsoukou A, Kyriakopoulou M, Petrochilou K, Kompoti M, Michalia M, Clouva-Molyvdas F-M, Gkiokas G, Nikolakopoulos F, Psychogiou V, Malliotakis P, Akoumianaki E, Lilitsis E, Koulouras V, Nakos G, Kalogirou M, Komnos A, Zafeiridis T, Chaintoutis C, Arvaniti K, Matamis D, Chaintoutis C, Kydona C, Gritsi-Gerogianni N, Giasnetsova T, Giannakou M, Soultati I, Chytas I, Antoniadou E, Antipa E, Lathyris D, Koukoubani T, Paraforou T, Spiropoulou K, Bekos V, Spring A, Kalatzi T, Nikolaou H, Laskou M, Strouvalis I, Aloizos S, Kapogiannis S, Soldatou O, Bassetti M, Adembri C, Villa G, Giarratano A, Maurizio Raineri S, Cortegiani A, Montalto F, Strano MT, Ranieri VM, Sandroni C, De Pascale G, Molin A, Pelosi P, Montagnani L, Urbino R, Mastromauro I, De Rosa FG, Ranieri VM, Cardoso T, Afonso S, Goncalves-Pereira J, Baptista JP, Akova M, Ozveren A. DALI: defining antibiotic levels in intensive care unit patients: are current -lactam antibiotic doses sufficient for critically ill patients? Clin Infect Dis. 2014;58:1072–83. https://doi.org/10.1093/cid/ciu027.

Advanced Adsorption Technologies and Selective Cytokine Removal

4

Francesco Guzzi and Vincenzo Pota

4.1 Background

Over the past two decades, extracorporeal therapies for sepsis, systemic inflammation, and organ dysfunction have undergone substantial evolution. While early blood purification strategies were primarily developed for renal replacement therapy, advances in the understanding of inflammatory pathobiology have shifted the focus toward both selective and nonselective adsorption platforms capable of modulating the host immune response. This shift is clinically justified: sepsis and related inflammatory states are driven by a complex interplay of pathogen-associated molecular patterns (PAMPs), damage-associated molecular patterns (DAMPs), and a vast network of cytokines that collectively sustain an uncontrolled cycle of immune activation and organ injury. Advanced adsorption technologies refer to engineered systems designed to efficiently and selectively remove specific molecules—such as cytokines—from blood or plasma, typically through extracorporeal hemoperfusion or filtration. These systems employ adsorbents with tailored pore sizes, surface chemistries, and functionalization strategies (e.g., antibodies or nanobodies) to enhance both selectivity and adsorption capacity. Selective cytokine removal involves the targeted elimination of pathogenic cytokines (e.g., TNF-α, IL-6, IL-1β, IL-17A) with the goal of restoring immune homeostasis in conditions such as sepsis, cytokine release syndrome, or severe systemic inflammation.

F. Guzzi
Nephrology and Dialysis Unit, Department of Medical Specialties, Azienda USL Toscana Centro, Prato, Italy
e-mail: francesco.guzzi@uslcentro.toscana.it

V. Pota (✉)
Anesthesia and Intensive Care Unit, Department of Women, Child, General and Specialistic Surgery, University of Campania "L. Vanvitelli", Naples, Italy
e-mail: vincenzo.pota@unicampania.it

S. De Rosa, S. Lassola (eds.), *Next-Gen Blood Purification*,
https://doi.org/10.1007/978-3-032-27033-7_4

Selectivity may be achieved through ligand functionalization—using antibodies or nanobodies—or through engineering adsorbent structures that preferentially capture molecules of specific sizes or charges. This approach allows deleterious cytokines to be reduced while sparing beneficial plasma components and can be customized to remove multiple mediators simultaneously.

This chapter synthesizes these developments and discusses how adsorption technologies are reshaping the management of inflammation in critical care.

4.2 Engineering Framework of Adsorption Technologies

To frame these developments from an engineering perspective, adsorptive blood purification technologies can be classified into two fundamentally different generations. First-generation systems rely on passive, nonselective physisorption within porous materials integrated into extracorporeal circuits. These platforms are designed to broadly remove middle-molecular-weight solutes through hydrophobic and electrostatic interactions, with limited control over molecular specificity or adsorption kinetics.

In contrast, next-generation adsorption systems are being engineered as active, molecularly selective modules in which surface chemistry, ligand specificity, and hydrodynamic design are co-optimized to control which mediators are removed, when, and at what rate. Rather than functioning as passive filters, these platforms behave as programmable extracorporeal reactors capable of interacting with the immune system at the molecular level. This conceptual shift, from bulk cytokine removal to precision immunomodulation, provides the technological framework underlying both the limitations of current devices and the promise of emerging selective adsorption strategies discussed in this chapter.

4.3 Biological Rationale for Cytokine Removal

The biological rationale for cytokine removal in sepsis, cytokine release syndrome (CRS), and other hyperinflammatory conditions is grounded in the dysregulated and excessive immune response characteristic of these states. In both sepsis and CRS, PAMPs and DAMPs activate innate immune cells, leading to the release of large quantities of pro-inflammatory cytokines such as TNF-α, IL-1β, and IL-6. This generates a self-amplifying "*cytokine storm*", which drives endothelial dysfunction, capillary leak, coagulopathy, and ultimately multiorgan failure [1–4].

Cytokine removal therapies—such as hemoadsorption, high-volume hemofiltration, and other blood purification techniques—aim to attenuate this hyperinflammatory state by physically removing circulating cytokines and inflammatory mediators. The goal is to interrupt the vicious cycle of immune activation, reduce collateral tissue injury, and restore immune homeostasis [1, 5]. Elevated cytokine levels correlate with disease severity and poor outcomes in both sepsis and CRS [2, 6].

However, these syndromes often progress from early hyperinflammation to later immunosuppression, with rising anti-inflammatory cytokines and regulatory mediators. Indiscriminate cytokine removal may therefore risk exacerbating immunoparalysis and impairing pathogen clearance [4, 7]. Thus, cytokine removal may be beneficial during early hyperinflammation, but clinical application requires careful patient selection and precise timing [1, 4, 7].

4.4 Physiochemical Principles and Mechanisms

Unlike chemisorption—which involves the formation of chemical bonds—nonselective adsorption relies largely on physical adsorption (physisorption), a nonspecific process mediated mainly by hydrophobic interactions between the solute and the sorbent material [8].

Other mechanisms contributing to physisorption include the following:

- Ionic interactions
- van der Waals forces
- Bioaffinity-like interactions

The efficiency of adsorption depends strongly on the structural characteristics of the sorbent, including surface area, pore architecture, and polymer chemistry. In hemoperfusion cartridges using porous polymer beads (e.g., CytoSorb®), the extremely large internal surface area facilitates the capture of specific molecular classes and enables the removal of substantial amounts of solutes compared with other modalities [8]. A crucial aspect of physical adsorption is that, while binding occurs at high rates, it is also relatively weak and highly reversible. This introduces a potential disadvantage: the high rate of desorption or displacement of the target solute by competitive solutes in the bloodstream.

The Hemoadsorption can be applied using several approaches:

Direct hemoadsorption (stand-alone): blood passes directly through a dedicated sorbent cartridge.

Combined techniques: the sorbent cartridge is integrated into existing extracorporeal circuits such as intermittent hemodialysis (IHD), continuous renal replacement therapy (CRRT), extracorporeal membrane oxygenation (ECMO), or cardiopulmonary bypass (CPB) [A].

Plasma adsorption: plasma is separated, circulated through the sorbent cartridge, and reinfused.

A key limitation of physical adsorption is that binding, though rapid, is weak and reversible. Consequently, target molecules may undergo desorption or be displaced by competing solutes in blood.

4.4.1 Nonselective Adsorption Technologies

Nonselective adsorption technologies remove a wide range of cytokines and inflammatory mediators using porous polymer beads, activated carbon, or silica-based sorbents. These modalities are primarily used in severe systemic inflammation such as sepsis or septic shock, where elevated cytokines contribute to organ dysfunction [1–3, 9, 10].

Their broad activity allows rapid reduction of multiple mediators (e.g., TNF-α, IL-6, IL-8, IL-1β), PAMPs, DAMPs, and mycotoxins, but may also result in the removal of protective molecules.

4.5 First-Generation Adsorptive Membranes (PMMA)

Brand name: Hemofeel™
Producer: Toray Medical Co., Ltd., Tokyo, Japan
Material: Polymethyl methacrylate (symmetric, synthetic polymer of acrylic acid)
Surface area: CH-1.8 W (1.8 m^2, 130 mL), CH-1.3 W (1.3 m^2, 94 mL)
Target: inflammatory mediators—IL-6
Treatment duration: 48–72 h
Optimal operational blood flow: 100–300 mL/min
Anticoagulation: Heparin/RCA
Approval: Filtryzer®, Japan, 1977—Hemofeel™, FDA approval, 2000

Enhanced adsorption properties combined with filtration capability, mechanical stability, and biocompatibility make Polymethyl methacrylate (PMMA) membranes particularly suitable for the treatment of chronic and acute renal patients. Large surface area and high porosity grant elevated water and solute permeability, while adsorption targets inflammatory mediators (e.g., IL-6, immunocomplexes), and medium/high molecular weight proteins (e.g., β2-microglobulin, albumin) [11]. In vitro and animal studies demonstrated efficient cytokine removal by adsorption and modulation of immunological LPS-driven dysfunction, thus encouraging the choice of PMMA membranes for extracorporeal blood purification in the context of sepsis-associated AKI [12, 13]. Although largely and increasingly utilized since the early nineties, the available clinical studies are few and limited in the study design and sample size [11, 14]. Conflicting results emerged from the earliest RCT studies describing the use of PMMA versus cuprophane membranes [15, 16]. Later, a meta-analysis addressing this controversy established that a significant survival advantage existed for all synthetic membranes over unsubstituted cellulose [17], paving the way for its subsequent abandonment in the mid-2000s [18, 19]. A clear superiority of one particular synthetic membrane over the others (PMMA, polysulfone (PS), polyacrylonitrile (PAN), and polyamide (PA)) was not identified, particularly in terms of hard outcomes, although electron microscopy studies showed differences in the adsorption properties of proteins and cells by each membrane [17, 19, 20]. Thanks to its chemical and structural characteristics, PMMA is particularly suitable for unstable patients, reducing the risk of adverse reactions, thus contributing to treatment safety. Together with septic shock patients, subsequent studies targeted particular populations such as patients affected by tumor lysis syndrome and severe acute pancreatitis, all showing that PMMA could exert beneficial effects not only as a renal replacement therapy but also as an immune modulator [21–23]. A recent RCT among sepsis patients demonstrated a different profile of cytokine adsorption between PMMA and AN69-ST, with the former reaching the best adsorption clearance of IL-6, suggesting that the two membranes could be alternatively used based on the target cytokine [24]. In the same trial, which included 52 patients, 28-day mortality was lower, even if not significantly, in the PMMA group (30.8%) versus the AN69-ST group (50%, $p = 0.26$) [24]. The effect of cytokine modulation, and in particular IL-6 adsorption, of the PMMA membrane has also been investigated in the treatment of ARDS patients [11, 25]. In summary, PMMA, a historical membrane in use for more than 40 years, characterized by elevated biocompatibility, high-flux permeability, and notable adsorptive capacity, through cytokine and immune modulation, is gaining a new role for sepsis and systemic inflammatory response syndrome treatment in the ICU.

4.6 Charge-Engineered Adsorptive Membranes (AN69-ST, oXiris)

Brand name: oXiris®
Producer: Baxter, Deerfield, IL, USA
Material: Acrylonitrile and sodium methallyl sulfonate copolymer + PolyethyleneImine (surface treatment agent) + heparin graft (4500 +/− 1500 IU/m^2)
Surface area: 1.5 m^2
Target: endotoxin and cytokines
Treatment duration: 24–72 h
Optimal operational blood flow: 100–450 mL/min
Anticoagulation: Heparin/RCA
Approval: AN69 France, 1969—oXiris CE mark in December 2007, EU market in December 2008

The AN69 membrane, a copolymer combining acrylonitrile and sodium methallyl sulfonate, is characterized by numerous negative charges distributed in a microporous hydrogel structure with high potential for cytokine adsorption [26]. Advantages of AN69 versus polysulfone appeared soon in early animal models and clinical studies [27, 28]. The AN69 membrane was later improved with a surface treatment (ST) consisting of a polyethyleneimine (PEI) coating, which interposes a layer of positive charges at the blood-membrane interface and offers an adsorption site for heparin [29]. The AN69-ST membrane overcomes the generation and release of bradykinin, which caused episodes of severe hypotension at treatment initiation, and it enhances antithrombogenic properties, reducing the need for systemic anticoagulation and ameliorating clinical results [30–33]. A further improvement appeared in 2009 with oXiris®, an AN69-ST membrane already grafted with 4500 +/− 1500 IU/m^2 heparin and containing multiple PEI layers ready to adsorb endotoxins [34]. Together with the ability to remove solutes via diffusion and convection (cut-off 40 kDa), the absorptive properties of oXiris are confirmed by in vitro, animal, and clinical studies [35–38]. However, clinical studies with this membrane are scarce and limited in design and sample size. Direct comparison between the old and new membranes showed reduced cytokine levels but no significant differences in hard outcomes [39]. In a single-center open-label RCT, among 52 sepsis patients undergoing CRRT, the adsorption clearance of HMGB1, TNF, IL-8, CXCL9, and macrophage inflammatory protein was significantly higher compared to PMMA, which instead expressed a significantly higher IL-6 adsorption clearance [24]. The 28-day mortality, although lower in the PMMA group, was not significantly different [24]. Improvements in hemodynamic stability and cardiac performance were most evident in patients affected by abdominal sepsis complicated by septic shock and AKI, particularly those with Gram-negative bacilli infection, but the best algorithm for patient selection for the treatment is still debated. In 2020, the FDA issued an Emergency Use Authorization for the use of oXiris to treat COVID-19 patients admitted to the ICU with confirmed or imminent respiratory failure [40, 41]. In 2023, a Swiss multi-arm, randomized, controlled trial, the ENDoX study, compared oXiris, Toramyxin, and a control group in a 1:1:1 design and failed to identify a reduction in endotoxin or cytokine levels 72 h after treatment initiation in patients with highly endotoxemic, severe, and refractory septic shock [42]. The 2024 Asia-Pacific oXiris expert meeting consensus recommended, despite low-grade evidence, oXiris filters to be utilized in "sepsis or septic shock patients requiring CRRT with hemodynamic instability, hyperinflammatory state, severe lactic acidosis, or coagulation dysfunction" [43]. Careful consideration of antibiotic unintentional adsorption and removal by the oXiris membrane was also discussed and reported as an important practice point [43]. This topic has been recently explored in a comprehensive review [44]. The most recent systematic review found that patients treated with oXiris achieve a significant reduction in IL-6 levels, vasoactive inotropic score, norepinephrine dose, SOFA score, PCT, and CRP and show significant clinical improvement [45]. In summary, the use of oXiris was reported to be safe, showed improvement in clinical parameters, a reduction in inflammatory indexes, endotoxin activity, and cytokines, while its best target population and benefits on hard outcomes are yet to be investigated and are the objective of ongoing registries and clinical trials [46, 47].

4.7 Bulk Porous Sorbent Cartridges (CytoSorb®)

Brand name: CytoSorb®
Producer: CytoSorbents Corporation, Princeton, NJ, USA

Material/Mechanism: Cartridge containing polystyrene–divinylbenzene beads with a biocompatible polyvinylpyrrolidone coating, capable of adsorbing hydrophobic molecules up to approximately ~60 kDa via surface adsorption.
Target: Pro- and anti-inflammatory cytokines (e.g., IL-6, TNF-α, IL-1β), other inflammatory mediators, bilirubin, myoglobin, and selected lipophilic drugs.
Surface area: Studies report an extremely large adsorptive surface area (e.g., >40,000 m^2 theoretical adsorption surface within microporosities).
Treatment duration: Typically up to 24 h per cartridge.
Optimal operational blood flow: Reported in the literature as approximately 100–700 mL/min, depending on circuit configuration.
Anticoagulation: Can be integrated into CRRT and ECMO circuits, requiring standard anticoagulation (e.g., heparin or regional citrate anticoagulation), similar to other extracorporeal circuits (not always specified in publicly available data).
Approval: CE-marked.

The structure of the CytoSorb hemoadsorption device consists of a cartridge filled with highly porous polymer beads specifically engineered to maximize surface area and facilitate the adsorption of molecules from whole blood. These beads are composed of a biocompatible polystyrene–divinylbenzene copolymer, with pore sizes optimized to capture molecules in the 5–60 kDa range, encompassing most clinically relevant cytokines and other inflammatory mediators [48, 49].

The mechanism of action is based on nonselective adsorption: as blood passes through the cartridge, cytokines and other molecules are captured by the beads via hydrophobic interactions and size exclusion. This process allows the device to remove both pro-inflammatory and anti-inflammatory cytokines, as well as pathogen-associated molecular patterns (PAMPs), damage-associated molecular patterns (DAMPs), mycotoxins, and certain metabolic byproducts. The device is typically integrated into extracorporeal circuits such as continuous renal replacement therapy (CRRT) or extracorporeal membrane oxygenation (ECMO) [48, 50].

The cytokine adsorption profile of CytoSorb is broad. It efficiently adsorbs a wide array of cytokines, including but not limited to IL-6, TNF-α, IL-8, and IL-10, with significant reductions in plasma concentrations reported in both experimental and clinical settings. For example, in a human endotoxemia model, CytoSorb hemoperfusion resulted in a 71% reduction in IL-6, a 58% reduction in TNF-α, a 48% reduction in IL-8, and a 26% reduction in IL-10 compared with controls [51]. The device also removes other inflammatory mediators such as procalcitonin and C-reactive protein and has shown utility in conditions characterized by cytokine storm, sepsis, and acute-on-chronic liver failure [48, 51–54].

However, current clinical evidence indicates that CytoSorb hemoadsorption does not improve patient-centered outcomes such as mortality, organ dysfunction, or length of stay in the intensive care unit in conditions like sepsis or cytokine storm. Multiple systematic reviews and meta-analyses of randomized controlled trials and observational studies have consistently found no significant reduction in mortality with CytoSorb across a range of critical illnesses, including sepsis, septic shock, and COVID-19–associated cytokine storm [55–59].

Although CytoSorb therapy reliably reduces circulating cytokine levels (e.g., IL-6, TNF-α) and may transiently improve hemodynamic parameters such as mean arterial pressure and vasopressor requirements, these biochemical and physiological improvements have not translated into enhanced survival or reduced ICU length of stay in high-quality studies [53, 55, 58, 60].

Some retrospective and single-center studies have reported possible reductions in observed-versus-predicted mortality or improvements in organ dysfunction scores, but these findings are limited by methodological bias and have not been confirmed in randomized trials [54, 61, 62].

Several ongoing and upcoming randomized controlled trials are investigating the impact of CytoSorb hemoadsorption on patient-centered outcomes in sepsis and cytokine storm, aiming to provide more robust evidence regarding its clinical utility.

The DECRISS trial (NCT04742764) is a prospective, randomized, multicenter phase III study comparing standard medical therapy with CytoSorb therapy in patients with early refractory septic shock. This trial specifically evaluates shock reversal and time to shock reversal, as well as different dosing regimens (device exchange every 12 vs. 24 h), and is designed to address previous limitations in study design and sample size [63].

4.8 Resin-Based Hemoadsorption Platforms (HA330/HA380)

Brand name: HA330/HA380 (Jafron Biomedical Co., Ltd., Zhuhai, China)

Producer: Jafron Biomedical Co., Ltd., Guangdong, China

Material/Mechanism: Macroporous sorbent resin composed of styrene–divinylbenzene copolymer beads with a biocompatible surface, capable of adsorbing solutes and inflammatory mediators through hydrophobic interactions and other adsorption mechanisms.

Target: Inflammatory cytokines (e.g., IL-6, IL-10, TNF-α), other inflammatory mediators, and metabolic toxins in the blood; may also adsorb drugs and other middle-molecular-weight compounds (10–60 kDa).

Surface area: Public technical specifications do not report a defined numerical adsorptive surface area, unlike other adsorption devices.

Treatment duration: Typically ~2–2.5 h per hemoperfusion session; may be adapted in combination with other extracorporeal therapies.

Optimal operational blood flow: Generally comparable to CRRT blood flow rates (e.g., ~150–250 mL/min in standard protocols).

Anticoagulation: Can be integrated into CRRT or ECMO circuits, requiring standard anticoagulation (e.g., heparin or citrate).

Approval: CE-marked.

The Jafron HA330 and HA380 hemoadsorption cartridges are extracorporeal blood purification devices designed for the removal of inflammatory mediators in conditions such as sepsis and cytokine storm. Both cartridges contain highly porous resin beads made from a styrene–divinylbenzene copolymer, providing a large internal surface area with pore sizes optimized for the adsorption of middle-molecular-weight substances (typically 5000–60,000 Da), which include most clinically relevant cytokines [64–66].

Their mechanism of action is based on nonselective adsorption: as blood flows through the cartridge, cytokines and other inflammatory mediators are captured by the resin beads via hydrophobic and van der Waals interactions. This process effectively removes both pro-inflammatory and anti-inflammatory cytokines, along with other molecules such as C-reactive protein (CRP) and procalcitonin (PCT). The cartridges are typically integrated into continuous renal replacement therapy (CRRT) or continuous venovenous hemodiafiltration (CVVHDF) circuits [64, 65, 67].

The cytokine adsorption characteristics of the HA330 and HA380 include marked reductions in circulating concentrations of key cytokines—particularly interleukin-6 (IL-6)—with mean posttreatment decreases of approximately 70% reported in pediatric cytokine storm and sepsis cohorts. CRP and PCT levels also decline substantially after treatment. Clinical studies have demonstrated improvements in organ dysfunction scores and a favorable safety profile, with no device-related adverse events [64, 65, 67, 68]. Comparative studies have shown efficacy similar to that of CytoSorb in reducing inflammatory markers in pediatric sepsis [65, 67].

However, current clinical evidence indicates that Jafron hemoadsorption cartridges (HA330/HA380) have not consistently improved patient-centered outcomes such as mortality, organ dysfunction, or length of stay in the intensive care unit in sepsis or cytokine storm. The most recent systematic review and network meta-analysis of randomized controlled trials found that HA330 had the highest probability of reducing hospital mortality and ICU stay among adsorptive blood purification modalities; however, the authors reported substantial heterogeneity across studies and emphasized the need for large-scale, high-quality trials to validate these findings [69].

Pediatric data, although limited, suggest that HA330/HA380 can reduce inflammatory markers (e.g., IL-6, CRP, PCT) and improve organ dysfunction scores, with high survival rates and no device-related adverse events. Nonetheless, these studies are generally small and lack control groups, limiting the strength of the conclusions [64, 67]. In adult populations, comparative studies with CytoSorb demonstrate similar efficacy in reducing cytokine levels but no statistically significant differences in clinical outcomes [67].

During COVID-19, large propensity-matched cohort studies found that hemoadsorption (including Jafron devices) was associated with increased in-hospital mortality and a higher incidence of complications such as coagulopathy and arrhythmias, with no survival benefit in septic shock and no influence of treatment timing on outcomes [59]. Meta-analyses in severe COVID-19 have suggested a possible reduction in mortality among patients not requiring ECMO, but the evidence is of very low quality and is not specific to Jafron devices [70].

4.9 Nanobodies

Advanced adsorption technologies for blood purification in sepsis and cytokine storm are engineered to achieve selective cytokine removal by combining molecular recognition elements—such as nanobodies or antibodies—with functionalized adsorbent surfaces. Unlike traditional nonselective hemoadsorption systems (e.g., CytoSorb, HA330/380), which rely on size exclusion and hydrophobic interactions to broadly remove middle–molecular-weight molecules, these advanced platforms exploit specific ligand–cytokine interactions to target and capture individual cytokines or defined cytokine groups with high affinity and selectivity [9, 71].

One approach involves conjugating nanobodies (single-domain antibody fragments) to functionalized polymer resins, such as L-arginine-modified polystyrene beads. This design provides abundant and specific binding sites for both cytokines (e.g., TNF-α, IL-6) and endotoxins, enabling efficient and simultaneous removal of these mediators while maintaining excellent biocompatibility [9].

This material integrates three functional components within a single platform: a high-affinity anti–TNF-α nanobody, a mesoporous polystyrene (PS) resin, and an L-arginine functional arm. Together, these elements provide a synergistic strategy to simultaneously target two central drivers of sepsis pathophysiology: bacterial endotoxins and major pro-inflammatory cytokines. The use of nanobodies—single-domain antibody fragments derived from heavy-chain-only antibodies naturally found in camelids—represents a significant technological advance. Their compact structure, exceptional physicochemical stability, and strong antigen-binding properties make them highly suitable ligands for hemoperfusion applications. In this system, the anti–TNF-α nanobody displays nanomolar affinity and retains its binding capability even in the presence of interfering molecules, a crucial feature when operating within the biochemical complexity of whole blood.

Meanwhile, the mesoporous PS matrix provides a stable, high-surface-area scaffold capable of adsorbing medium–molecular-weight cytokines such as IL-6 and IL-8. Its porous architecture enables efficient physical trapping and hydrophobic interactions, essential for broad-spectrum cytokine capture. The incorporation of L-arginine adds an additional functional advantage: the amino acid's positively charged guanidine group enhances electrostatic interactions with negatively charged endotoxin molecules, markedly improving endotoxin removal. The integration of these three mechanisms results in a truly multitarget immunosorbent capable of operating across a diverse molecular spectrum, effectively overcoming the single-target limitations of many current biomaterials.

Experimental results in vitro confirm the multitarget nature of PS-Arg-Nb. In human plasma, the material demonstrated markedly superior removal of TNF-α compared with both pure PS resin and the commercial CytoSorb® device, achieving clearance rates exceeding 90%. Its performance in removing IL-6 and IL-8 was similarly high, matching or slightly surpassing that of established hemoadsorption systems due to the shared PS matrix. The improvement in endotoxin clearance was particularly striking: adsorption capacity more than doubled compared with control materials, highlighting the impact of arginine functionalization. Another important characteristic is its rapid adsorption kinetics, with most mediators substantially reduced within the first hour—an aspect of clear clinical relevance given the time-sensitive nature of septic shock [9].

The in vivo application of the immunosorbent in a rat model of lipopolysaccharide-induced sepsis further strengthened evidence of therapeutic potential. A single 1-hour hemoperfusion session resulted in marked reductions in circulating LPS and key inflammatory cytokines, accompanied by distinct improvements in liver, lung, and kidney histopathology. Perhaps the most notable finding was the survival benefit: more than 40% of treated animals survived, and all survivors recovered fully. Equally important, the device exhibited no adverse effects on blood cell counts, coagulation markers, or biochemical parameters, and in vitro studies confirmed the absence of cytotoxicity. Long-term stability testing demonstrated that PS-Arg-Nb maintains its adsorption performance for at least 12 months at 4 °C, underscoring its practical feasibility.

Overall, PS-Arg-Nb emerges as an advanced technological platform capable of combining immunological specificity, physical adsorption, and biological safety. Its ability to simultaneously target endotoxins and cytokines distinguishes it from currently available hemoperfusion technologies and provides a strong foundation for future clinical development.

Another highly innovative blood-purification platform, in which the geometry of the conduit itself becomes an active component of cytokine removal, has recently been proposed [1]. The authors designed a nanobody-functionalized static-mixer conduit (Nb-SMC) that combines ligand-based molecular recognition with enhanced mass transfer generated by hydrodynamic mixing. This hybrid device represents a novel class of immunoadsorption technology—neither a traditional cartridge nor a passive tubular segment—but rather a functionalized flow-reactor engineered to extract cytokines with high specificity at physiological concentrations.

The technological concept relies on three integrated components. The first is the polydimethylsiloxane (PDMS) conduit, chosen for its biocompatibility and compatibility with standard clinical tubing diameters. To transform its hydrophobic lumen into a reactive, hydrophilic, ligand-friendly surface, the authors grafted poly(2-hydroxyethyl methacrylate) (pHEMA) brushes using surface-initiated RAFT polymerization. This modification markedly altered the surface chemistry and morphology—reducing water contact angle by approximately 60% and increasing nanoscale roughness—thereby facilitating stable covalent immobilization of nanobodies.

The second component is the incorporation of low-pressure-drop (LPD) static mixers into the conduit wall. Each mixer unit consists of two crossed blades at 90°, arranged in a tessellated pattern along the lumen. Computational fluid dynamics (CFD) simulations demonstrated that these geometric elements generate local vortices and strong transverse velocity fields, disrupting the laminar boundary layer that normally restricts cytokine access to immobilized ligands. Optimizing the spacing between mixer units was crucial: CFD identified an optimal H/G ratio of 2.5, which maximizes mixing without inducing excessive turbulence or shear.

The third component is the nanobody ligand itself. Nanobodies offer several advantages over conventional antibodies, including superior stability, low molecular weight, high bacterial expression yields, and strong affinity for target cytokines. In this study, an anti-IL-17A nanobody was used to develop a proof-of-concept device.

Once assembled, the Nb-SMC exhibited remarkable capacity for cytokine removal under biomimetic conditions. Surface-immobilized nanobodies bound IL-17A with a maximal surface loading of approximately 7 $\mu g/cm^2$, and static adsorption tests demonstrated efficient depletion of IL-17A even at physiological concentrations (~200 pg/mL). Importantly, adsorption capacity remained stable across multiple regeneration cycles, supporting the potential for cost-effective clinical use.

The most compelling results emerged from dynamic in vitro hemoperfusion experiments. When blood was circulated through conduits lacking mixers, IL-17A removal did not exceed 30%. By contrast, Nb-SMCs incorporating mixers achieved consistent clearance exceeding 85%, confirming that hydrodynamic mixing dramatically accelerates cytokine–ligand interactions. These results closely matched CFD predictions: particle-tracking simulations revealed swirling trajectories induced by the mixer blades, repeatedly driving cytokines toward the conduit wall and enhancing binding probability. The device maintained strong performance even under continuous cytokine infusion, effectively preventing IL-17A accumulation and maintaining near-baseline concentrations. Variations in flow rate and blood volume resulted in only modest reductions in efficiency, underscoring the robustness of this mass-transfer-enhanced design.

Beyond efficacy, biocompatibility was rigorously evaluated. Hemolysis remained well below ISO 10993 thresholds, platelet activation and thrombin generation markers (PF4, TAT) were essentially unchanged, and complement activation (C3a, C5a) was negligible. Complete blood counts and plasma protein analyses demonstrated no significant nonspecific adsorption—an essential property for a selective immunoadsorption device. These findings confirm that the optimized mixing structures did not introduce excessive shear or turbulence capable of damaging blood components.

A particularly promising extension of this technology is its multitarget capability. By incorporating multiple nanobodies during the ligand-coupling process, the authors created a single conduit capable of simultaneously removing IL-17A, IL-6, and TNF-α. Each cytokine was efficiently adsorbed, with postregeneration removal rates still exceeding 60–80%. This modularity offers a powerful platform for treating complex inflammatory syndromes driven by multiple mediators, such as sepsis, CAR-T-associated cytokine release syndrome, and severe viral infections.

Nanobody-based adsorbents therefore herald the transition from passive sorbents to precision immunotherapeutic extracorporeal devices.

4.10 Conclusion

Over the past decade, adsorption-based blood purification technologies have evolved substantially, spanning from conventional dialysis membranes with intrinsic adsorptive properties to dedicated hemoperfusion cartridges and, more recently, selective immunoadsorptive platforms. Systems such as polymethyl methacrylate (PMMA) membranes and AN69-based filters, including oXiris®, represent a clinically relevant intermediate step in this evolution, combining diffusion and convection with meaningful adsorption. These technologies allow simultaneous renal support and immunomodulation in critically ill patients with acute kidney injury and systemic inflammation.

PMMA membranes have demonstrated consistent adsorption of inflammatory mediators—particularly interleukin-6—together with high biocompatibility and hemodynamic stability, making them suitable for prolonged use in unstable patients. Similarly, the AN69-ST membrane and its heparin-grafted evolution, oXiris®, extend adsorption capabilities to endotoxins in addition to cytokines while mitigating adverse reactions associated with earlier AN69 formulations. Although clinical studies have shown improvements in inflammatory biomarkers and hemodynamic parameters, evidence for a definitive benefit on hard outcomes such as mortality remains limited and heterogeneous.

Dedicated nonselective hemoadsorption devices, including CytoSorb® and HA330/HA380 resin cartridges, further enhance the capacity to rapidly reduce a broad spectrum of circulating cytokines and inflammatory mediators. Despite consistent biochemical effects and occasional transient improvements in physiological parameters, randomized trials and meta-analyses have not demonstrated a consistent impact on patient-centered outcomes, highlighting the intrinsic limitations of broadly acting adsorption strategies in highly heterogeneous inflammatory conditions.

In parallel, a new generation of adsorption technologies is emerging, aiming to overcome these limitations through increased molecular specificity. Nanobody-based immunosorbents and functionalized conduits with enhanced mass-transfer properties exemplify a shift toward selective extracorporeal immunomodulation, enabling targeted removal of key pathogenic mediators—such as TNF-α, IL-6, IL-17A, and endotoxins—while preserving protective plasma components.

Overall, extracorporeal adsorption therapies are transitioning from broadly supportive interventions toward precision-oriented immunotherapeutic strategies. Further progress will require robust randomized clinical trials, refined patient phenotyping, optimal timing of intervention, and clear treatment algorithms tailored to specific inflammatory endotypes. As selective and multitarget platforms advance toward clinical translation, they may become integral components of personalized immunomodulatory therapy in sepsis, cytokine storm, and related hyperinflammatory states.

Selective, ligand-based adsorption platforms have the potential to transform extracorporeal blood purification from a supportive therapy into a programmable immunomodulatory technology.

References

1. Moriyama K, Nishida O. Targeting cytokines, pathogen-associated molecular patterns, and damage-associated molecular patterns in sepsis via blood purification. Int J Mol Sci. 2021;22(16):8882. https://doi.org/10.3390/ijms22168882. PMID: 34445610; PMCID: PMC8396222.
2. Fajgenbaum DC, June CH. Cytokine storm. N Engl J Med. 2020;383(23):2255–73. https://doi.org/10.1056/NEJMra2026131. PMID: 33264547; PMCID: PMC7727315.
3. You W. Roles of cytokine storm in sepsis progression: biomarkers, and emerging therapeutic strategies. Front Immunol. 2025;16:1696366. https://doi.org/10.3389/fimmu.2025.1696366. PMID: 41262247; PMCID: PMC12623314.
4. Vella R, Panci D, Carini F, Malta G, Vieni S, David S, Albano GD, Puntarello M, Zerbo S, Argo A. Cytokines in sepsis: a critical review of the literature on systemic inflammation and multiple organ dysfunction. Front Immunol. 2025;16:1682306. https://doi.org/10.3389/fimmu.2025.1682306. PMID: 41268545; PMCID: PMC12626998.
5. Jarczak D, Kluge S, Nierhaus A. Septic hyperinflammation-is there a role for extracorporeal blood purification techniques? Int J Mol Sci. 2024;25(6):3120. https://doi.org/10.3390/ijms25063120. PMID: 38542094; PMCID: PMC10970398.
6. Blackwell TS, Christman JW. Sepsis and cytokines: current status. Br J Anaesth. 1996;77(1):110–7. https://doi.org/10.1093/bja/77.1.110. PMID: 8703620.
7. Volk HD, Reinke P, Krausch D, Zuckermann H, Asadullah K, Müller JM, Döcke WD, Kox WJ. Monocyte deactivation--rationale for a new therapeutic strategy in sepsis. Intensive Care Med. 1996;22(Suppl 4):S474–81. https://doi.org/10.1007/BF01743727. PMID: 8923092.
8. Bellomo R, Ankawi G, Bagshaw SM, et al. Hemoadsorption: consensus report of the 30th Acute Disease Quality Initiative Workgroup. Nephrol Dial Transplant. 2024;39(11):1945–64.
9. Wang L, Ding Y, Xue F, et al. Nanobody-based high-performance multitarget immunosorbents protect against sepsis by concurrently adsorbing endotoxins and inflammatory cytokines. Acta Biomater. 2025:S1742-7061(25)00840-2. https://doi.org/10.1016/j.actbio.2025.11.016.
10. Gruda MC, Ruggeberg K-G, O'Sullivan P, Guliashvili T, Scheirer AR, Golobish TD, et al. Broad adsorption of sepsis-related PAMP and DAMP molecules, mycotoxins, and cytokines from whole blood using CytoSorb® sorbent porous polymer beads. PLoS One. 2018;13(1):e0191676.
11. Balzani E, Lassola S, Wozniak H, Bellani G, De Rosa S. Advances in renal replacement therapy: the role of polymethyl methacrylate membranes in acute critically ill patients. Blood Purif. 2025:1–11.
12. Kishikawa T, Fujieda H, Sakaguchi H. Comprehensive analysis of cytokine adsorption properties of polymethyl methacrylate (PMMA) membrane material. J Artif Organs. 2022;25(4):343–9.
13. Stasi A, Franzin R, Divella C, Sallustio F, Curci C, Picerno A, et al. PMMA-based continuous hemofiltration modulated complement activation and renal dysfunction in LPS-induced acute kidney injury. Front Immunol. 2021;12:605212.
14. Thadhani R, Pascual M, Bonventre JV. Acute renal failure. N Engl J Med. 1996;334(22):1448–60.
15. Hakim RM, Wingard RL, Parker RA. Effect of the dialysis membrane in the treatment of patients with acute renal failure. N Engl J Med. 1994;331(20):1338–42.
16. Jörres A, Gahl GM, Dobis C, Polenakovic MH, Cakalaroski K, Rutkowski B, et al. Haemodialysis-membrane biocompatibility and mortality of patients with dialysis-dependent acute renal failure: a prospective randomised multicentre trial. International Multicentre Study Group. Lancet. 1999;354(9187):1337–41.
17. Subramanian S, Venkataraman R, Kellum JA. Influence of dialysis membranes on outcomes in acute renal failure: a meta-analysis. Kidney Int. 2002;62(5):1819–23.
18. Pannu N, Klarenbach S, Wiebe N, Manns B, Tonelli M, Alberta Kidney Disease Network. Renal replacement therapy in patients with acute renal failure: a systematic review. JAMA. 2008;299(7):793–805.

19. Khwaja A. KDIGO clinical practice guidelines for acute kidney injury. Nephron Clin Pract. 2012;120(4):c179–84.
20. Michikoshi J, Matsumoto S, Miyawaki H, Morita M, Niu H, Seo K, et al. Evaluation of proteins and cells that adsorb to dialysis membranes used in continuous hemodiafiltration: comparison of AN69ST, polymethylmethacrylate, and polysulfone membranes. Blood Purif. 2019;48(4):358–67.
21. Nakada TA, Oda S, Matsuda KI, Sadahiro T, Nakamura M, Abe R, et al. Continuous hemodiafiltration with PMMA Hemofilter in the treatment of patients with septic shock. Mol Med. 2008;14(5–6):257–63.
22. Nakamura M, Oda S, Sadahiro T, Hirayama Y, Tateishi Y, Abe R, et al. The role of hypercytokinemia in the pathophysiology of tumor lysis syndrome (TLS) and the treatment with continuous hemodiafiltration using a polymethylmethacrylate membrane hemofilter (PMMA-CHDF). Transfus Apher Sci. 2009;40(1):41–7.
23. Abe R, Oda S, Shinozaki K, Hirasawa H. Continuous hemodiafiltration using a polymethyl methacrylate membrane hemofilter for severe acute pancreatitis. Contrib Nephrol. 2010;166:54–63.
24. Nakamura Y, Hatomoto H, Yamasaki S, Yamauchi K, Kiyomi F, Hoshino K, et al. Comparison of the cytokine adsorption ability in continuous renal replacement therapy using polyethyleneimine-coated polyacrylonitrile (AN69ST) or polymethylmethacrylate (PMMA) hemofilters: a pilot single-center open-label randomized control trial. Eur J Med Res. 2023;28(1):208.
25. Matsuda K, Moriguchi T, Oda S, Hirasawa H. Efficacy of continuous hemodiafiltration with a cytokine-adsorbing hemofilter in the treatment of acute respiratory distress syndrome. Contrib Nephrol. 2010;166:83–92.
26. Monard C, Rimmelé T, Ronco C. Extracorporeal blood purification therapies for sepsis. Blood Purif. 2019;47(Suppl 3):1–14.
27. Klouche K, Cavadore P, Portales P, Clot J, Canaud B, Béraud JJ. Continuous veno-venous hemofiltration improves hemodynamics in septic shock with acute renal failure without modifying TNFalpha and IL6 plasma concentrations. J Nephrol. 2002;15(2):150–7.
28. Rogiers P, Zhang H, Pauwels D, Vincent JL. Comparison of polyacrylonitrile (AN69) and polysulphone membrane during hemofiltration in canine endotoxic shock. Crit Care Med. 2003;31(4):1219–25.
29. Chanard J, Lavaud S, Paris B, Toure F, Rieu P, Renaux JL, et al. Assessment of heparin binding to the AN69 ST hemodialysis membrane: I. Preclinical studies. ASAIO J. 2005;51(4):342–7.
30. Verresen L, Fink E, Lemke HD, Vanrenterghem Y. Bradykinin is a mediator of anaphylactoid reactions during hemodialysis with AN69 membranes. Kidney Int. 1994;45(5):1497–503.
31. Chanard J, Lavaud S, Maheut H, Kazes I, Vitry F, Rieu P. The clinical evaluation of low-dose heparin in haemodialysis: a prospective study using the heparin-coated AN69 ST membrane. Nephrol Dial Transplant. 2008;23(6):2003–9.
32. Shiga H, Hirasawa H, Nishida O, Oda S, Nakamura M, Mashiko K, et al. Continuous hemodiafiltration with a cytokine-adsorbing hemofilter in patients with septic shock: a preliminary report. Blood Purif. 2014;38(3–4):211–8.
33. Doi K, Iwagami M, Yoshida E, Marshall MR. Associations of polyethylenimine-coated AN69ST membrane in continuous renal replacement therapy with the intensive care outcomes: observations from a claims database from Japan. Blood Purif. 2017;44(3):184–92.
34. Cecchi M, Ulsamer A, Villa G. Oxiris membrane in sepsis and multiple organ failure. Contrib Nephrol. 2023;200:55–65.
35. Malard B, Lambert C, Kellum JA. In vitro comparison of the adsorption of inflammatory mediators by blood purification devices. Intensive Care Med Exp. 2018;6(1):12.
36. Turani F, Barchetta R, Falco M, Busatti S, Weltert L. Continuous renal replacement therapy with the adsorbing filter oXiris in septic patients: a case series. Blood Purif. 2019;47(Suppl 3):1–5.
37. Broman ME, Hansson F, Vincent JL, Bodelsson M. Endotoxin and cytokine reducing properties of the oXiris membrane in patients with septic shock: a randomized crossover double-blind study. PLoS One. 2019;14(8):e0220444.

38. Kalenka A, Arens P, Müllenbach RM, Weigand MA, Brune M, Fiedler-Kalenka MO. Effects of Oxiris® therapy on cytokine elimination after a LPS infusion—an experimental animal study. Int J Mol Sci. 2024;25(17):9283.
39. Zang S, Chen Q, Zhang Y, Xu L, Chen J. Comparison of the clinical effectiveness of AN69-oXiris versus AN69-ST filter in septic patients: a single-centre study. Blood Purif. 2022;51(7):617–29.
40. Schwindenhammer V, Girardot T, Chaulier K, Grégoire A, Monard C, Huriaux L, et al. oXiris® use in septic shock: experience of two French centres. Blood Purif. 2019;47(Suppl 3):1–7.
41. https://www.fda.gov/medical-devices/covid-19-emergency-use-authorizations-medical-devices/blood-purification-devices-euas.
42. Wendel-Garcia PD, Eberle B, Kleinert EM, Hilty MP, Blumenthal S, Spanaus K, et al. Effects of enhanced adsorption haemofiltration versus haemoadsorption in severe, refractory septic shock with high levels of endotoxemia: the ENDoX bicentric, randomized, controlled trial. Ann Intensive Care. 2023;13(1):127.
43. Zhang L, Srisawat N, Lee CC, Lee DH, Lee K, Liu Z, et al. Extracorporeal blood purification with the oXiris® filter for patients with sepsis and hyperinflammatory conditions: the Asia-Pacific oXiris expert meeting 2024 consensus statements. Blood Purif. 2025;54(11):621–38.
44. Paul R, Ansari AS, Ballesteros D, Klaus T, Honoré PM. Current knowledge on the impact of extracorporeal blood purification devices on drug clearance – systematic search & narrative review. Blood Purif. 2025;54(12):1–22.
45. Ulsamer A, Pomarè Montin D, Bocciero V, Parra Morales TJ, Tofani L, di Girolamo L, et al. Interleukin-6 removal and clinical effects of Oxiris: a systematic review and meta-analysis. Blood Purif. 2025:1–10.
46. Villa G, Fioccola A, Cecchi M, Scirè Calabrisotto C, Pomarè Montin D, De Rosa S, et al. Use of Oxiris membrane in real-world clinical practice in critical care patients: a multicenter observational study. J Anesth Analg Crit Care. 2025;5(1):91.
47. Chen J, Zhang Z, Gao J, Liu Y, Zhu B, Gao Y, et al. A multicentre, randomised controlled clinical trial evaluating the effect of the adsorptive filter oXiris on haemodynamics in abdominal septic shock patients requiring continuous renal replacement therapy (Oxiris for Abdominal SEptic Shock study). BMJ Open. 2025;15(7):e094792.
48. Gruda MC, Ruggeberg KG, O'Sullivan P, Guliashvili T, Scheirer AR, Golobish TD, Capponi VJ, Chan PP. Broad adsorption of sepsis-related PAMP and DAMP molecules, mycotoxins, and cytokines from whole blood using CytoSorb® sorbent porous polymer beads. PLoS One. 2018;13(1):e0191676. https://doi.org/10.1371/journal.pone.0191676. PMID: 29370247; PMCID: PMC5784931.
49. Calabrò MG, Febres D, Recca G, Lembo R, Fominskiy E, Scandroglio AM, Zangrillo A, Pappalardo F. Blood purification with CytoSorb in critically ill patients: single-center preliminary experience. Artif Organs. 2019;43(2):189–94. https://doi.org/10.1111/aor.13327. Epub 2018 Aug 29. PMID: 30156308.
50. Lei K, Chen A, An X, Guo J, Su B, Li Y. The use of CytoSorb hemoadsorption in critically ill patients: a narrative review. Front Med (Lausanne). 2025;12:1628241. https://doi.org/10.3389/fmed.2025.1628241. PMID: 41058625; PMCID: PMC12497824.
51. Jansen A, Waalders NJB, van Lier DPT, Kox M, Pickkers P. CytoSorb hemoperfusion markedly attenuates circulating cytokine concentrations during systemic inflammation in humans in vivo. Crit Care. 2023;27(1):117. https://doi.org/10.1186/s13054-023-04391-z. PMID: 36945034; PMCID: PMC10029173.
52. Haselwanter P, Scheiner B, Balcar L, Semmler G, Riedl-Wewalka M, Schmid M, Reiberger T, Zauner C, Schneeweiss-Gleixner M. Use of the CytoSorb adsorber in patients with acute-on-chronic liver failure. Sci Rep. 2024;14(1):11309. https://doi.org/10.1038/s41598-024-61658-3. PMID: 38760460; PMCID: PMC11101465.
53. Persic V, Jerman A, Malgaj Vrecko M, Berden J, Gorjup V, Stecher A, Lukic M, Jereb M, Taleska Stupica G, Gubensek J. Effect of CytoSorb coupled with hemodialysis on interleukin-6 and hemodynamic parameters in patients with systemic inflammatory

response syndrome: a retrospective cohort study. J Clin Med. 2022;11(24):7500. https://doi.org/10.3390/jcm11247500. PMID: 36556116; PMCID: PMC9788171.
54. Hawchar F, Tomescu D, Träger K, Joskowiak D, Kogelmann K, Soukup J, Friesecke S, Jacob D, Gummert J, Faltlhauser A, Aucella F, van Tellingen M, Malbrain MLNG, Bogdanski R, Weiss G, Herbrich A, Utzolino S, Nierhaus A, Baumann A, Hartjes A, Henzler D, Grigoryev E, Fritz H, Bach F, Schröder S, Weyland A, Gottschaldt U, Menzel M, Zachariae O, Novak R, Berden J, Haake H, Quintel M, Kloesel S, Kortgen A, Stecher S, Torti P, Nestler F, Nitsch M, Olboeter D, Muck P, Findeisen M, Bitzinger D, Kraßler J, Benad M, Schott M, Schumacher U, Molnar Z, Brunkhorst FM. Hemoadsorption in the critically ill-final results of the International CytoSorb Registry. PLoS One. 2022;17(10):e0274315. https://doi.org/10.1371/journal.pone.0274315. PMID: 36282800; PMCID: PMC9595535.
55. Becker S, Lang H, Vollmer Barbosa C, Tian Z, Melk A, Schmidt BMW. Efficacy of CytoSorb®: a systematic review and meta-analysis. Crit Care. 2023;27(1):215. https://doi.org/10.1186/s13054-023-04492-9. PMID: 37259160; PMCID: PMC10230475.
56. Heymann M, Schorer R, Putzu A. Mortality and adverse events of hemoadsorption with CytoSorb® in critically ill patients: a systematic review and meta-analysis of randomized controlled trials. Acta Anaesthesiol Scand. 2022;66(9):1037–50. https://doi.org/10.1111/aas.14115. Epub 2022 Jul 18. PMID: 35788557; PMCID: PMC9541789.
57. Goetz G, Hawlik K, Wild C. Extracorporeal cytokine adsorption therapy as a preventive measure in cardiac surgery and as a therapeutic add-on treatment in sepsis: an updated systematic review of comparative efficacy and safety. Crit Care Med. 2021;49(8):1347–57. https://doi.org/10.1097/CCM.0000000000005023. PMID: 33935160.
58. Stockmann H, Thelen P, Stroben F, Pigorsch M, Keller T, Krannich A, Spies C, Treskatsch S, Ocken M, Kunz JV, Krüger A, Khadzhynov D, Kron S, Budde K, Eckardt KU, Enghard P, Lehner LJ. CytoSorb rescue for COVID-19 patients with vasoplegic shock and multiple organ failure: a prospective, open-label, randomized controlled pilot study. Crit Care Med. 2022;50(6):964–76. https://doi.org/10.1097/CCM.0000000000005493. Epub 2022 Feb 9. PMID: 35135967; PMCID: PMC9112514.
59. Kloka JA, Jasny T, Old O, Nürenberg-Goloub E, Scharf C, Meybohm P, Supady A, Zacharowski K, Friedrichson B. Critical risks of haemoadsorption for COVID-19 patients and directions for future evaluations: a nationwide propensity score matched cohort study. Sci Rep. 2025;15(1):29184. https://doi.org/10.1038/s41598-025-13860-0. PMID: 40783423; PMCID: PMC12335523.
60. Jerman A, Gubenšek J, Berden J, Peršič V. A matched case-control study on the effectiveness of extracorporeal cytokine adsorption in critically ill patients. Sci Rep. 2023;13(1):13464. https://doi.org/10.1038/s41598-023-40719-z. PMID: 37596304; PMCID: PMC10439174.
61. Brouwer WP, Duran S, Kuijper M, Ince C. Hemoadsorption with CytoSorb shows a decreased observed versus expected 28-day all-cause mortality in ICU patients with septic shock: a propensity-score-weighted retrospective study. Crit Care. 2019;23(1):317. https://doi.org/10.1186/s13054-019-2588-1. PMID: 31533846; PMCID: PMC6749645.
62. Berlot G, Carocci P, Votrico V, Iacoviello B, Taverna N, Gerini U, di Maso V, Tomasini A. Real-world outcomes of hemoadsorption with CytoSorb® in patients with septic shock: insights from a single-center study. J Intensive Care Med. 2025;40(9):993–1000. https://doi.org/10.1177/08850666251331905. Epub 2025 Apr 1. PMID: 40170437.
63. Kanjo A, Molnar Z, Zádori N, Gede N, Erőss B, Szakó L, Kiss T, Márton Z, Malbrain MLNG, Szuldrzynski K, Szrama J, Kusza K, Kogelmann K, Hegyi P. Dosing of Extracorporeal Cytokine Removal In Septic Shock (DECRISS): protocol of a prospective, randomised, adaptive, multicentre clinical trial. BMJ Open. 2021;11(8):e050464. https://doi.org/10.1136/bmjopen-2021-050464. PMID: 34446497; PMCID: PMC8395301.
64. Azenova K, Sazonov V. Hemoadsorption in children with cytokine storm using the Jafron HA330 and HA380 cartridges. J Clin Med. 2025;14(18):6359. https://doi.org/10.3390/jcm14186359. PMID: 41010563; PMCID: PMC12470262.
65. Lesbekov T, Nurmykhametova Z, Kaliyev R, Kuanyshbek A, Faizov L, Bekishev B, Jabayeva N, Samalavicius R, Pya Y. Hemadsorption in patients requiring V-A ECMO support: com-

parison of Cytosorb versus Jafron HA330. Artif Organs. 2023;47(4):721–30. https://doi.org/10.1111/aor.14457. Epub 2022 Nov 25. PMID: 36398369.
66. Yildiz AB, Copur S, Tanriover C, Yavuz F, Vehbi S, Hasbal NB, Kanbay M. A potential approach toward the management of sepsis: the extracorporeal cytokine hemadsorption therapy. Semin Dial. 2024;37(2):117–21. https://doi.org/10.1111/sdi.13188. Epub 2023 Dec 12. PMID: 38084784.
67. Ryazanova D, Tobylbayeva Z, Mironova O, Kakenov E, Sazonov V. Comparison of CytoSorb and Jafron HA330 hemoadsorption devices in pediatric oncological patients with sepsis: retrospective observational study. J Clin Med. 2024;13(24):7694. https://doi.org/10.3390/jcm13247694. PMID: 39768616; PMCID: PMC11676993.
68. Erkurt MA, Sarici A, Özer AB, Kuku I, Biçim S, Aydogan MS, Kose A, Memisoglu F, Ince V, Otan E, Kaya E, Berber I, Özgül M, Keser MF. The effect of HA330 hemoperfusion adsorbent method on inflammatory markers and end-organ damage levels in sepsis: a retrospective single center study. Eur Rev Med Pharmacol Sci. 2022;26(21):8112–7. https://doi.org/10.26355/eurrev_202211_30165. PMID: 36394761.
69. Xing H, Wei Y, Zhang D, Jiang Z, Qin J, Ou S, Wu W. Comparing adsorptive blood purification modalities for sepsis patients: a systematic review and network meta-analysis. Respir Med. 2025;239:107994. https://doi.org/10.1016/j.rmed.2025.107994. Epub 2025 Feb 12. PMID: 39952412.
70. He J, Lin Y, Cai W, Lin Y, Qin W, Shao Y, Liu Q. Efficacy of supplemental hemoadsorption therapy on severe and critical patients with COVID-19: an evidence-based analysis. Shock. 2023;60(3):333–44. https://doi.org/10.1097/SHK.0000000000002189. Epub 2023 Aug 4. PMID: 37548606; PMCID: PMC10510838.
71. Yao G, Ji F, Chen J, Dai B, Jia L. Nanobody-functionalized conduit with built-in static mixer for specific elimination of cytokines in hemoperfusion. Acta Biomater. 2023;172:260–71. https://doi.org/10.1016/j.actbio.2023.09.050. Epub 2023 Oct 6. PMID: 37806373.

Sepsis and Cytokine Storm: A New Approach to Extracorporeal Therapy

5

Gabriella Bottari

5.1 Introduction

Sepsis remains one of the leading causes of mortality in intensive care units (ICUs) worldwide. Despite advances in antimicrobial therapy, fluid resuscitation, and organ support, the mortality rate of septic shock continues to exceed 30–40%. A hallmark of severe sepsis and septic shock is the dysregulated host immune response to infection, characterized by the uncontrolled release of pro- and anti-inflammatory mediators, commonly referred to as a cytokine storm (CS). The term cytokine storm was first used by James Ferrara to describe acute graft-versus-host disease in the setting of engraftment syndrome following allogenic stem-cell transplantation [1]. CS is usually understood to mean the overwhelming immune response characterized by the release of cytokines, including interleukins, interferons, chemokines, and other mediators. This hyperinflammatory reaction leads to endothelial injury, capillary leakage, hemodynamic instability, and multiple organ dysfunction syndrome (MODS). This dysregulated response leads to self-reinforcing feedback and may, ultimately, be life-threatening to the host [1].

While conventional management focuses on source control and supportive therapy, these approaches are frequently insufficient to restore immune homeostasis once a cytokine storm is established. Over the past decade, extracorporeal blood purification (EBP) techniques have emerged as promising adjuncts in the

G. Bottari (✉)
Pediatric Intensive Care Unit, Children Hospital Bambno Gesù, Rome, Italy
e-mail: gabriella.bottari@opbg.net

S. De Rosa, S. Lassola (eds.), *Next-Gen Blood Purification*,
https://doi.org/10.1007/978-3-032-27033-7_5

management of sepsis, aimed at modulating the systemic inflammatory response through the removal of circulating mediators, endotoxins, and other soluble pathogenic factors [2, 3].

The transition from renal replacement therapy (RRT) to targeted extracorporeal immunomodulation represents a paradigm shift in critical care. Originally conceived to replace renal function in acute kidney injury (AKI), continuous kidney replacement therapy (CKRT) has evolved into a platform for multi-target blood purification. Techniques such as hemofilter with enhanced adsorption capacity, high cut-off (HCO) filtration, hemo-adsorption, and plasma exchange (PEX) are now being integrated in sequential or combined strategies to modulate both pro- and anti-inflammatory pathways [4, 5].

The central concept driving these interventions is the restoration of immune balance—not the complete suppression of inflammation, but the attenuation of excessive mediator release and the prevention of immune-paralysis. Recent advances in device engineering, sorbent materials, and adsorption kinetics have greatly expanded the clinical applicability of extracorporeal blood purification, moving from experimental approaches to evidence-based, protocolized therapies in selected patient populations [4–6].

5.2 Pathophysiology of Sepsis and Cytokine Storm

Sepsis is now recognized as a *complex syndrome of immune dysregulation* rather than a simple infection-driven inflammatory process. The host response to invading pathogens is mediated by pattern recognition receptors (PRRs) that detect *pathogen-associated molecular patterns (PAMPs)* and *damage-associated molecular patterns (DAMPs)*. Once activated, these receptors trigger intracellular signaling cascades that result in the release of numerous cytokines and chemokines—including tumor necrosis factor-α (TNF-α), interleukin-1β (IL-1β), IL-6, IL-8, interferon-γ (IFN-γ), and anti-inflammatory mediators such as IL-10 and transforming growth factor-β (TGF-β) [1, 7].

Cytokines exert pleiotropic effects on vascular tone, permeability, and coagulation [1]. IL-6, one of the key mediators, acts as a central amplifier of the acute phase response, correlating strongly with disease severity and outcome [8]. Elevated IL-6 levels have been shown to parallel hemodynamic instability and predict mortality in septic patients [8]. Similarly, IL-8 and TNF-α drive neutrophil recruitment and oxidative stress, while IL-10 suppresses antigen presentation and adaptive immune responses [1]. Several reports confirm that high concentrations of IL-10 in septic patients were correlated with high mortality [9–11]. Recently, a retrospective analysis in critically ill pediatric patients confirmed that high levels of cytokines were predictive of organ injury; in particular, IL-6 and IL-10 predict cardiac arrest, and IL-17A was a good predictor of the incidence of acute liver failure [12].

A balanced protective inflammatory response consists of diverse mechanisms and involves activation of both pro- and anti-inflammatory pathways within the innate and the acquired immune systems. After a successful defense and initiation of healing, the immune system returns to a state of homeostasis and assumes a wait-and-see role [1]. Clinical and experimental data suggest that mortality in sepsis is linked not only to the intensity but also to the persistence of inflammatory activation and the failure to regain immune equilibrium [11]. Therapeutic strategies must aim to modulate, rather than abolish, the inflammatory cascade [13]. However is difficult to distinguish between adequate cytokine production to fight systemic infection and dysregulated cytokine production.

Several studies have demonstrated that cytokine kinetics can guide prognosis and therapeutic decisions. For instance, persistently high IL-6 or IL-8 levels during the first 48 h are associated with poor outcomes, while rapid declines after extracorporeal blood purification therapies correlate with hemodynamic stabilization [14, 15]. Biomarkers, including IL-6/IL-10 ratios and endotoxin activity assays (EAA), are being increasingly used to define specific inflammatory phenotypes that could benefit from targeted extracorporeal interventions [16]. The practical implementation of cytokine-guided therapy requires rapid and reliable assays; furthermore, because cytokine dynamics are highly time-dependent, serial measurements are recommended every 12–24 h during active therapy [17].

Post-mortem and genomic analyses have revealed profound heterogeneity in immune gene expression among septic patients, identifying distinct immune trajectories. Some patients remain locked in a hyperinflammatory state, while others transition rapidly into immune suppression, characterized by low HLA-DR expression and reduced cytokine production [18]. This heterogeneity underlies the growing interest in immunophenotyping and precision extracorporeal therapy, where the selection of the appropriate device and timing is tailored to the individual's cytokine and immune profile. In this context, extracorporeal therapies act not merely as supportive measures but as immunomodulatory tools that can dynamically shape the host response to infection [19]. The integration of these biomarkers with clinical parameters (vasopressor index, SOFA score, lactate clearance) forms the cornerstone of precision extracorporeal immunomodulation [17].

Given the pathophysiological background now well understood in septic shock, both the exaggerated, dysregulated, and persistent inflammatory response can become a therapeutic target for EBPT. EBPT plays a role in this setting by removing mediators through different mechanisms, including diffusion, convection, adsorption, and plasma separation (Table 5.1). All these mechanisms contribute to modulating the high concentrations of sepsis mediators, not only by mechanically reducing their levels but also by modulating the immune system and promoting immune homeostasis. Indeed, by reducing high concentrations of cytokines and other mediators, it is possible to interrupt the vicious cycle that sustains the cytokine storm and ultimately prevent organ damage.

Table 5.1 Mechanism of sepsis mediator removal during EBPT

Mechanism	Transport principle	Molecular weight range	Impact on immune response
Diffusion	Concentration-gradient–dependent solute transport across a semipermeable membrane	Low molecular weight (<500 Da) and selected middle molecules	Marginal contribution to cytokine clearance
Convection	Pressure-driven ultrafiltration with solvent drag	Middle and large molecules (up to membrane cut-off)	Sustained reduction of circulating cytokines
Adsorption	Electrostatic and hydrophobic binding to membrane or cartridge surface	Cytokines, endotoxins, DAMPs, PAMPs	Immune modulation and restoration of immune homeostasis
Plasma separation	Physical separation and removal of plasma, with replacement by albumin or plasma	Protein-bound mediators, large cytokines, immune complexes	Nonselective reduction of circulating inflammatory mediators

Da Dalton, *DAMPs* damage-associated molecular patterns, *PAMPs* pathogen-associated molecular patterns

5.3 Rationale for Extracorporeal Therapy in Sepsis

Given the complexity of the inflammatory process and its impact on the immune system during hyperinflammatory states of both septic and nonseptic origin, it is evident that—particularly in the "cytokine storm" phase, characterized by dysregulation of the coagulation and complement systems—an ideal therapy should aim to attenuate the pro-inflammatory state through a nonselective mechanism, rather than targeting a single mediator of the process. Therefore, both the pro-inflammatory and anti-inflammatory pathways represent therapeutic targets [13].

Extracorporeal blood purification techniques have been proposed as potential therapeutic strategies designed to nonspecifically remove mediators of the inflammatory process. Through the nonselective removal of both pro- and anti-inflammatory mediators—without completely abolishing their physiological effects [20, 21]—these methods may interrupt the pathological "redundancy" and cytokine "cross talk" processes that can ultimately lead to multiple organ failure (MOF) [5].

Several theories have been proposed to explain the mechanisms underlying extracorporeal blood purification. Initially, Ronco [13] hypothesized that cytokine removal systems could reduce the peak plasma concentrations of these molecules during sepsis, thereby limiting organ damage and decreasing the incidence of MOF [13]. Subsequently, Honoré [22] proposed the "immunomodulation threshold" theory, suggesting that the removal of circulating cytokines leads, in turn, to the removal of tissue cytokines, resulting in a new equilibrium between the two compartments. A third theory, proposed by Di Carlo and Alexander [23], suggests that hemodialysis with an adequate effluent flow may enhance lymphatic drainage and thus improve clearance of inflammatory mediators. More recently, Peng [24] proposed that extracorporeal blood purification may exert an immunomodulatory effect by promoting immune "reprogramming" of deactivated monocytes, neutrophils, and lymphocytes [24].

The potential benefits of such extracorporeal blood purification therapies have been further emphasized by recognition of the importance of "organ cross talk" during sepsis, in which dysfunction of one organ can affect other organ systems, particularly in the context of multiple organ dysfunction syndrome (MODS). Ronco and Bellomo first introduced the concept of multi-organ support therapy (MOST) in 2002 [4, 6], which later evolved into the concept of extracorporeal organ support (ECOS) [5], based on the premise that malfunctioning organs are still perfused with blood, which is thus a valid target for interventions.

The Sequential Extracorporeal Therapy (SET) model, proposed by Ronco and colleagues (2023), offers a conceptual framework for integrating multiple blood purification modalities according to the patient's clinical stage and immune profile [25]. SET combines hemoadsorption, high cut-off filtration, and plasma exchange in a stepwise approach to address distinct pathogenic pathways: removal of endotoxins, reduction of circulating cytokines, and replacement of plasma components such as complement or coagulation factors. By addressing both different targets, SET represents a personalized and adaptive approach.

5.4 Extracorporeal Blood Purification Techniques

Extracorporeal blood purification (EBP) encompasses a group of techniques designed to remove circulating toxins, inflammatory mediators, and pathogenic molecules from the bloodstream. Although originally developed for renal replacement therapy (RRT), EBP has evolved to target immune modulation rather than mere solute clearance. Among the available modalities, three principal strategies are currently used in septic shock and cytokine storm syndromes: hemoadsorption, including hemofilters with enhanced adsorption properties; high cut-off (HCO) filtration; and therapeutic plasma exchange (TPE). Table 5.2 includes a concise summary of extracorporeal techniques and associated modalities.

5.4.1 Hemoadsorption

Hemoadsorption (HA) is based on the principle of adsorption, in which solutes are removed from plasma by physical and chemical interactions with a solid sorbent surface. Commercially available devices, such as **CytoSorb®**, **Jafron® HA330/HA380**, and **oXiris®**, use porous polymer beads or membranes capable of binding hydrophobic molecules in the 5–60 kDa range, including a wide spectrum of cytokines (IL-1β, IL-6, IL-8, TNF-α), myoglobin, bilirubin, and other middle molecules [26].

The **CytoSorb cartridge**, composed of polystyrene divinylbenzene copolymer beads with a large surface area (~40,000 m^2), has been the most extensively studied in septic shock. In the DECRISS trial [27], a structured dosing protocol

Table 5.2 Main extracorporeal blood purification modalities by mechanism

Main principle	Technique/ modality	How it works	Key notes
Diffusion	CVVHD	Conventional CKRT Dialysate-based diffusion across a semipermeable membrane	Continuous veno-venous hemodialysis (dose depends on dialysate flow)
Convection	CVVH	Conventional CKRT Ultrafiltration with solvent drag; replacement fluid	Continuous veno-venous hemofiltration (higher effluent → higher clearance)
Diffusion + convection	CVVHDF	Conventional CKRT Combined dialysate diffusion + convective clearance	Continuous veno-venous hemodiafiltration (flexible balance of dialysate/ replacement)
Enhanced adsorption (± diffusion/convection)	Hemofilter with enhanced adsorption properties	Conventional CKRT membrane with higher adsorptive capacity	Often used within CVVHD/CVVH/ CVVHDF circuits; performance depends on membrane chemistry and saturation
Large-pore clearance (mainly convection)	High cut-off (HCO) hemofilter	Larger pore size increases clearance of larger middle molecules	CVVHD to limit protein/albumin loss
Adsorption	Cartridge-based adsorption (stand-alone or in-line with CKRT)	Blood passes through a sorbent cartridge; mediators bind to the sorbent surface	Broad cytokine adsorption Selective cartridges (e.g., endotoxin adsorption)
Plasma separation	Therapeutic plasma exchange (TPE)	Separation and removal of plasma, replaced with albumin/fresh frozen plasma; can be coupled to adsorption (CPFA-like concepts)	Higher 'bulk' removal of plasma constituents; replacement strategy influences coagulation and volume status

CVVHD continuous veno-venous hemodialysis, *CVVH* continuous veno-venous hemofiltration, *CVVHDF* continuous veno-venous hemodiafiltration, *CKRT* continuous kidney replacement therapy, *HCO* high cut off, *TPE* therapeutic plasma exchange, *CPFA* coupled plasma filtration adsorption demonstrated improved hemodynamic stability and decreased vasopressor demand in patients receiving early, repeated hemoadsorption sessions. Similarly, Boss et al. [28] reported a significant reduction in catecholamine requirements in postoperative septic patients with AKI treated with CytoSorb in combination with CKRT.

A proof-of-concept randomized study by Hawchar et al. [15] showed that hemoadsorption led to rapid decreases in IL-6 and IL-8 levels, accompanied by improved mean arterial pressure and reduced lactate, although without a statistically significant mortality benefit. More recent pediatric studies have expanded these findings: Bottari et al. [17] demonstrated that combined CytoSorb plus CKRT therapy in children with septic shock improved hemodynamics and reduced vasoactive support requirements without major adverse effects [29].

Newer HA330 and HA380 cartridges employ neutral macroporous resin sorbents with broader adsorption spectra and have shown favorable cytokine clearance in children and adults with hyperinflammatory syndromes and viral sepsis [30, 31]. These results suggest that hemoadsorption is not limited to cytokine removal but also facilitates stabilization of the vascular endothelium and microcirculation, leading to more rapid reversal of shock.

In parallel, the oXiris® membrane—an AN69-based hemodiafilter modified with a polyethyleneimine (PEI) surface and preheparinization—combines cytokine adsorption, endotoxin removal, and renal support within a single device. This triple-action profile makes it particularly suited for septic shock with concomitant AKI [32]. Clinical studies have reported reductions in circulating endotoxin activity and pro-inflammatory cytokines, along with improved hemodynamic stability and decreased vasopressor requirements in adults and children undergoing CKRT with oXiris®. Although evidence remains heterogeneous and predominantly observational, current data support its role as an integrated adsorptive–renal therapy that may enhance early shock control in hyperinflammatory states [16, 33].

Although current evidence supports significant improvements in hemodynamics and inflammatory markers, large randomized controlled trials (RCTs) are still limited. The Goetz et al. systematic review confirmed that hemoadsorption is safe and can reduce vasopressor requirements, but mortality benefit remains uncertain due to heterogeneity of study designs [34].

5.4.2 Therapeutic Plasma Exchange

Therapeutic plasma exchange (TPE) differs fundamentally from adsorption or filtration in that it removes plasma nonselectively, replacing it with donor plasma or albumin solution. This approach enables simultaneous elimination of a wide range of injurious circulating factors—cytokines, endotoxins, DAMPs/PAMPs, immune complexes, and autoantibodies—while replenishing protective plasma components often depleted in severe sepsis, including antithrombin III, ADAMTS-13, complement proteins, and endogenous anticoagulants.

The meta-analysis by Kuklin et al. (2024), including over 500 patients with sepsis-induced organ dysfunction, reported a significant reduction in short-term mortality with TPE compared to standard care, particularly when initiated early and applied in repeated daily sessions [35]. The benefit was attributed to both the detoxification effect and the restoration of key homeostatic factors.

Preliminary data from a recent randomized controlled trial highlight the role of TPE in septic shock: the *EXCHANGE-S* trial (2023), a multicenter RCT enrolling adults with early septic shock and severe coagulopathy, reported a reduction in 28-day mortality from 54% (standard care) to 36% (TPE) when plasma exchange was initiated within the first 12 hours of shock onset. Treated patients showed faster lactate clearance, improved hemodynamics, and a significant rise in ADAMTS-13 activity after the first exchange session. Similarly, the *PEPAS* pediatric RCT [36] evaluating early TPE in children with sepsis-associated multiple organ dysfunction demonstrated improved organ failure scores at 48 h and a reduction in vasoactive requirements, although the study was underpowered for mortality outcomes. A smaller single-center RCT [37] focusing on patients with hyperinflammatory septic phenotypes showed that two consecutive daily TPE sessions resulted in marked decreases in IL-6, IL-8, and endotoxin activity, along with improved mean arterial pressure and fewer days of organ support.

5.5 Limitations of Current Evidence and Future Perspectives

Despite compelling mechanistic rationale and consistent physiological improvements, robust mortality data remain elusive. Most studies are single-center, non-blinded, and underpowered to detect survival differences. Heterogeneity in patient selection, timing, device choice, and treatment intensity complicates interpretation. In addition, extracorporeal blood purification carries procedure-related risks, including excessive mediator removal, protein loss, and hemodynamic instability. These risks can be mitigated through careful patient selection, appropriate timing, and tailoring of modality and dose (Table 5.3).

Table 5.3 Risks and mitigation strategies associated with extracorporeal blood purification techniques

Risk	Main mechanism involved	Mitigation strategy
Excessive mediators removal including nutrients and drugs	Diffusion/convection/adsorption	Appropriate patient selection, dose prescription, and timing; drug adjustment
Protein and albumin loss	High cut-off membranes, plasma separation	Prefer CVVHD when applicable; monitor and replace albumin
Hemodynamic instability	Rapid solute and fluid shifts	Gradual initiation; close hemodynamic monitoring
Filter or cartridge saturation	Adsorption-based techniques	Timely filter/cartridge replacement
Coagulation disturbances	Plasma separation, anticoagulation	Individualized anticoagulation and laboratory monitoring

Furthermore, the lack of standardized cytokine monitoring limits our ability to identify responders. The cost and technical complexity of integrating multiple devices also hinder widespread adoption. Future research must emphasize phenotype-based randomization, standardized dosing algorithms, and adaptive trial designs to validate efficacy in clearly defined patient subsets.

The next frontier of extracorporeal therapy lies in personalization and integration with real-time immune monitoring [17]. The advent of multiplex cytokine assays and bedside biosensors enables dynamic tracking of inflammatory markers. In parallel, artificial intelligence (AI) and machine-learning algorithms are being trained to predict cytokine trajectories and recommend optimal intervention windows.

Hybrid devices that combine adsorption, filtration, and sensing functions are under development, capable of adjusting flow rates and cartridge exchanges automatically in response to cytokine concentrations. Advances in sorbent nanotechnology and surface modification are improving selectivity and minimizing albumin loss, addressing previous limitations.

In the near future, clinicians may rely on integrated platforms where extracorporeal therapy is guided by continuous feedback loops linking cytokine sensors, hemodynamic monitors, and AI-driven decision support systems. Such systems could personalize not only whether to intervene but also how intensely and for how long, optimizing benefit while minimizing resource use.

5.6 Conclusions

Extracorporeal blood purification has evolved from a supportive renal replacement technique into a cornerstone of immunomodulatory therapy for sepsis and cytokine storm. The integration of hemoadsorption, high cut-off filtration, and plasma exchange within the Sequential Extracorporeal Therapy (SET) framework provides a rational, physiology-based approach to restore immune homeostasis.

Key lessons from current evidence include the following:

1. Timing is critical—early initiation during the hyperinflammatory phase yields the best outcomes.
2. Patient phenotyping matters—cytokine and endotoxin profiles should guide modality selection.
3. Combination therapy enhances efficacy—SET allows complementary removal of mediators and plasma reconstitution.
4. Monitoring is essential—serial IL-6, IL-10, and EAA measurements enable adaptive therapy control.

While a survival benefit remains to be conclusively proven, the accumulating body of evidence demonstrates consistent physiological improvement, suggesting that extracorporeal therapies can meaningfully alter the course of septic shock when used judiciously and in the right patients.

Ongoing advances in precision medicine, biomarker integration, and intelligent extracorporeal systems will likely transform sepsis management from empiric resuscitation to targeted immune modulation, marking the dawn of a new era in critical care.

References

1. Jarczak D, Nierhaus A. Cytokine storm-definition, causes, and implications. Int J Mol Sci. 2022;23(19):11740.
2. Kellum J, Bellomo R, Metha R, Ronco C. Blood purification in non-renal critical illness. Blood Purif. 2003;21:6–13.
3. Ostermann M, Ankawi G, Cantaluppi V, et al. Nomenclature of extra-corporeal blood purification therapies for acute indications: the nomenclature standardization conference. Blood Purif. 2024;53:358–72.
4. Ronco C, Bellomo R. Acute renal failure and multiple organ dysfunction in the ICU: from renal replacement therapy (RRT) to multiple organ support therapy (MOST). Int J Artif Organs. 2022;25:733–47.
5. Husain-Syed F, Ricci Z, Brodie D, et al. Extarcorporeal organ support (ECOS) in critical illness and acute kidney injury: from native to artificial organ crosstalk. Intensive Care Med. 2018;44:1447–59.
6. Ronco C, Ricci Z, Husain-Syed F. From multiple organ support therapy to extracorporeal organ support in critically ill patients. Blood Purif. 2019;48:99–105.
7. Moriyama K, Nishida O. Targeting cytokines, pathogen-associated molecular patterns, and damage-associated molecular patterns in sepsis via blood purification. Int J Mol Sci. 2021;22(16):8882. https://doi.org/10.3390/ijms22168882.
8. Ruiz-Rodríguez JC, Chiscano-Camón L, Ruiz-Sanmartin A, et al. Cytokine hemoadsorption as rescue therapy for critically ill patients with SARS-CoV-2 pneumonia with severe respiratory failure and hypercytokinemia. Front Med. 2021;8:779038. https://doi.org/10.3389/fmed.2021.779038.
9. Gogos C, Drosou E, Bassaris H, et al. Pro-versus anti-inflammatory cytokine profile in patients with severe sepsis: a marker for prognosis and future therapeutic options. J Infect Dis. 2000;181(1):176–80.
10. Pinsky M, Vinent JL, Deviere J, et al. Serum cytokine levels in human septic shock. Chest. 1992;103(2):565–74.
11. Kellum J, Kong L, Fink M, et al. Understanding the inflammatory cytokine response in pneumonia and sepsis. Arch Intern Med. 2007;167(15):1655–63.
12. Zhu R, Cao L, Wu T, et al. The evolution of cytokines in predicting the organ injury of critically pediatric patients: a retrospective study. Transl Pediatr. 2024;13(7):1169–78.
13. Ronco C, Bonello M, Bordoni V, et al. Extracoporeal therapies in non-renal disease: treatment of sepsis and the peak concentration hypothesis. Blood Purif. 2004;22:164–74.
14. Hellman T, Uusalo P, Järvisalo MJ. Renal replacement techniques in septic shock. Int J Mol Sci. 2021;22(19):10238. https://doi.org/10.3390/ijms221910238.
15. Hawchar F, László I, Öveges N, et al. Extracorporeal cytokine adsorption in septic shock: a proof of concept randomized, controlled pilot study. J Crit Care. 2019;49:172–8. https://doi.org/10.1016/j.jcrc.2018.11.003.
16. Theisen BE, Lichtenstern C, Nusshag C, et al. Simultaneous removal of endotoxins, inflammatory mediators and uremic toxins in ICU patients with septic shock: a retrospective cohort study. Sci Rep. 2024;14(1):19645. https://doi.org/10.1038/s41598-024-70522-3.
17. Bottari G, Ranieri VM, Ince C, et al. Use of extra-corporeal blood purification therapies in sepsis: the current paradigm, available evidence, and future perspectives. Crit Care. 2024;28:432.
18. Vincent JL, van der Poll T, Marshall JC. The end of "one size fits all" sepsis therapies: toward an individualized approach. Biomedicines. 2022;10(9):2260.

19. Bottari, G., Ranieri, V.M., Ince, C. et al. Use of extracorporeal blood purification therapies in sepsis: the current paradigm, available evidence, and future perspectives. Crit Care 2024;28:432. https://doi.org/10.1186/s13054-024-05220-7.
20. Yildiz AB, Copur S, Tanriover C, et al. A potential approach toward the management of sepsis: the extracorporeal cytokine hemadsorption therapy. Semin Dial. 2024;37(2):117–21. https://doi.org/10.1111/sdi.13188.
21. Jarczak D, Kluge S, Nierhaus A. Septic hyperinflammation – is there a role for extracorporeal blood purification techniques? Int J Mol Sci. 2024;25(6):3120. https://doi.org/10.3390/ijms25063120.
22. Honorè P, Matson J. Extracoporeal removal for sepsis: acting at the tissue level-the beginningof a new era for this treatment modality in septic shock. Crit Care Med. 2004;32(3):896–7.
23. Di Carlo JV, Alexander SR. Hemofiltration for cytokine-driven illnesses: the mediator delivery hypothesis. Int J Artif Organs. 2005;28(8):777–86.
24. Peng Z, et al. Blood purification in sepsis: a new paradigm. Contrib Nephrol. 2010;165:322–8.
25. Ronco C, Chawla L, Husain-Syed F, Kellum JA. Rationale for Sequential Extracorporeal Therapy (SET) in sepsis. Crit Care. 2023;27(1):50. https://doi.org/10.1186/s13054-023-04310-2. (Leading Journal)
26. Neri M, Villa G, Garzotto F, et al. New frontiers in extracorporeal blood purification for sepsis and septic shock: from RRT to multimodal immunotherapy. Blood Purif. 2020;49(1–2):1–9. https://doi.org/10.1159/000505574.
27. Kanjo A, Molnar Z, Zádori N, et al. Dosing of extracorporeal cytokine removal in septic shock (DECRISS): protocol of a prospective, randomised, adaptive, multicentre clinical trial. BMJ Open. 2021;11(8):e050464. https://doi.org/10.1136/bmjopen-2021-050464.
28. Boss K, Jahn M, Wendt D, et al. Extracorporeal cytokine adsorption after cardiac surgery: clinical experience and mechanistic insights. Crit Care Res Pract. 2023;2023:1–9. https://doi.org/10.1155/2023/8569423.
29. Bottari G, Guzzo I, Cappoli A, et al. Impact of CytoSorb and CKRT on hemodynamics in pediatric patients with septic shock: the PedCyto study. Front Pediatr. 2023;11:1259384. https://doi.org/10.3389/fped.2023.1259384.
30. Azenova K, Sazonov V. Hemoadsorption in children with cytokine storm using the Jafron HA330 and HA380 cartridges. J Clin Med. 2025;14(18):6359. https://doi.org/10.3390/jcm14186359.
31. Hui WF, Chan RWY, Wong CK, et al. The sequential use of extracorporeal cytokine removal devices in an adolescent With COVID-19 receiving continuous renal replacement therapy. ASAIO J. 2022;68(12):e230–4.
32. Broman ME, Hansson F, Vincent JL, Bodelsson M. Endotoxin and cytokine reducing properties of the oXiris membrane in patients with septic shock: a randomized crossover double-blind study. PLoS One. 2019;14:e0220444.
33. Pérez-Fernández X, Ulsamer A, Cámara-Rosell M, et al. SIRAKI02 Study Group. Extracorporeal blood purification and acute kidney injury in cardiac surgery: the SIRAKI02 randomized clinical trial. JAMA. 2024;332(17):1446–54. https://doi.org/10.1001/jama.2024.20630.
34. Goetz G, Hawlik K, Wild C. Extracorporeal cytokine adsorption therapy as a preventive measure in cardiac surgery and as a therapeutic add-on treatment in sepsis: an updated systematic review of comparative efficacy and safety. Crit Care Med. 2021;49(8):1347–57.
35. Kuklin V, Sovershaev M, Bjerner J, et al. Influence of therapeutic plasma exchange treatment on short-term mortality of critically ill adult patients with sepsis-induced organ dysfunction: a systematic review and meta-analysis. Crit Care. 2024;28(1):12.
36. PEPAS Study Group. Pediatric early plasma exchange for sepsis-associated multiple organ dysfunction: randomized controlled trial results. Abstract presented at the 2024 Society of Critical Care Medicine (SCCM) Congress; 2024.
37. Hassan M, El-Masry A, Youssef S. Early therapeutic plasma exchange in hyperinflammatory septic shock: a randomized controlled pilot study. Crit Care Explor. 2023;5(7):e0920.

6 Extracorporeal Blood Purification in Infectious Diseases and COVID-19

Vedran Premuzic

6.1 Introduction

Source control is a cornerstone of effective sepsis management. It encompasses the prompt administration of broad-spectrum antimicrobials to target the underlying infection, alongside supportive measures to restore tissue perfusion and maintain organ function [1, 2]. The primary objectives are to reduce the microbial burden at the infection site, prevent the spread of infection, and interrupt the dysregulated immune response that characterizes sepsis [3]. A significant challenge in achieving adequate source control is the persistent use of antibiotics, which contributes to the development of antimicrobial resistance—a growing concern, particularly in intensive care units (ICUs). Infections caused by multidrug-resistant organisms are linked to prolonged ICU and hospital stays, increased mortality, and higher healthcare costs [4]. Patients with COVID-19 in the ICU are particularly susceptible to bacterial superinfections, largely due to prolonged hospital stays and the frequent use of mechanical ventilation. This increased vulnerability has been linked to higher mortality rates compared to those seen in previous acute viral infections [5, 6]. Bacterial superinfections, along with the presence of bacterial endotoxins, can exacerbate viral dissemination and amplify the host's systemic inflammatory response—significantly increasing the risk of sepsis [7, 8]. Early identification of patients with elevated bacterial loads enables timely and targeted interventions, which can meaningfully improve sepsis outcomes in this high-risk population.

V. Premuzic (✉)
Department of Nephrology, Hypertension, Dialysis and Transplantation, School of Medicine, University Hospital Center Zagreb, Zagreb, Croatia

S. De Rosa, S. Lassola (eds.), *Next-Gen Blood Purification*,
https://doi.org/10.1007/978-3-032-27033-7_6

6.2 Clinical Implications of Uncontrolled Infection and the Possible Role of EBP

Monitoring viral load has long been a cornerstone in the management of infections such as human immunodeficiency virus (HIV) and hepatitis C, where it serves as a key indicator of disease progression and treatment efficacy. Limaye et al. demonstrated that cytomegalovirus (CMV) viremia is independently associated with increased risk of hospitalization or death within 30 days in ICU patients [9]. Similar patterns have been observed with Epstein-Barr virus (EBV) in the context of allogeneic hematopoietic stem cell transplantation [10]. In the setting of COVID-19, Bermejo-Martin et al. reported that SARS-CoV-2 RNAemia and elevated plasma viral RNA loads correlate strongly with critical illness. The heightened immune dysregulation associated with high viral burden may contribute to disease severity, underscoring the value of viral load monitoring in guiding clinical management and prognostication in immunocompromised individuals, particularly those undergoing solid organ or hematopoietic cell transplantation, as well as patients with HIV [11–17]. In this context, extracorporeal blood purification (EBP) has emerged as a promising adjunctive strategy for immunosuppressed ICU patients with high viral loads. EBP may aid in reducing circulating pathogen and toxin levels, thereby potentially mitigating the inflammatory cascade and improving outcomes. An open-label, randomized controlled trial suggested that early initiation of blood purification therapy is associated with significantly improved survival in patients with COVID-19 infection [18].

6.2.1 EBP in Infectious Diseases

In a study by Andermatt et al., EBP technology demonstrated in vivo effectiveness in reducing viral loads of herpes simplex virus type 2 (HSV-2) and Epstein-Barr virus (EBV) [19]. The study found that therapeutic plasma exchange (TPE) reduced circulating HSV-2 copies by approximately 25% and EBV copies by 40% in patients with acute liver failure. Notably, the Seraph-100 outperformed TPE in removing EBV, highlighting its potential as a targeted intervention for EBV-associated pathologies. Similar positive effects were observed in an experimental device-based experience on a patient undergoing immunosuppression due to a kidney graft and with disseminated adenovirus infection [20]. Data reported by Monard et al. demonstrated promising outcomes with the intraoperative use of the Seraph-100® in patients undergoing surgery for aortic vascular or endovascular graft infections [21]. Their findings included improved intraoperative hemodynamic stability and the achievement of negative intraoperative blood cultures, suggesting a potential role for the device in managing high-risk surgical infections. The Seraph-100® Microbind® Affinity Blood Filter (Seraph-100®; Exthera Medical Corporation, Martinez, CA) is an extracorporeal hemoperfusion device engineered to remove a broad spectrum of pathogens—including bacteria, viruses, and fungi—from the bloodstream. Its clinical application has been described in a prospective, multicenter, nonrandomized interventional study and in individual case reports [22, 23].

The Hemopurifier® (Aethlon Medical, San Diego, CA, USA) is an extracorporeal device that combines plasmapheresis and adsorption-based mechanisms to facilitate the reported in-vitro removal of viruses from the bloodstream [24]. In clinical use, integration of the Hemopurifier® with dialysis led to a 75% reduction in hepatitis C viral load within one week, as reported in an experimental device-based safety study protocol [25]. Furthermore, the device has shown potential in the management of severe viral infections, with case reports indicating a marked decrease in viral burden in a patient with severe Ebola virus disease [26]. Clinicians should be aware that the reported efficacy of the Hemopurifier® is based on early or low-powered data, highlighting the need for future randomized controlled studies with larger sample sizes.

In many cases, EBP is not a direct treatment for different pathogens and infection itself but a method to manage consequences of the overactive immune response and to improve hemodynamic stability, reduce inflammatory markers, and support organ function in critically ill patients. Fluher et al. [27] described a case report of a patient with severe leptospirosis, complicated by multiorgan failure and profound circulatory collapse of both distributive and cardiogenic etiology. The patient was managed with comprehensive supportive care and continuous veno-venous hemodiafiltration (CVVHDF) combined with extracorporeal cytokine removal, which managed to improve the patient's clinical features. CytoSorb® (CytoSorbents Corporation, Monmouth Junction, NJ, USA) is a cytokine adsorber approved for infectious and noninfectious conditions. EBP with Cytosorb has been shown in several studies to reduce the need for vasopressor drugs, inflammatory parameters, and mortality in patients with septic shock, with a trend indicating that more severely ill patients (assessed by the APACHE II score) benefited more, although there are studies reporting no such relationship [28–30].

COVID-19 represents a unique phenotype for EBP because it combines intense immune dysregulation characterized by elevated circulating cytokines, prolonged viral activity, and high rates of secondary infection, creating multiple simultaneous therapeutic targets within the bloodstream. Hyperinflammation contributes directly to acute respiratory distress syndrome (ARDS), shock, and multiorgan failure—pathophysiological processes that EBP technologies are designed to modulate by removing inflammatory mediators. Devices capable of binding or removing viral particles or viral-associated pathogen-associated molecular patterns (PAMPs) may offer a mechanistic benefit in reducing ongoing immune activation. Critically ill patients with COVID-19 have a substantial risk of bacterial and fungal superinfections due to immune exhaustion, prolonged mechanical ventilation, and extensive use of immunomodulatory therapies. This creates a mixed inflammatory milieu driven by both viral and nonviral pathogens, making broad-spectrum blood purification approaches potentially relevant.

Together, these features distinguish COVID-19 from classical bacterial sepsis or isolated viral infections and provide a strong biological rationale for investigating EBP as an adjunctive therapy in selected patients.

6.2.2 EBP in COVID-19

EBP in COVID-19 is a treatment that uses specialized filters to remove inflammatory mediators from the blood to manage the hyperinflammatory response in severe cases of COVID-19. Studies suggest it may reduce mortality, shorten ICU stays, and decrease the need for life support like extracorporeal membrane oxygenation (ECMO) [31–33]. In a meta-analysis of COVID-19 patients, EBP has been shown to be associated with improved outcomes, which in turn correlates with the decrease of inflammatory parameters [34].

On the other hand, some authors concluded that randomized clinical trials did not provide conclusive evidence for benefits and even suggest risks in COVID-19 patients [35]. The reasons for these conclusions were that the timing of the hemoadsorption therapy had no effect on patients' outcomes, further suggesting that, due to inconclusive evidence for benefit and potential harm, EBP should be limited to thoroughly designed clinical trials before being introduced into clinical routine in the context of COVID-19.

The oXiris® membrane (Baxter, IL, USA) is a modified hemodiafilter primarily used in septic patients with acute kidney injury (AKI), and has also been employed in the management of COVID-19 patients [33, 36, 37]. Similarly, the Jafron HA330 cartridge (Jafron Medical, Zhuhai, China), a synthetic resin hemofilter composed of polystyrene divinylbenzene copolymer, a nonselective hemoadsorption device designed to nonselectively eliminate molecules ranging from 10 to 60 kDa, and for use in clinical conditions associated with elevated cytokine levels, such as sepsis and other cytokine release syndromes [38], has also been employed in the management of COVID-19 patients.

As demonstrated in previous observational and prospective cohort studies involving patients with severe COVID-19 [39, 40], the early implementation of HA-330 hemoperfusion, in conjunction with standard therapy, was associated with improved organ function outcomes and may also contribute to a reduction in mortality.

Most studies involving the Seraph-100® have focused on its use in patients with COVID-19 and sepsis. The PURIFY-OBS study with preliminary observational data, which assessed the safety and efficacy of the Seraph-100 in patients with severe COVID-19, has shown potential in physically removing bacterial and viral pathogens in patients with concurrent COVID-19 infection and reported a 3.5-fold increase in the odds of survival among treated patients. However, the ability to draw definitive conclusions was limited by a small sample size and loss of statistical power due to propensity score matching [41]. In addition, the COSA study, a multicenter observational study conducted across 12 hospitals, demonstrated that early initiation of Seraph-100 treatment, specifically within the first 60 h of ICU admission, was associated with a significant mortality benefit compared to delayed use [42].

The concept of sequential extracorporeal blood purification involves the targeted removal of specific circulating molecules, such as endotoxins and cytokines, in the management of sepsis and septic shock [43]. Originally developed prior to the COVID-19 pandemic, this approach has been applied in carefully selected patient populations [44]. In a study by Premuzic et al., a sequential blood purification strategy—combining the Seraph-100® device with nonselective hemoadsorbers—was evaluated in ICU patients with COVID-19 and confirmed bacterial superinfection [45].

Overall, this sequential blood purification strategy represents a promising therapeutic approach for optimizing the management of patients with sepsis and septic shock, particularly in those with complex clinical presentations, such as COVID-19 complicated by bacterial superinfection.

6.3 Practical Considerations for EBP in Infectious Diseases and COVID-19

EBP may be considered in patients with septic shock who are failing standard therapy, including adequate fluid resuscitation, vasopressor support, and appropriate antimicrobial treatment, and who exhibit ongoing or worsening organ dysfunction. Patients most likely to benefit from EBP are those demonstrating a hyperinflammatory phenotype, characterized by: elevated inflammatory biomarkers (e.g., IL-6, TNF-α, C-reactive protein), high lactate levels (e.g., >6.5 mmol/L), significant vasopressor requirements (e.g., norepinephrine >0.5 μg/kg/min), and high illness severity scores (e.g., SOFA or APACHE II) [46–48]. The therapeutic goal of EBP in this population is the removal of excessive circulating cytokines, pathogen-associated molecular patterns (PAMPs), and damage-associated molecular patterns (DAMPs) to mitigate immune dysregulation and restore immunologic balance. EBP should be considered after the implementation of standard-of-care interventions when hemodynamic instability and organ dysfunction persist.

EBP appears to be most effective when initiated early and before the development of irreversible organ damage. Available evidence suggests that earlier initiation of EBP—particularly within 24 h of sepsis onset—is associated with improved hemodynamic stabilization and may confer a survival benefit, although high-quality randomized controlled trials are still needed to confirm these findings [46, 47, 49]. Treatment duration and exchange intervals vary by device. For example, CytoSorb® cartridges have a maximum approved treatment duration of 24 hours per device and are often exchanged every 12 h during the initial treatment phase, followed by 24-h exchanges as clinical stability improves [47, 49]. EBP is typically continued until clinical stabilization is achieved or until a predefined treatment duration is reached. Therapy should be discontinued when no further benefit is anticipated, balancing efficacy with device limitations and patient safety.

Continuous assessment of hemodynamic status is essential, including mean arterial pressure, vasopressor requirements (e.g., norepinephrine dose reduction), cardiac output when available, and overall perfusion. Markers of end-organ recovery, such as urine output and improvement in organ dysfunction scores (e.g., SOFA), should be closely followed. Serial measurement of inflammatory and metabolic biomarkers can help assess response to therapy. Given the potential for nonselective adsorption, serum concentrations of essential medications—particularly antimicrobials—should be monitored when feasible. Device-specific parameters should be routinely assessed, including blood flow rates, total blood volume processed, cartridge lifespan, clearance efficiency, and anticoagulation adequacy to ensure optimal performance and minimize complications [46–49].

Treatment endpoints should include reduction of circulating inflammatory mediators or pathogen load, stabilization of hemodynamics, evidenced by reduced vasopressor requirements, improvement of organ function, as reflected by better lactate clearance, improved urine output, reductions in SOFA or APACHE scores, and potential improvement in ICU and hospital survival, though definitive evidence from randomized controlled trials remains limited [46–50].

6.4 Conclusions

In sepsis, an overactive and dysregulated immune response leads to the release of a wide array of pro- and anti-inflammatory mediators, cytokines, and pathogen-associated molecular patterns (PAMPs). The incorporation of EBP offers a promising adjunctive strategy for critically ill ICU patients, particularly those with high pathogen burdens unresponsive to conventional therapies. These interventions aim to remove circulating inflammatory mediators and microbial toxins, thereby contributing to pathogen source control and potentially improving clinical outcomes. This approach may be especially valuable in cases where standard treatments prove insufficient, underscoring the urgent need for further research and clinical trials to better define the role and timing of EBP. Nevertheless, the current body of evidence has several important limitations, including small sample sizes, heterogeneous patient populations, a lack of randomized controlled trials, and reliance on surrogate endpoints. In addition, the included studies on EBP in COVID-19 were conducted at different stages of the pandemic and involved a variety of concomitant anti-inflammatory therapies used in combination with hemoadsorption, complicating the interpretation of results. At present, EBP as an adjunctive therapy for critically ill patients with infectious diseases or with COVID-19 remains unproven and should be considered investigational. Large, prospective randomized trials with well-defined inclusion criteria and standardized treatment protocols are needed to determine the true clinical benefit of EBP.

References

1. Evans L, Rhodes A, Alhazzani W, Antonelli M, Coopersmith CM, French C, et al. Surviving sepsis campaign: international guidelines for management of sepsis and septic shock 2021. Intensive Care Med. 2021;47:1181–247. https://doi.org/10.1007/s00134-021-06506-y.
2. Timsit JF, Bassetti M, Cremer O, Daikos G, de Waele J, Kallil A, et al. Rationalizing antimicrobial therapy in the ICU: a narrative review. Intensive Care Med. 2019;45:172–89. https://doi.org/10.1007/s00134-019-05520-5.
3. De Waele JJ. Importance of timely and adequate source control in sepsis and septic shock. J Intensive Med. 2024;4(3):281–6. https://doi.org/10.1016/j.jointm.2024.01.002.

4. Karukappadath RM, Sirbu D, Zaky A. Drug-resistant bacteria in the critically ill: patterns and mechanisms of resistance and potential remedies. Front Antibiot. 2023;2:1145190. https://doi.org/10.3389/frabi.2023.1145190.
5. Zhou P, Liu Z, Chen Y, Xiao Y, Huang X, Fan X-G. Bacterial and fungal infections in COVID-19 patients: a matter of concern. Infect Control Hosp Epidemiol. 2020;41:1124–5.
6. Li R, Pei S, Chen B, Song Y, Zhang T, Yang W, et al. Substantial undocumented infection facilitates the rapid dissemination of novel coronavirus (SARS-CoV-). Science. 2020;368(6490):489–93.
7. Kruglikov IL. Scherer PE (2021) Preexisting and inducible endotoxemia as crucial contributors to the severity of COVID-19 outcomes. PLoS Pathog. 2021;17:e1009306.
8. Khan S, Bolotova O, Sahib H, Foster D, Mallipattu SK. Endotoxemia in critically ill patients with COVID-19. Blood Purif; 2021. p. 1–7.
9. Limaye AP, Kirby KA, Rubenfeld GD, Leisenring WM, Bulger EM, Neff MJ, Gibran NS, Huang ML, Santo Hayes TK, Corey L, Boeckh M. Cytomegalovirus reactivation in critically ill immunocompetent patients. JAMA. 2008;300(4):413–22.
10. Tsushima T, Masuda SI, Yoda N, Kainuma S, Kimeda C, Konno S, Tanaka K, Matsuo K, Shimoji S, Kimura K, Arai H, Utsu Y, Imadome KI, Aotsuka N. Clinical characteristics and outcomes of Epstein-Barr virus viral load after allogeneic hematopoietic stem cell transplantation. Ann Hematol. 2024;103(3):935–46.
11. Bermejo-Martin JF, González-Rivera M, Almansa R, Micheloud D, Tedim AP, Domínguez-Gil M, et al. Viral RNA load in plasma is associated with critical illness and a dysregulated host response in COVID-19. Crit Care. 2020;24(1):691.
12. Hakimi Z, et al. Burden of cytomegalovirus disease in solid organ transplant recipients: a national matched cohort study in an inpatient setting. Transpl Infect Dis. 2017;19:3.
13. Avery RK, et al. Cytomegalovirus infections in lung and hematopoietic cell transplant recipeints in the Organ Transplant Infection Prevention and Detection Study: a multi-year, multicenter prospective cohort study. Transpl Infect Dis. 2018;E12877
14. Allen U, Alfieri C, Preiksaitis J, et al. Epstein-Barr virus infection in transplant recipients: summary of a workshop on surveillance, prevention and treatment. Can J Infect Dis Med Microbiol. 2002;13(2):89–99.
15. Wingfield T, Dearden L, Calvert P, Osanlou O, Johnston B, Chawla A, Hart I, Thompson C, Turtle L, Wenstone R. Adenovirus Type 7 causing severe lower respiratory tract infection in immunocompetent adults: a comparison of two contrasting cases from an intensive care unit in North West England. Clin Infect Pract. 2019;2:100007.
16. Allen UD, Preiksaitis JK. AST Infectious Diseases Community of Practice. Epstein-Barr virus and posttransplant lymphoproliferative disorder in solid organ transplantation. Am J Transplant. 2019;33(9):e13652.
17. Boucher HW, Talbot GH, Bradley JS, Edwards JE, Gilbert D, Rice LB, et al. Bad bugs, no drugs: no ESKAPE! An update from the Infectious Diseases Society of America. Clin Infect Dis. 2009;48(1):1–12.
18. Surasit K, Srisawat N. The role of early hemoadsorption in severe COVID-19 treatment: a pilot randomized controlled trial. Blood Purif. 2024;53(10):793–803. https://doi.org/10.1159/000540584.
19. Andermatt R, Bloemberg GV, Ganter CC, Mueller NJ, Mueller AMS, Muellhaupt B, Kielstein JT, David S. Elimination of Herpes Simplex Virus-2 and Epstein-Barr Virus with Seraph 100 microbind affinity blood filter and therapeutic plasma exchange: an explorative study in a patient with acute liver failure. Crit Care Explor. 2022;4(8):e0745.
20. Li DS, Burke TM, Smith JM, Reed RC, Okamura DM, Menon S. Use of the Seraph® 100 Microbind® Affinity Blood Filter in an adolescent patient with disseminated adenoviral disease. Pediatr Nephrol. 2024;39(1):331–5.
21. Monard C, Tresson P, Lamblin A, Benatir F, Taverna XJ, Rimmelé T. Intraoperative extracorporeal blood purification therapy during major septic vascular surgery. Crit Care. 2022;26(1):404.

22. Eden G, Schmidt JJ, Büttner S, et al. Safety and efficacy of the Seraph® 100 Microbind® Affinity Blood Filter to remove bacteria from the blood stream: results of the first in human study. Crit Care. 2022;26:181.
23. Seffer MT, Eden G, Engelmann S, Kielstein JT. Elimination of Staphylococcus aureus from the bloodstream using a novel biomimetic sorbent haemoperfusion device. BMJ Case Rep. 2020;13:e235262.
24. Koch B, Schult-Dietrich P, Büttner S, Dilmaghani B, Lohmann D, Baer PC, et al. Lectin affinity plasmapheresis for middle east respiratory syndrome-coronavirus and marburg virus glycoprotein elimination. Blood Purif. 2018;46(2):126–33.
25. Tullis RH, Duffin RP, Handley HH, Sodhi P, Menon J, Joyce JA, et al. Reduction of hepatitis C virus using lectin affinity plasmapheresis in dialysis patients. Blood Purif. 2009;27(1):64–9.
26. Büttner S, Koch B, Dolnik O, Eickmann M, Freiwald T, Rudolf S, et al. Extracorporeal virus elimination for the treatment of severe Ebola virus disease: first experience with lectin affinity plasmapheresis. Blood Purif. 2014;38(3–4):286–91.
27. Fluher J, Cestar I, Jerenec K, Kalamar Ž, Baklan Z, Markota A. A patient with severe leptospirosis treated with cytokine removal and high-dose corticosteroids. Infect Dis Rep. 2022;14(5):635–40. https://doi.org/10.3390/idr14050068.
28. Hawchar F, Lászlő I, Öveges N, Trásy D, Ondrik Z, Molnar Z. Extracorporeal cytokine adsorption in septic shock: a proof of concept randomized, controlled pilot study. J Crit Care. 2019;49:172–8.
29. Friesecke S, Träger K, Schittek GA, Molnar Z, Bach F, Kogelmann K, et al. International registry on the use of the CytoSorb® adsorber in ICU patients: study protocol and pre-liminary results. Med Klin Intensivmed Notfmed. 2019;114(8):699–707.
30. Friesecke S, Stecher S-S, Gross S, Felix SB, Nierhaus A. Extracorporeal cytokine elimination as rescue therapy in refractory septic shock: a prospective single-center study. J Artif Organs. 2017;20(3):252–9.
31. Niazi NS, Nassar TI, Stewart IJ, Honore PM, Sharma K, Chung KK. A review of extracorporeal blood purification techniques for the treatment of critically ill coronavirus disease 2019 patients. ASAIO J. 2022;68:1219–27. https://doi.org/10.1097/MAT.0000000000001761.
32. Rampino T, Gregorini M, Perotti L, Ferrari F, Pattonieri EF, Grignano MA, et al. Hemoperfusion with CytoSorb as adjuvant therapy in critically ill patients with SARS-CoV2 pneumonia. Blood Purif. 2021;50(4–5):566–71.
33. Villa G, Romagnoli S, De Rosa S, Greco M, Resta M, Pomarè Montin D, et al. Blood purification therapy with a hemodiafilter featuring enhanced adsorptive properties for cytokine removal in patients presenting COVID-19: a pilot study. Crit Care. 2020;24(1):605.
34. Merad M, Martin JC. Pathological inflammation in patients with COVID-19: a key role for monocytes and macrophages. Nat Rev Immunol. 2020;20(6):355–62.
35. Kloka JA, Jasny T, Old O, et al. Critical risks of haemoadsorption for COVID-19 patients and directions for future evaluations: a nationwide propensity score matched cohort study. Sci Rep. 2025;15:29184.
36. Premužić V, Babel J, Gardijan D, Lapić I, Gabelica R, Ostojić Z, et al. Extracorporeal blood purification is associated with improvement in biochemical and clinical variables in the critically-ill COVID-19 patients. Ther Apher Dial. 2022;26(2):316–29.
37. Broman ME, Hansson F, Vincent J-L, Bodelsson M. Endotoxin and cytokine reducing properties of the oXiris membrane in patients with septic shock: a randomized crossover double-blind study. PLoS One. 2019;14(8):e0220444.
38. Lorenzin A, de Cal M, Marcello M, Sorbo D, Copelli S, Ronco C, et al. Vancomycin Ad-sorption during in vitro Model of Hemoperfusion with Mini-Module of HA380 Cartridge. Blood Purif. 2023;52(2):174–82.
39. Mikaeili H, Taghizadieh AP, Nazemiyeh M, Rezaeifar P, Zununi Vahed S, Safiri S, et al. The early start of hemoperfusion decreases the mortality rate among severe COVID-19 patients: a preliminary study. Hemodial Int. 2021;26(2):176–82.
40. Surasit K, Srisawat N. The efficacy of early additional hemoperfusion therapy for severe COVID-19 patients: a prospective cohort study. Blood Purif. 2022;51(11):879–88.

41. Chitty SA, Mobbs S, Rifkin BS, et al. A multicenter evaluation of the Seraph 100 Microbind Affinity Blood Filter for the treatment of severe COVID-19. Crit Care Explor J. 2022;4(4):1–11.
42. Schmidt JJ, Borchina D, van't Klooster M, et al. Interim analysis of the COSA (COVID-19 patients treated with the Seraph 100 Microbind Affinity Filter) registry. Nephrol Dial Transplant. 2022;37(4):673–80.
43. Ruiz-Rodríguez JC, Chiscano-Camón L, Palmada C, Ruiz-Sanmartin A, Pérez-Carrasco M, Larrosa N. Endotoxin and cytokine sequential hemoadsorption in septic shock and multi-organ failure. Blood Purif. 2022;51(7):630–3.
44. Ronco C, Chawla L, Husain-Syed F, et al. Rationale for sequential extracorporeal therapy (SET) in sepsis. Crit Care. 2023;27:50.
45. Premuzic V, Situm I, Lovric D, et al. Sequential extracorporeal blood purification is associated with prolonged survival among ICU patients with COVID-19 and confirmed bacterial superinfection. Blood Purif. 2023;52(7-8):642–51.
46. Zhang L, Srisawat N, Lee CC, et al. Extracorporeal Blood Purification with the oXiris® filter for patients with sepsis and hyperinflammatory conditions: the Asia-Pacific oXiris expert meeting 2024 consensus statements. Blood Purif. 2025;54(11):621–38. https://doi.org/10.1159/000548214.
47. Guarino M, Costanzini A, Luppi F, et al. Extracorporeal cytokine adsorption in sepsis: current evidence and future perspectives. Biomedicines. 2025;13(7):1684. https://doi.org/10.3390/biomedicines13071684.
48. Mehta Y, Paul R, Ansari AS, et al. Extracorporeal blood purification strategies in sepsis and septic shock: an insight into recent advancements. World J Crit Care Med. 2023;12(2):71–88. https://doi.org/10.5492/wjccm.v12.i2.71.
49. Romagnoli S, Villa G, Barbani F, Ricci Z. Hemoadsorption: one name, varied techniques. Blood Purif. 2025:1–9. https://doi.org/10.1159/000545741.
50. Forni LG, Premuzic V. Endotoxin, virus, and bacterial removal: why, when, and how? Blood Purif. 2025:1–8. https://doi.org/10.1159/000546923.

7 Extracorporeal Therapies in Chronic Kidney Disease

Federica Pellecchia and Marco Fiorentino

7.1 Introduction

Chronic kidney disease (CKD) is defined by the presence of kidney damage or a persistent reduction in the estimated glomerular filtration rate (eGFR) <60 mL/min/1.73 m^2 for at least 3 months. It affects over 70 million people worldwide, and its prevalence is steadily increasing, mainly due to the rising incidence of several clinical conditions such as diabetes, hypertension, and cardiovascular diseases. CKD is associated with a progressive and irreversible decline in kidney function, leading to end-stage kidney disease (ESKD) and the need for renal replacement therapies, such as dialysis or kidney transplantation [1].

Enhancing awareness of the global burden of CKD is essential to improve disease management and treatment strategies. Substantial evidence highlights the significant clinical, social, and economic impact of CKD, leading to a persistent need for novel therapeutic approaches. As the disease progresses, patients show a progressive deterioration in health-related quality of life, and, despite existing therapies, nearly fifty percent of affected individuals experience adverse renal and cardiovascular outcomes. Despite several emerging treatments showing promise in slowing disease progression, the future development of novel curative options capable of halting kidney damage remains an urgent goal [2].

Although kidney transplantation is universally recognized as the best option for patients with ESKD, offering superior survival rates, improved quality of life, and reduced long-term healthcare costs, only a subgroup of CKD patients has access to and can benefit from this therapeutic option due to organ shortage and comorbidities/eligibility criteria. In this scenario, dialysis treatment remains a cornerstone of

F. Pellecchia · M. Fiorentino (✉)
Department of Precision and Regenerative Medicine and Ionian Area, University of Bari Aldo Moro, Bari, Italy
e-mail: f.pellecchia4@studenti.uniba.it

S. De Rosa, S. Lassola (eds.), *Next-Gen Blood Purification*,
https://doi.org/10.1007/978-3-032-27033-7_7

renal replacement therapy in patients who are not eligible for transplantation or for those on the waiting list; however, while it provides life-sustaining treatment, it is associated with cardiovascular complications, infection risks, and impaired quality of life.

This chapter reviews the classification of uremic toxins, the mechanisms of conventional dialysis modalities, and recent advances in extracorporeal therapies designed to target middle molecules and protein-bound solutes. The rationale behind current extracorporeal approaches and their impact on inflammation, nutrition, and patient-centered outcomes is also discussed.

7.2 Uremic Toxins Classification and Rationale for Extracorporeal Blood Purification

In the setting of kidney failure and uremia, solutes accumulate, exhibiting distinct physicochemical characteristics and specific biological effects [3]. Uremic toxins derive mainly from protein metabolism and can increase in the blood during renal dysfunction, reaching multiple organs (including kidneys and heart) and impairing their biological functions. The uremic syndrome is therefore characterized by the accumulation of toxic compounds that play a central role in inducing endothelial dysfunction [6].

According to the European Uremic Toxins Work Group (EUTox), over 150 uremic toxins have been identified and classified into three main groups (Fig. 7.1) [4]:

1. Small water-soluble molecules (<500 Da), such as urea and creatinine, which are easily removed by conventional hemodialysis (HD).
2. Middle molecules (>500 Da), including β2-microglobulin and leptin, which are only partially removed by high-permeability membranes.
3. Protein-bound compounds (phenols, indoles), which are derived from amino acid metabolism, and they are not removed since only the free fraction is dialyzable.

The accumulation of these toxins is implicated in the development of immune dysfunction, chronic inflammation, anorexia, malnutrition, atherosclerosis, and cardiac hypertrophy, as well as cognitive impairment [5–7].

The removal of protein-bound uremic toxins (PBUTs) remains one of the main challenges in the treatment of patients with renal failure. HD is still the most widely used extracorporeal blood purification therapy and is highly effective in removing small water-soluble molecules. However, the efficacy of such treatment is limited when considering middle molecules and PBUTs, due to both the protein binding and the small pore size of HD membranes, which are specifically designed to prevent albumin loss [8, 9].

Modifying dialysis settings and parameters, such as increasing frequency and treatment duration, can enhance small and middle molecule removal, although it does not significantly affect the elimination of protein-bound toxins [10]. To

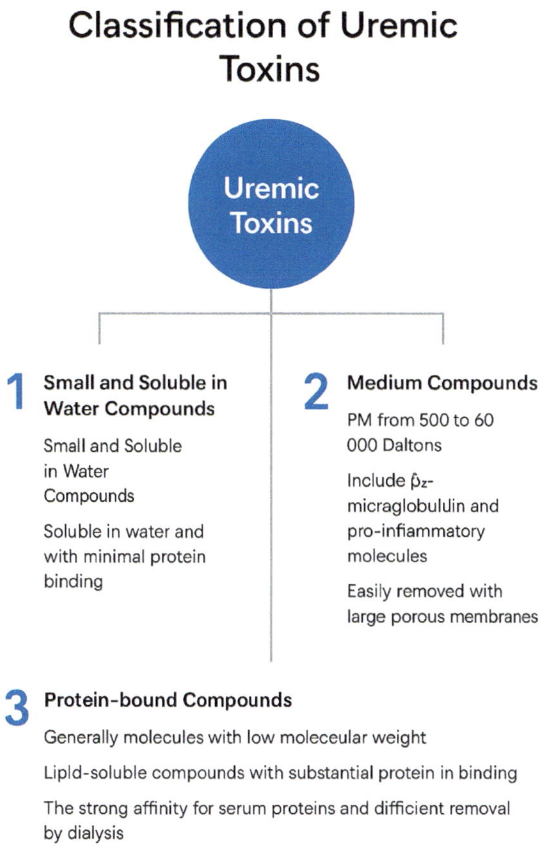

Fig. 7.1 Classification of uremic toxins and their characteristics

overcome these limitations, the introduction of high-flux membranes has improved the clearance of middle-molecular-weight solutes compared to standard HD. This improvement is achieved through a larger pore size and an enhanced convective component of the treatment [11]. However, despite these advantages, albumin and micronutrient loss remain a concern. During the last years, innovations in dialysis have been mainly focused on the possibility to enhance the clearance of toxins that are not typically removed by standard dialysis techniques and membranes. This technological evolution reflects the sequential need to address each toxin category identified by the EUTox classification. In this scenario, while HD is effective for removing small water-soluble molecules, the development and application of hemodiafiltration (HDF) enhances convective removal of middle molecules; lastly, adsorptive membranes and devices have been recently designed and introduced in clinical practice to address the unmet need for PBUTs removal. In the next sections, a detailed description of the evolution of extracorporeal treatments beyond conventional diffusive HD to improve clinical outcomes.

7.3 Conventional Dialysis Modalities in ESKD

HD techniques involve extracorporeal blood circulation through a semipermeable membrane that selectively removes uremic toxins and excessive fluid, as well as corrects electrolyte imbalances and reduces serum potassium, making it the preferred modality for the management of acute refractory hyperkalemia [12, 13]. The properties of the dialysis membrane and the solute transport mechanisms are the main determinants of HD effectiveness. Combinations of treatment intensity, use of diffusive and convective forces can further enhance HD treatment dose administration, enabling a notable reduction in the concentrations of a wide range of uremic compounds [12]. Conventional HD removes small water-soluble molecules mainly through diffusion, but this treatment is less effective in clearing middle- to large-molecular-weight toxins, which are mostly implicated in chronic inflammation, atherosclerosis, and dialysis-related amyloidosis. HDF represents an advancement of conventional HD, combining both diffusion and convection to enhance the removal of middle- and large-molecular-weight solutes [14]. HDF exploits convective transport by generating a water flow through the membrane that drags solutes along ("solvent drag"), leading to an increased removal of middle and large molecules. HDF may reduce inflammatory complications, improve hemodynamic stability, and potentially prolong survival [14]. Postdilution hemofiltration shows similar safety profiles to conventional hemodialysis regarding neurocognitive function [15]. Patients' outcomes are greatly impacted by the frequency and intensity of dialysis administration, and HD must be tailored to individual patient needs, including electrolyte composition, dialysate buffer concentration, and anticoagulation strategy. Convective therapies, particularly HDF, may reduce cardiovascular mortality and improve hemodynamic stability, but strong evidence of an effect on all-cause mortality or other clinically relevant outcomes is still missing. A recent multicenter randomized controlled trial testing the impact on all-cause mortality between high-volume online HDF and conventional high-flux HD described a significant reduction of mortality risk in patients assigned and treated with high-volume HDF, associated with fewer cardiovascular deaths, lower infection-related mortality, and lower risk of hospitalization [14].

The enhanced removal observed with HDF represents the first technological step beyond conventional HD toward broader solute clearance, especially for middle molecules.

Compared to in-center HD, peritoneal dialysis (PD) represents an alternative modality of renal replacement therapy, enhancing patients' autonomy and treatment flexibility [16]. PD utilizes the peritoneum as a semipermeable membrane for solute and fluid exchange, with dialysate instilled into the peritoneal cavity through a specific peritoneal catheter and exchanged periodically. The main treatment for PD is continuous ambulatory peritoneal dialysis (CAPD), which involves doing several manual exchanges every day and night, usually four to five times a day. CAPD greatly enhances quality of life and job prospects by enabling patients to perform dialysis at home with flexibility in schedule and location. Automated peritoneal dialysis (APD) represents an alternative involving night-time exchanges using a mechanical cycler, providing options for patients who prefer overnight dialysis. Stepwise beginning of peritoneal dialysis (SIPD), which involves introducing PD gradually with long break-in periods, is one of the novel techniques for PD initiation [17]. The extended break-in period in SIPD, averaging 176 days compared to 27 days in conventional PD, reduces infectious complications, including peritonitis and catheter-related infections. In terms of overall survival, PD was not inferior to HD, according to a prospective randomized trial that compared the survival rates between treatments: the hazard ratio for death on PD compared to HD was 0.76 (95% CI 0.47–1.24) [18].

Finally, home hemodialysis (HHD) provides an alternative delivery method associated with decreased cardiovascular risk compared to peritoneal dialysis, including 42% lower risk of stroke and 17% lower risk of acute coronary syndrome [19].

7.4 Innovations in Hemodialysis Technologies

7.4.1 High Cut-Off and Medium Cut-Off Membranes for Expanded Hemodialysis

The development of advanced dialysis membranes has been driven by the need to overcome small solute removal and better address middle molecules and PBUTs removal, which mostly contribute to chronic inflammation and long-term complications in dialysis patients. Early high–cut off (HCO) membranes enabled the removal of large solutes but raised concerns regarding albumin loss, whereas medium–cut off (MCO) membranes enabled expanded hemodialysis (HDx) with improved cytokine and free-light chain removal and long-term safety profile.

HCO membranes have shown promising results in removing high molecular weight solutes, as their larger pores can clear molecules up to 60 kDa. These membranes have been used mainly in specific settings, such as acute kidney injury (AKI) in the context of multiple myeloma or severe sepsis, to enhance cytokine and inflammatory mediator removal [20]. However, the risk of albumin loss limits their routine use in chronic patients. The concept of HDx, a dialysis technique intended to enhance the removal of middle- and large-sized molecules, has been developed more recently thanks to the introduction of MCO membranes. This approach may help to improve chronic inflammation and overall clinical outcomes, limiting albumin loss [21]. Expanded HD with MCO membranes represents one of the most significant innovations in the treatment of ESKD. They are typically composed of polyarylethersulfone and polyvinylpyrrolidone and have a surface area of at least 1.6 m^2. They feature a more uniform and larger pore distribution compared to conventional membranes. Their pore radius (≈5 nm, reduced to ≈3.5 nm upon contact with blood) allows removal of toxins up to 45 kDa. Structural modifications (reduction of fiber wall thickness to 180 μm and increase in fiber number) enhance permeability, blood flow, and dialysis efficiency [21]. MCO dialyzers are able to remove a wide spectrum of toxins (β2-microglobulin, kappa, and lambda free light chains) using standard parameters (Qb ≥ 300 mL/min, Qd = 500 mL/min) and without the need for substitution fluid [22]. In addition, MCO membranes may provide benefits in the removal of inflammatory cytokines (IL-6, TNF-α), potentially improving the inflammatory state [23, 24].

Numerous studies have confirmed the safety and efficacy of such membranes compared with high-flux HD, demonstrating superior clearance of β2-microglobulin and free light chains [25]. A recent meta-analysis including 18 studies and 853 patients showed that HDx is superior to high-flux HD in terms of clearance of these molecules, although no clinically significant advantages over HDF were observed [25]. Albumin loss is comparable to that described in the context of HDF, which is crucial for long-term safety. The reduction in serum β2-microglobulin levels was particularly significant, and free light chains, known to be associated with worse outcomes in dialysis patients, were also more effectively removed [21].

Beyond solute clearance, HDx also appears to improve patient-reported outcomes. In a multicenter prospective study involving 992 patients, switching from high-flux HD to HDx for 12 months, a significant reduction of the prevalence of restless leg syndrome was observed, in association with improvements in the symptoms of uremic pruritus and scratching frequency during sleep [26]. From an economic perspective, HDx may offer cost advantages, as it does not require large volumes of substitution fluid as in HDF, thereby reducing logistical costs. Moreover, a reduction in the use of erythropoiesis-stimulating agents and iron supplementation has been reported, possibly due to improved removal of inflammatory mediators, better iron metabolism, and reduced ESA resistance [27].

7.4.2 Targeting Inflammatory Mediators and Cytokines Removal

Since middle molecules and PBUTs play a central role in the inflammatory state of CKD, innovations have increasingly focused on adsorption-based approaches capable of targeting cytokines and other immune mediators beyond simple diffusion and convection.

Chronic inflammation is a hallmark of CKD, associated with disease progression to ESKD. Biomarkers of inflammatory status, such as interleukin-6 (IL-6) and C-reactive protein (CRP), are typically elevated in patients with advanced CKD and even more frequently in those on chronic dialysis. The pathogenesis of this hyperinflammatory state is multifactorial, involving cytokine overproduction, oxidative stress, chronic infections, fluid and sodium overload, intestinal dysbiosis, and dialysis procedures themselves. Monitoring inflammatory markers is clinically crucial, as their levels strongly correlate with mortality. However, no standardized therapeutic approach currently exists for chronic inflammation in CKD and ESKD. Lifestyle interventions such as a balanced diet and physical exercise may have positive effects, but are insufficient to control systemic inflammation. Increasing attention has recently been given to middle molecules, which account for about 23% of identified uremic toxins, including cytokines and pro-inflammatory mediators. These compounds tend to accumulate during renal dysfunction, contributing to the inflammatory vicious cycle and consequent complications such as atherosclerosis, osteoporosis, sarcopenia, diabetes, depression, and increased cardiovascular risk.

Patients treated with MCO membranes exhibited diminished expression of tumor necrosis factor-α (TNF-α) and IL-6 mRNA in peripheral leukocytes compared to conventional HD, indicating a potential anti-inflammatory effect [21]. Research on oxidative stress has produced inconclusive findings, and a recent clinical trial demonstrated no significant differences in cardiovascular parameters, including echocardiography and brachial-ankle pulse wave velocity, when compared to online HDF [27].

Among available approaches, adsorption-based therapies have gained increasing attention due to their capacity to remove middle- to large-molecular-weight substances independent of concentration gradients. Some dialysis membranes exhibit adsorptive properties in addition to diffusion and convection. Polymethylmethacrylate (PMMA) dialysis membranes represent an important advance in the management of inflammatory uremia. Unlike standard polysulfone (PS) membranes and MCO membranes, PMMA membranes combine different purification mechanisms, introducing the concept of adsorption, which relies on direct binding of targeted molecules (cytokines and other pro-inflammatory proteins) to the membrane surface through multiple interactions. Several studies demonstrated a more pronounced reduction of IL-6, interleukin-8 (IL-8), and CRP levels progressively in patients treated with PMMA membranes compared to PS dialyzers [28]. The adsorption mechanism is thought to be induced by the hydrophobic properties of PMMA and by the presence of nanopores that selectively trap molecules with molecular weights between 8 and 30 kDa, including many cytokines [29]. In addition, PMMA membranes have shown the ability not to activate the complement system. Compared with MCO membranes, PMMA provides a more targeted approach to reducing the inflammatory burden, with minimal impact on albumin loss, an especially relevant factor in malnourished or hypoalbuminemic patients. Conversely, MCO membranes are better suited for maximizing β2-microglobulin and free light chain removal, with benefits in preventing long-term complications such as dialysis-related amyloidosis, albeit with a higher risk of protein loss.

All these features together suggest the immunoprotective effects of PMMA membranes are particularly relevant in patients with persistent chronic inflammation. The association between inflammation down-regulation and the prevention of systemic complications makes these membranes a promising therapeutic option to reduce overall mortality, particularly in patients with treatment-resistant inflammatory uremia [30].

7.4.3 Sorbent-Based Dialysis Systems

These techniques complement conventional dialysis by improving the removal of inflammatory mediators and protein-bound solutes, with measurable effects on uremic symptoms, pruritus, nutritional markers, and inflammatory burden. In the context of adsorption-based extracorporeal therapy, a promising strategy for uremic toxins removal is related to the use of sorbents; while the use of such devices is widely studied in the setting of AKI and sepsis, this approach has been proposed even for patients on chronic hemodialysis [31]. A resin-based sorbent, composed of styrene and divinylbenzene, has been utilized as an add-on therapy to improve inflammatory burden and uremic symptom control in chronic dialysis patients. It consists of synthetic macroporous resin beads designed to adsorb molecules primarily in the molecular weight range of approximately 500 Da to 50 kDa (inflammatory cytokines, β2-microglobulin, parathyroid hormone fragments, protein-bound uremic toxins, advanced glycation end products). The cartridge represents a novel hemoadsorption device specifically designed to enhance the removal of protein-bound and middle-molecular-weight uremic toxins from blood. Recent clinical evidence demonstrates its substantial efficacy in this regard. In a randomized controlled trial comparing hemoadsorption combined with hemodialysis (HAHD) versus online hemodiafiltration (HDF), the combined HAHD approach demonstrated significantly superior removal of indoxyl sulfate (IS) and p-cresyl sulfate (PCS)—two prototypical protein-bound uremic toxins [32]. Specifically, the HAHD group achieved a single-session reduction ratio of IS of 46.9% compared to 31.8% in the HDF-q2w group ($p = 0.044$), and demonstrated superior PCS clearance at 44.6% versus 31.4% ($p = 0.003$) [32]. These improvements in toxin clearance translated into clinical benefits: patients treated with weekly HAHD reported greater relief from pruritus and improved sleep quality compared to those receiving HDF alone, with comparable adverse event profiles across all treatment groups [32].

When examined in comparative studies with standard hemodialysis (HD) and hemodiafiltration (HDF), the performance profile of HAHD reveals interesting patterns of complementarity. In one comprehensive analysis comparing low-flux HD (LFHD), LFHD with HA (LFHD-HA), high-flux HD (HFHD), HFHD with HA (HFHD-HA), HDF, and HDF-HA, the addition of hemoadsorption to low-flux hemodialysis significantly enhanced the removal of middle-molecular-weight markers [33]. Specifically, LFHD-HA demonstrated increased reduction ratios for beta-2 microglobulin, myoglobin, prolactin, and lambda-free immunoglobulin light chains compared with LFHD alone. Similarly, HFHD-HA showed enhanced removal of myoglobin, alpha-1 microglobulin, and free light chains relative to HFHD [33].

Several observational studies in ESKD patients show that the addition of hemoadsorption in series to the standard hemofilter (one treatment/week) was educes systemic inflammatory markers (e.g., CRP, IL-6), improves nutritional markers such as serum albumin, alleviating fatigue and anorexia associated with inflammation; in addition, a significant reduction in uremic symptoms, such as uremic pruritus, has been widely reported, as well as reductions in parathyroid hormone levels and calcium-phosphate product [34]. The incorporation of sorbents within dialysis membranes as mixed matrix membranes represents a promising approach to reduce the complexity and costs of hemoadsorption therapy while potentially improving efficacy.

7.5 Conclusions

Extracorporeal therapies in CKD have evolved from simple diffusion-based HD toward multimodal approaches incorporating convection and adsorption to target a broader spectrum of uremic solutes, including middle molecules and protein-bound toxins. Technological innovation—moving from HDF to MCO membranes and sorbent-based membranes and devices—reflects the increasing understanding of the biological role of inflammatory mediators, oxidative stress, and toxin–protein interactions. While these advances demonstrate meaningful improvements in solute clearance, inflammatory control, and patient-reported outcomes, ongoing research is still needed to determine the long-term impact on mortality, cardiovascular risk, and quality of life. The tailored integration of such options for a personalized dialysis delivery is expected to play a central role in the future management of chronic kidney disease.

References

1. Vaidya SR, Aeddula NR. Chronic kidney disease. In: StatPearls. Treasure Island: StatPearls Publishing LLC. StatPearls Publishing Copyright © 2025; 2025.
2. Braun L, Sood V, Hogue S, Lieberman B, Copley-Merriman C. High burden and unmet patient needs in chronic kidney disease. Int J Nephrol Renov Dis. 2012;5:151–63.
3. Vanholder R, Meert N, Schepers E, Glorieux G, Argiles A, Brunet P, et al. Review on uraemic solutes II – variability in reported concentrations: causes and consequences. Nephrol Dial Transplant. 2007;22(11):3115–21.
4. Rosner MH, Reis T, Husain-Syed F, Vanholder R, Hutchison C, Stenvinkel P, et al. Classification of uremic toxins and their role in kidney failure. Clin J Am Soc Nephrol. 2021;16(12):1918–28.
5. Glassock RJ. Uremic toxins: what are they? An integrated overview of pathobiology and classification. J Ren Nutr. 2008;18(1):2–6.
6. Vanholder R, De Smet R, Glorieux G, Argiles A, Baurmeister U, Brunet P, et al. Review on uremic toxins: classification, concentration, and interindividual variability. Kidney Int. 2003;63(5):1934–43.
7. Vanholder R, Glorieux G, De Smet R, Lameire N, European Uremic Toxin Work G. New insights in uremic toxins. Kidney Int Suppl. 2003;84:S6–10.
8. Lesaffer G, De Smet R, Lameire N, Dhondt A, Duym P, Vanholder R. Intradialytic removal of protein-bound uraemic toxins: role of solute characteristics and of dialyser membrane. Nephrol Dial Transplant. 2000;15(1):50–7.
9. Yamamoto S, Kazama JJ, Wakamatsu T, Takahashi Y, Kaneko Y, Goto S, et al. Removal of uremic toxins by renal replacement therapies: a review of current progress and future perspectives. Ren Replace Ther. 2016;2(1):43.
10. Basile C, Libutti P, Di Turo AL, Casino FG, Vernaglione L, Tundo S, et al. Removal of uraemic retention solutes in standard bicarbonate haemodialysis and long-hour slow-flow bicarbonate haemodialysis. Nephrol Dial Transplant. 2011;26(4):1296–303.
11. Krieter DH, Hackl A, Rodriguez A, Chenine L, Moragues HL, Lemke HD, et al. Protein-bound uraemic toxin removal in haemodialysis and post-dilution haemodiafiltration. Nephrol Dial Transplant. 2010;25(1):212–8.
12. Bowry SK, Chazot C. The scientific principles and technological determinants of haemodialysis membranes. Clin Kidney J. 2021;14(Suppl 4):i5–i16.

13. Alcantar-Vallin L, Zaragoza JJ, Ruíz-Ochoa FO, Sánchez-Alvarez JE, Chávez-Alonso G, Navarro-Viramontes Y, et al. Urgent initiation of hemodialysis versus peritoneal dialysis in severe hyperkalemia: a prospective study. Clin Kidney J. 2025;
14. Blankestijn PJ, Vernooij RWM, Hockham C, Strippoli GFM, Canaud B, Hegbrant J, et al. Effect of hemodiafiltration or hemodialysis on mortality in kidney failure. N Engl J Med. 2023;389(8):700–9.
15. Jimenez EV, Nuñez GC, Lerma A, Lerma C, Gonzalez AM, Perez-Grovas H, et al. Neurocognitive function with conventional hemodialysis versus post-dilution hemofiltration as initial treatment in ESKD patients: a randomized controlled trial – the DA-VINCI study. Blood Purif. 2023;53(2):130–7.
16. Legendre B, Lobbedez T, Couchoud C, Lanot A, Kolko A, Courivaud C, et al. The diversity of peritoneal dialysis care trajectories: a study based on the REIN registry and SNDS database. PLoS One. 2025;20(8):e0326745.
17. Hsiao P-K, Wong W-J, Hsieh S-I, Lin H-Y, Chen T-J, Cheng C-Y. Unveiling the intricacies: exploring stepwise initiation of peritoneal dialysis in a single-center setting. Medicina. 2024;60(10):1723.
18. Fan L, Yang X, Shen H, Chen M, Zhang H, Ni Z, et al. A prospective, randomized, multicenter, open-label trial comparing survival in subjects receiving peritoneal dialysis or conventional in-center hemodialysis. Med Adv. 2024;2(2):112–22.
19. Shah S, Weinhandl E, Gupta N, Leonard AC, Christianson AL, Thakar CV. Cardiovascular outcomes in patients on home hemodialysis and peritoneal dialysis. Kidney360. 2024;5(2):205–15.
20. Gondouin B, Hutchison CA. High cut-off dialysis membranes: current uses and future potential. Adv Chronic Kidney Dis. 2011;18(3):180–7.
21. Fiorentino M, La Fergola F, De Rosa S. Medium cut-off dialyzer for middle molecular uremic toxins in AKI and chronic dialysis. J Nephrol. 2024;37(1):23–37.
22. Cozzolino M, Magagnoli L, Ciceri P, Conte F, Galassi A. Effects of a medium cut-off (Theranova®) dialyser on haemodialysis patients: a prospective, cross-over study. Clin Kidney J. 2019;14(1):382–9.
23. Yeter HH, Korucu B, Akcay OF, Derici K, Derici U, Arinsoy T. Effects of medium cut-off dialysis membranes on inflammation and oxidative stress in patients on maintenance hemodialysis. Int Urol Nephrol. 2020;52(9):1779–89.
24. Zickler D, Schindler R, Willy K, Martus P, Pawlak M, Storr M, et al. Medium Cut-Off (MCO) membranes reduce inflammation in chronic dialysis patients – a randomized controlled clinical trial. PLoS One. 2017;12(1):e0169024.
25. Zhao Y, Gan L, Niu Q, Ni M, Zuo L. Efficacy and safety of expanded hemodialysis in hemodialysis patients: a meta-analysis and systematic review. Ren Fail. 2022;44(1):541–50.
26. Alarcon JC, Bunch A, Ardila F, Zuniga E, Vesga JI, Rivera A, et al. Impact of medium cut-off dialyzers on patient-reported outcomes: COREXH Registry. Blood Purif. 2021;50(1):110–8.
27. Sanabria RM, Hutchison CA, Vesga JI, Ariza JG, Sanchez R, Suarez AM. Expanded hemodialysis and its effects on hospitalizations and medication usage: a cohort study. Nephron. 2021;145(2):179–87.
28. Kishikawa T, Fujieda H, Sakaguchi H. Comprehensive analysis of cytokine adsorption properties of polymethyl methacrylate (PMMA) membrane material. J Artif Organs. 2022;25(4):343–9.
29. Maduell F, Broseta JJ, Rodriguez-Espinosa D, Hermida-Lama E, Rodas LM, Gomez M, et al. Evaluation and comparison of polysulfone TS-UL and PMMA NF-U dialyzers versus expanded hemodialysis and postdilution hemodiafiltration. Artif Organs. 2021;45(9):E317–E23.
30. Yoshida S, Yamamoto S, Miyauchi D, Terashima R, Hashimoto A, Miyazawa H, et al. Removal of alpha1-microglobulin using post-dilution online hemodiafiltration with polymethylmethacrylate membrane: an open-label, single-arm study. Blood Purif. 2024;53(2):123–9.
31. De Rosa S, Marengo M, Fiorentino M, Fanelli V, Brienza N, Fiaccadori E, et al. Extracorporeal blood purification therapies for sepsis-associated acute kidney injury in critically ill patients: expert opinion from the SIAARTI-SIN joint commission. J Nephrol. 2023;36(7):1731–42.

32. Yu S, Yuan H, Xiong X, Zhu Y, Fu P. Comparative efficacy of pHA130 haemoadsorption combined with haemodialysis versus online haemodiafiltration in removing protein-bound and middle-molecular-weight uraemic toxins: a randomized controlled trial. Toxins. 2025;17(8):392.
33. Maduell F, Escudero-Saiz VJ, Cuadrado-Payán E, Rodriguez-Garcia M, Rodas LM, Fontseré N, et al. Comparing hemodialysis and hemodiafiltration performance with and without hemoadsorption. Clin Kidney J. 2025;18(5)
34. Chen SJ, Jiang GR, Shan JP, Lu W, Huang HD, Ji G, et al. Combination of maintenance hemodialysis with hemoperfusion: a safe and effective model of artificial kidney. Int J Artif Organs. 2011;34(4):339–47.

8 Multi-Organ Extracorporeal Support: ECMO, CRRT, and Liver Support Integration

Luisa Cueva-Castro, Miriam Montero-Estopiñá, Desirée Catalán-García, Valentina M. Blanco-Fernández, and Gregorio Romero-González

8.1 Multi-Organ Failure, Shock, and the Physiological Rationale for Extracorporeal Organ Support

8.1.1 Definition and Clinical Relevance of Multi-Organ Failure

Multi-organ failure (MOF), often conceptualized as multiple organ dysfunction syndrome (MODS), marks the point at which the body can no longer maintain internal equilibrium in the face of severe systemic injury. It is defined as the simultaneous or sequential failure of at least two vital organ systems resulting from a dysregulated host response to infection, ischemia–reperfusion, trauma, or other catastrophic insults [1]. Despite major advances in critical care, MOF remains the leading cause of death in intensive care units (ICUs) worldwide and a principal determinant of long-term disability among survivors. The epidemiology of MOF reflects its broad clinical reach. In their seminal review, Angus and van der Poll

L. Cueva-Castro
Anesthesiology Department, San Pau University Hospital, Barcelona, Spain
e-mail: lcuevac@santpau.cat

M. Montero-Estopiñá · D. Catalán-García · V. M. Blanco-Fernández
Nephrology Department, Germans Trias i Pujol University Hospital (HUGTiP), Badalona, Spain
e-mail: mmonteroe.germanstrias@gencat.cat; dcatalang.germanstrias@gencat.cat; vmblanco.germanstrias@gencat.cat

G. Romero-González (✉)
Nephrology Department, Germans Trias i Pujol University Hospital (HUGTiP), Badalona, Spain

REMAR Research Group, Germans Trias i Pujol Research Institute (IGTP), Badalona, Spain

Department of Medicine, Universitat Autònoma de Barcelona (UAB), Badalona, Spain

International Renal Research Institute of Vicenza (IRRIV), Vicenza, Italy

S. De Rosa, S. Lassola (eds.), *Next-Gen Blood Purification*, https://doi.org/10.1007/978-3-032-27033-7_8

estimated that severe sepsis accounts for nearly 2% of all hospital admissions and 10% of ICU admissions in the United States, affecting more than 750,000 patients annually, with global incidence exceeding 19 million cases per year [2].

Contemporary data confirm that sepsis-related hospitalizations and associated organ dysfunction have steadily increased due to population aging, higher comorbidity burdens, improved survival from acute illnesses previously considered lethal, and greater diagnostic sensitivity [3]. Mortality rises sharply with increasing numbers of failing organs. Cohort studies consistently show that mortality is approximately 5% with no organ failure, surpasses 50% when two organs fail, and exceeds 90% when three or more organs fail persistently. Five-organ failure approaches universal mortality [4–6]. Beyond its biological impact, MOF imposes a profound economic burden. Based on national estimates of approximately 1.7 million sepsis hospitalizations each year and contemporary per-episode hospitalization costs, sepsis-related hospital expenditures in the United States exceed USD 50 billion annually [7, 8], and European economic analyses estimate that the direct hospital cost of treating severe sepsis or septic shock ranges between EUR 23,000 and 29,000 per admission, largely driven by prolonged ICU length of stay [8–10].

Yet these figures, while striking, only capture the administrative surface of a deeper clinical reality, one in which the lungs can no longer oxygenate, the heart can no longer perfuse, the kidneys can no longer maintain solute and fluid balance, and the liver becomes overwhelmed by toxins. When these physiological pillars begin to collapse simultaneously, the clinical trajectory accelerates dramatically toward irreversible organ dysfunction.

8.2 The Shock Continuum as the Pathway to Organ Failure

Shock represents the dynamic physiological continuum from which MOF emerges. It is not a discrete event but a progressive collapse of circulatory integrity and cellular oxygen utilization. This collapse advances through recognizable phases, ranging from subtle hemodynamic compromise to refractory circulatory collapse [11]. In the earliest compensated stage, arterial pressure may remain deceptively normal because neurohumoral vasoconstriction temporarily preserves macrocirculatory flow. Despite this apparent stability, tissue-level hypoperfusion is already present. Clinical markers such as tachycardia, reduced urine output, modest lactate elevation, and subtle cognitive changes frequently precede hypotension and reflect the onset of impaired oxygen delivery at the cellular level [12, 13]. As compensatory mechanisms begin to fail, patients drift into a phase of mild shock. Cardiac output becomes insufficient for metabolic demands, peripheral perfusion deteriorates, and lactate rises further. Early organ dysfunction—most often renal or neurological—begins to appear. Bedside markers such as prolonged capillary refill time, cool extremities, and worsening oliguria signal that the balance between oxygen supply and demand is unraveling [12, 13]. Once overt shock develops, hypotension becomes sustained and organ injury becomes unmistakable. Reduced perfusion pressure, hyperlactatemia, and the onset of metabolic acidosis coexist with rapidly progressing renal dysfunction, altered mental status, and impaired skin perfusion [12].

In cases with a cardiogenic substrate, additional triggers such as arrhythmias or recurrent ischemia may accelerate the decline along this continuum [11]. Profound shock signifies a deeper collapse of both macro- and microcirculatory function. Vasoplegia, myocardial depression, capillary leak, and endothelial injury intensify, driving a precipitous fall in oxygen delivery. At the cellular level, disturbances in mitochondrial function result in impaired oxygen utilization, often termed "cytopathic hypoxia," a hallmark of this stage and a strong predictor of organ failure and mortality [12, 13]. Refractory shock occupies the terminal end of the trajectory. At this point, circulatory collapse persists despite maximal vasoactive therapy. Lactate climbs relentlessly, acidemia deepens, and oxygen extraction falls toward zero. Without rapid implementation of extracorporeal rescue strategies, survival is exceedingly unlikely [11–13].

Across all stages of this continuum, a unifying insight becomes clear: shock advances through the bloodstream. As perfusion fails, arterial oxygen content declines, carbon dioxide accumulates, lactate rises, pH drifts, inflammatory mediators proliferate, and hepatically cleared toxins accumulate [12]. Each organ becomes both a victim and an amplifier of this disordered internal environment. This systemic physiology provides the rationale for considering the bloodstream itself as the primary therapeutic target in multi-organ extracorporeal support.

8.3 Physiological Basis for Extracorporeal Organ Support

The systemic nature of shock explains why organ-support therapies must themselves be systemic. As multi-organ dysfunction accelerates, it is not the isolated failure of lungs, kidney, or liver that determines outcome, but the collapse of the circulation as an integrated physiological environment. The conceptual shift from organ-specific thinking to a circulation-centric model is captured by the evolution from Multiple Organ Support Therapy (MOST) to the broader framework of extracorporeal organ support (ECOS) [14–16]. Within this framework, extracorporeal therapies are no longer seen merely as mechanical substitutes for failing organs; they are deliberate interventions on the bloodstream—the medium that distributes oxygen, solutes, inflammatory mediators, and toxins. This is the essence of ECOS: the bloodstream becomes the organ to treat [14] (Fig. 8.1).

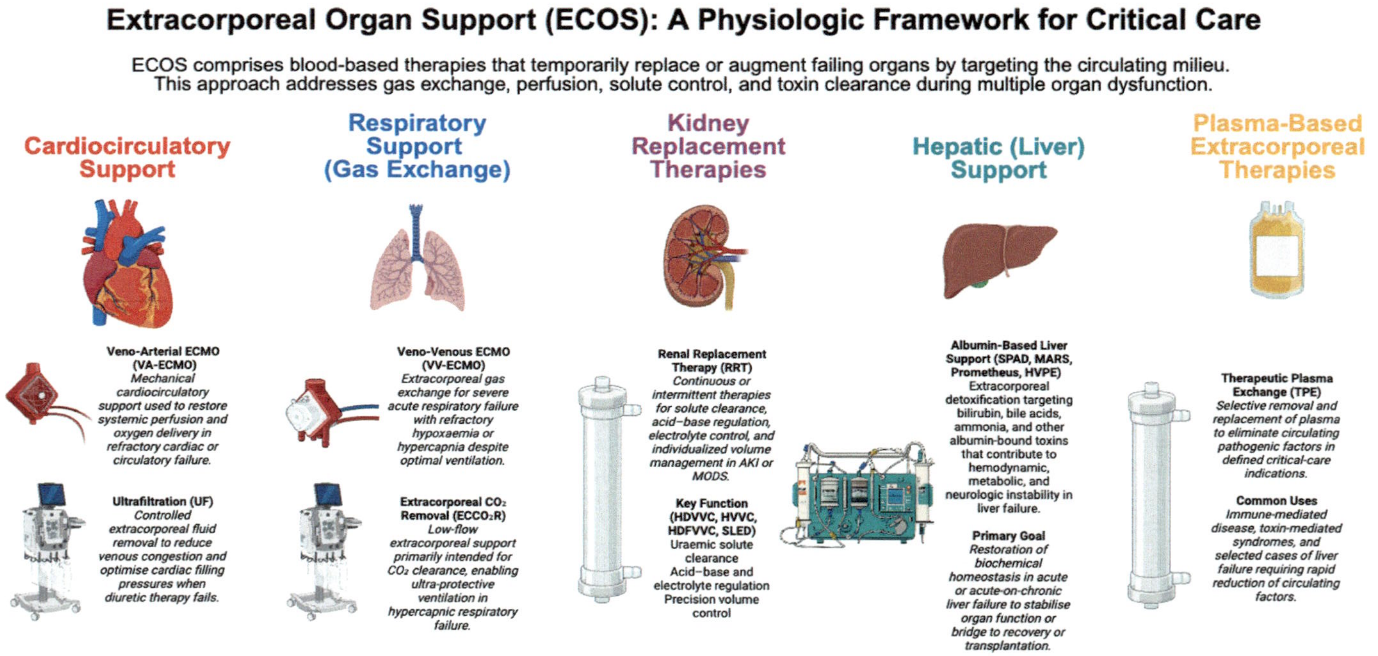

Fig. 8.1 Extracorporeal organ support modalities. Created in BioRender. Romero-González, G. (2026) https://BioRender.com/d8w8t4xOverview of the main modalities included within the extracorporeal organ support (ECOS) framework, grouped into circulatory, respiratory, renal, hepatic, and plasma-based therapies. *ECOS* extracorporeal organ support, *VA-ECMO* veno-arterial extracorporeal membrane oxygenation, VV-ECMO veno-venous extracorporeal membrane oxygenation, *ECCO$_2$R* extracorporeal carbon dioxide removal, *CRRT* continuous renal replacement therapy, *RRT* renal replacement therapy, *SPAD* single-pass albumin dialysis, *MARS* molecular adsorbent recirculating system, *HVPE* high-volume plasma exchange, *TPE* therapeutic plasma exchange

8.3.1 Integrated Physiological Rationale for Extracorporeal Organ Support

As perfusion deteriorates along the shock continuum, several abnormalities emerge simultaneously: falling oxygen content, carbon dioxide accumulation, progressive metabolic acidosis, electrolyte imbalance, and expansion of inflammatory signals. In parallel, albumin-bound toxins accumulate and further depress vascular tone, myocardial function, and cerebral activity [12, 13]. No single therapy can reverse this entire landscape. Instead, each extracorporeal modality addresses a distinct physiological domain:

- ECMO restores oxygen transport and systemic perfusion, interrupting the hemodynamic component of deterioration.
- CRRT stabilizes the metabolic and volumetric environment by correcting acidosis, electrolyte imbalance, fluid overload, and water-soluble toxins.
- Albumin dialysis (SPAD/MARS) removes protein-bound toxins-bilirubin, bile acids, aromatic amino acids, and hydrophobic mediators-that neither ECMO nor standard CRRT can clear.

The rationale for integrating these therapies is therefore inherently physiological:

- Oxygen delivery is ineffective without metabolic stability
- Metabolic stability remains insufficient if toxins continue to impair vascular, mitochondrial, and neurological function
- Detoxification cannot sustain life in the absence of adequate perfusion

Only the coordinated application of ECMO + CRRT + liver support can address the full spectrum of derangements defining advanced shock and MOF.

In the following sections, we describe each extracorporeal modality individually (ECMO, CRRT, and albumin-based liver support), outline their technical and physiological principles, and finally integrate them into a unified framework for multi-organ support.

8.4 Extracorporeal Organ Support Techniques: CRRT, ECMO, and Liver Support

Extracorporeal organ support in critical illness is not merely a set of technologies but an extension of physiology. Each modality: CRRT, ECMO, and albumin-based liver support, acts on a different aspect of the bloodstream, and understanding them individually is essential before attempting integration (Table 8.1). The following section describes each technique in detail, focusing on clinical indications, technical considerations, and the real-world challenges of anticoagulation [14–16].

Table 8.1 Physiological targets, clinical functions, and integration feasibility of extracorporeal organ support modalities

Modality	Primary physiological target	Main actions	Clinical goals	Integration with ECMO/CRRT
ECMO (VA/VV)	Oxygen transport and systemic perfusion	Extracorporeal oxygenation and CO_2 removal; circulatory assistance	Restore oxygen delivery; stabilize perfusion; bridge to recovery or decision-making	*Fully integrable*–cornerstone platform for multi-organ support
CRRT (CVVH/CVVHD/CVVHDF)	Metabolic and volumetric stability	Continuous correction of acidosis, electrolyte imbalance, uremia, and fluid overload	Maintain biochemical and fluid continuity; reduce venous congestion; support organ recovery	*Fully integrable*—routinely combined with ECMO
SPAD	Albumin-bound toxin removal	Albumin-enriched dialysate enabling diffusion of bilirubin, bile acids, and hydrophobic solutes	Reduce toxic burden; improve hemodynamics and neurological status	*Integrable via CRRT platform*; requires no separate circuit
MARS	High-efficiency albumin-bound toxin clearance	Albumin circuit with charcoal and anion-exchange resin regeneration	Stabilize ALF/ACLF physiology; bridge to transplant or recovery	*Integrable*, but requires independent vascular access; cannot run through ECMO limbs
Prometheus (FPSA)	Albumin-bound toxin clearance	Fractionated plasma separation with adsorption	Detoxification in liver failure	*Not compatible*—fractionator cannot tolerate ECMO pressures/flows
HVPE	Removal of plasma and circulating toxins	Large-volume plasma exchange with albumin or FFP replacement	Reduce inflammatory/toxic mediators	*Generally not compatible*—coagulopathy and large fluid shifts destabilize ECMO physiology; interaction with anticoagulation
Bioartificial liver systems	Metabolic support via hepatocytes	Extracorporeal bioreactors containing viable hepatocytes	Provide synthetic/metabolic liver functions	*Not compatible*—hepatocytes cannot tolerate ECMO shear stress, complement activation, cytokine load

ECMO extracorporeal membrane oxygenation, *VA ECMO* veno arterial ECMO, *VV ECMO* veno venous ECMO, *CRRT* continuous renal replacement therapy, *CVVH* continuous veno venous hemofiltration, *CVVHD* continuous veno venous hemodialysis, *CVVHDF* continuous veno venous hemodiafiltration, *SPAD* single pass albumin dialysis, *MARS* molecular adsorbent recirculating system, *FPSA* fractionated plasma separation and adsorption (Prometheus), *HVPE* high volume plasma exchange, *FFP* fresh frozen plasma, *ALF* acute liver failure, *ACLF* acute on chronic liver failure

8.4.1 Continuous Renal Replacement Therapy (CRRT)

CRRT is often the earliest modality initiated in the critically ill because the kidney is among the first organs to suffer the consequences of shock physiology. A combination of renal hypoperfusion, venous congestion, inflammatory activation, endothelial injury, and nephrotoxic exposure drives the development of acute kidney injury (AKI) [15, 17]. In patients receiving ECMO, these injuries are exacerbated by circuit-related shear stress, hemolysis, elevated venous pressures, and high catecholamine load [18]. Once renal function deteriorates, metabolic acidosis deepens, electrolytes drift from normal ranges, uremia progresses, and positive fluid balance worsens pulmonary and hepatic congestion, amplifying multi-organ dysfunction [19–21]. CRRT is therefore used to provide continuous solute, acid-base, and fluid management in hemodynamically unstable patients. Unlike intermittent hemodialysis, which imposes abrupt solute and volume shifts, CRRT maintains stability, allowing recovery in patients too hemodynamically fragile to tolerate alternative therapies [22, 23].

8.4.2 Indications and Contraindications

Clinicians typically initiate CRRT for progressive AKI with oliguria or anuria, fluid overload that compromises oxygenation or cardiovascular performance, metabolic acidosis unresponsive to medical therapy, or refractory electrolyte disturbances such as hyperkalemia [22, 24]. In liver failure, CRRT forms part of ammonia-lowering strategies aimed at preventing cerebral edema [25]. During ECMO support, CRRT becomes almost essential because AKI and fluid overload occur in the majority of ECMO patients, and continuous therapy allows precise control of solute balance and volume status [18, 26, 27]. Contraindications are few but significant. CRRT is withheld when anticoagulation is impossible due to uncontrolled bleeding, when multi-organ failure is clearly irreversible and therapy cannot meaningfully alter prognosis, or when the goals of care shift toward comfort [21, 22]. Even in these situations, decisions must be re-evaluated continuously, as the need for metabolic control may still outweigh risks in selected circumstances.

8.4.3 Modalities and Ultrafiltration

CRRT may be delivered by convection (CVVH), diffusion (CVVHD), or a hybrid method (CVVHDF). CVVHDF is generally preferred in multi-organ support because it allows balanced clearance of small and middle molecules alongside fine regulation of acid–base status [21, 22, 27]. Ultrafiltration, long considered simply a means of fluid removal, plays a far deeper physiological role. When applied gradually, it reduces venous congestion, lowers right ventricular afterload, improves renal perfusion, and reduces extravascular lung water. In ECMO patients, even modest ultrafiltration often improves gas exchange and enhances venous drainage to the circuit. Rates typically begin at low levels and are increased only as hemodynamic tolerance allows [28].

8.4.4 Anticoagulation in CRRT (Pragmatic Clinical Perspective)

Anticoagulation is one of the most consequential decisions in CRRT, especially when liver dysfunction, ECMO support, or coagulopathy complicate management. In real clinical practice, intensivists alternate between systemic unfractionated heparin (UFH) and regional citrate anticoagulation (RCA), depending on bleeding risk, hepatic function, and circuit behavior [29, 30]. UFH remains the most commonly used agent, particularly when the patient is already systemically anticoagulated for ECMO [21, 29]. It allows rapid titration, predictable monitoring, and immediate reversibility. However, UFH increases hemorrhagic risk, particularly in trauma, postoperative bleeding, coagulopathy, or thrombocytopenia [21, 29, 31]. A drop in hemoglobin, new surgical bleeding, or neurological symptoms may require immediate dose adjustment or temporary cessation [21, 29]. Heparin-induced thrombocytopenia, although uncommon, must always be considered in the presence of falling platelet counts [21, 31]. RCA, by contrast, anticoagulates the circuit without exposing the patient to systemic bleeding risk [29, 32]. Citrate chelates ionized calcium within the circuit, preventing clot formation; calcium is then replaced in the systemic circulation [21, 29]. Trials demonstrate longer filter life and reduced bleeding compared with heparin [29, 33]. Nevertheless, RCA depends heavily on adequate hepatic metabolism. In acute liver failure (ALF), acute-on-chronic liver failure (ACLF), severe ischemic hepatitis, or profound shock, citrate may accumulate, producing metabolic alkalosis, rising total calcium, and falling ionized calcium [34–36]. These signs demand immediate reassessment and often require transition to UFH. In ICU practice, decisions are pragmatic: when a patient is already anticoagulated for ECMO, CRRT often "rides" on that anticoagulation. When there is significant bleeding risk and liver function is preserved, RCA is preferable. When hepatic metabolism is uncertain, caution is essential, with frequent calcium monitoring guiding the choice. In unstable patients with severe hepatic dysfunction or coagulopathy, CRRT may need to run without anticoagulation entirely, accepting reduced filter lifespan in exchange for safety [31, 37]. Above all, anticoagulation during CRRT is not a fixed protocol but a continuous negotiation between physiology and risk. Every fluctuation in pH, lactate, oxygenation, or circuit pressure may indicate the need to adapt the strategy.

8.4.5 Extracorporeal Membrane Oxygenation (ECMO)

ECMO represents the most powerful form of temporary respiratory or circulatory support available in contemporary critical care. By diverting blood through a membrane oxygenator, ECMO facilitates extracorporeal gas exchange and temporary cardiopulmonary support. Its purpose is not to replace these organs indefinitely but to create time—time for recovery, for definitive intervention, or for meaningful decisions about the future [38, 39].

8.4.6 Indications and Contraindications

Veno-venous ECMO (VV-ECMO) is reserved for severe respiratory failure, most often ARDS. The EOLIA trial established ECMO as rescue therapy when refractory hypoxemia persists despite optimal mechanical ventilation, prone positioning, and adjunctive measures ($PaO_2/FiO_2 < 80$ mmHg) [40]. VV-ECMO is also indicated in hypercapnic respiratory failure with severe acidosis unresponsive to noninvasive or conventional mechanical ventilation [41, 42]. Veno-arterial ECMO (VA-ECMO) provides circulatory support and is indicated in cardiogenic shock refractory to medical and mechanical therapies. It is used in fulminant myocarditis, massive pulmonary embolism, acute myocardial infarction with mechanical complications, postcardiotomy failure, and selected cases of poisoning. In patients with witnessed cardiac arrest and potentially reversible etiology [43], VA-ECMO may support extracorporeal CPR [44]. Contraindications include irreversible multi-organ failure, severe neurological injury, catastrophic bleeding, end-stage malignancy without curative options, and prolonged unwitnessed arrest, although decisions always require individualized judgment [45–47].

8.4.7 Cannulation Strategies

Cannulation determines the stability of ECMO support and influences the feasibility of integrating CRRT or liver support. In VV-ECMO, femoro–jugular cannulation remains common because it provides robust drainage and reliable oxygenated return. Dual-lumen internal jugular cannulae offer single-site access, reduce recirculation when well positioned, and facilitate mobilization, although correct placement is technically demanding and often requires fluoroscopic or echocardiographic guidance [48–51]. VA-ECMO most commonly uses femoro–femoral access due to its speed and ease of deployment in cardiogenic shock [43]. However, this approach carries risks of limb ischemia and differential hypoxemia [43, 52]. Axillary artery cannulation provides antegrade aortic flow and may reduce cerebral hypoxia while allowing early mobilization, though it requires surgical expertise [53]. Central cannulation via sternotomy is reserved for postcardiotomy shock or situations where peripheral access is inadequate [54].

8.4.8 Anticoagulation in ECMO

Anticoagulation during ECMO represents a delicate equilibrium between preventing thrombosis within the circuit and minimizing bleeding in a patient who is already coagulopathic from shock, inflammation, and extracorporeal circulation. In everyday practice, UFH is the primary agent. It is widely available, rapidly titratable, and reversible [55]. Anti-Xa monitoring offers accuracy, whereas ACT remains useful intra-operatively or when frequent adjustments are necessary [56]. UFH dosing must be interpreted dynamically. Requirements may change hourly, depending on circuit performance, oxygenator pressures, surgical drains, cannulation sites, chest tubes, and subtle neurological signs. The clinician must constantly determine whether bleeding risk outweighs thrombosis risk or vice versa. This is not a static decision but a fluid, ongoing negotiation. When heparin-induced thrombocytopenia is suspected or confirmed, bivalirudin becomes the anticoagulant of choice because it directly inhibits thrombin without relying on antithrombin [57]. It provides stable anticoagulation but demands careful dosing, vigilant monitoring, and carries high cost. Citrate is never used for ECMO anticoagulation, given its hepatic metabolism and the risk of profound metabolic disturbance [55]. However, citrate anticoagulation can still be used safely in a separate CRRT circuit, provided that citrate is confined to that limb and ionized calcium is monitored closely [32, 36].

Ultimately, ECMO anticoagulation is not governed by formulas but by clinical proximity. Rising transmembrane pressures, falling sweep efficiency, new clot burden, fresh bleeding, hemoglobin decline, or neurological changes each signal the need to revisit anticoagulation targets. The art of ECMO lies in interpreting these signals early enough to prevent catastrophe.

8.4.9 Liver Support Systems: SPAD, MARS, and the Limitations of Alternative Modalities

Liver dysfunction in the critically ill, whether due to ALF, ACLF, or cholestatic injury during shock, contributes decisively to multi-organ failure [58]. The accumulation of bilirubin, bile acids, aromatic amino acids, ammonia, and hydrophobic inflammatory mediators disrupts vascular reactivity, mitochondrial function, cerebral autoregulation, and immune homeostasis [58]. Conventional CRRT can clear water-soluble toxins, but it is unable to remove protein-bound solutes, which represent the majority of hepatotoxic metabolites [59]. For this reason, albumin-based liver support systems have emerged as essential adjuncts when the liver becomes a central driver of systemic collapse [58, 59]. Among these technologies, SPAD and MARS are the only modalities realistically compatible with complex extracorporeal strategies such as ECMO and CRRT.

8.5 Single-Pass Albumin Dialysis (SPAD)

8.5.1 Concept, Technical Preparation, Delivery, and Evidence

SPAD is the simplest and most accessible form of albumin dialysis and is particularly valuable in critically ill patients who already require CRRT [60]. Its underlying principle is physiologically elegant: by enriching the dialysate with albumin, a diffusion gradient is created that allows protein-bound toxins to dissociate from plasma albumin and bind to albumin present in the dialysate [61, 62]. Because the dialysate is discarded after a single pass, toxin removal is continuous, predictable, and easy to control [61, 63].

8.5.2 Type of Albumin Required

SPAD requires 20% pharmaceutical-grade human serum albumin (HSA). This concentration ensures that a small volume of albumin can raise dialysate albumin concentration to the desired 2–4% without adding excess fluid or lowering oncotic pressure [62, 64]. Lower-concentration albumin solutions (e.g., 5%) are unsuitable because they require large infusion volumes and produce unstable concentrations [64]. Albumin bottles should be gently inverted (not shaken) to avoid foam formation, and warmed to room temperature to prevent precipitation during mixing [65].

8.5.3 Preparation of SPAD Dialysate

The key to effective SPAD is pre-mixing the dialysate bags. Albumin should never be injected directly into the CRRT machine or added to the dialysate line during treatment, as this creates unpredictable gradients, risks filter fouling, and leads to inconsistent therapy [62].

SPAD dialysate is prepared as follows:

- To prepare 2% albumin dialysate, mix 1 liter of 20% HSA with 9 liters of commercial dialysate (e.g., Prismasol or equivalent) [62, 64].
- To prepare 4% albumin dialysate, mix 1 liter of 20% HSA with 4 liters of commercial dialysate [62, 64].

These proportions can be scaled to match available bag sizes. Each bag must be prepared individually so that albumin concentration remains constant during the session. The mixture must be thoroughly homogenized by gentle inversion [62, 66].

8.5.4 Delivery and Circuit Parameters

SPAD is usually delivered via CVVHD or CVVHDF, using the existing CRRT circuit. Typical settings are as follows:

- Blood flow: 120–200 mL/min
- Dialysate flow: 1–2 L/h
- Duration: 6–12 h per session, depending on toxin burden
- Frequency: according to clinical response—often daily or every 48 h during acute deterioration [63, 64]

Ultrafiltration remains under CRRT control, which is a major advantage when SPAD is integrated with ECMO, as fluid balance can be maintained precisely.

8.5.5 Clinical Evidence for SPAD

Although large randomized trials are lacking, a growing number of observational studies and controlled comparisons support SPAD's biochemical efficacy [60]. Case reports and retrospective series in ALF and ACLF describe substantial reductions in bilirubin, bile acids, and ammonia, as well as improvement in encephalopathy, particularly in patients with concomitant AKI requiring dialysis [60, 63]. A randomized crossover study comparing SPAD and MARS in ICU patients with liver failure showed that both modalities significantly reduced bilirubin, conjugated bilirubin, and bile acids, with similar short-term biochemical efficacy [67]. Tolerance of SPAD was generally good, and no major adverse events attributable solely to the technique were reported [63, 67]. These data support the use of SPAD as a clinically effective, flexible, and economically accessible liver support modality, particularly suitable for centers without dedicated liver support devices or when integrating multiple extracorporeal systems [60].

8.5.6 Limitations

SPAD consumes substantial amounts of albumin, generating higher costs than standard CRRT [62, 64]. Its detoxification efficiency is lower than that of MARS because albumin is not regenerated [60, 67]. There is no clear evidence of survival benefit, and its efficacy depends on timing, toxin load, and overall physiological stability [60]. Nevertheless, its simplicity, safety, and compatibility with CRRT make it highly valuable in multi-organ support.

8.6 Molecular Adsorbent Recirculating System (MARS)

8.6.1 Mechanism, Technical Requirements, and Evidence

MARS is the most extensively studied form of extracorporeal liver support and provides more efficient and sustained detoxification than SPAD by regenerating albumin continuously within a closed-loop circuit [61]. In MARS, albumin in the dialysate compartment binds bilirubin, bile acids, and other protein-bound toxins, after which the albumin is passed through activated charcoal and anion-exchange columns; this allows sustained clearance of albumin-associated solutes. A second hemodialysis or hemofiltration circuit clears water-soluble toxins and maintains electrolyte balance. This dual-action approach allows prolonged clearance of albumin-bound toxins without large albumin consumption [68].

8.6.2 Technical Implementation

A typical MARS session uses the following:

- Blood flow: 150–250 mL/min
- Albumin circuit flow: 150–200 mL/min
- Session duration: 6–8 h
- Frequency: usually multiple sessions over several days [69, 70]

MARS is pressure-limited and cannot be connected to ECMO limbs due to high-flow, high-pressure fluctuations [68]. It therefore requires a dedicated double-lumen dialysis catheter, often in the right internal jugular vein. When CRRT is required simultaneously, it may run in parallel or intermittently depending on hemodynamic stability and extracorporeal load.

8.6.3 Clinical Evidence for MARS

A large body of observational and controlled studies describes the biochemical and clinical effects of MARS. Numerous reports demonstrate reductions in bilirubin, bile acids, ammonia, and aromatic amino acids, improvements in hepatic encephalopathy, resolution or delay of hepatorenal syndrome, and modest hemodynamic stabilization [71]. However, randomized controlled trials and meta-analyses have not consistently demonstrated survival benefit [72, 73]. Studies comparing MARS to standard therapy in ACLF found no significant survival advantage at preset treatment doses, despite robust detoxification effects [72, 73]. Survival benefits appear to be greatest in patients with ALF who are transplant candidates, where the goal is bridging to transplantation [71].

8.6.4 Limitations

MARS is resource-intensive, requiring specialized equipment, trained staff, and separate vascular access [68]. It demands close anticoagulation monitoring due to its circuit complexity [68, 69]. Its detoxification efficiency is higher than SPAD, but survival benefit is inconsistent [61, 71]. Nonetheless, it remains the most powerful albumin dialysis option available and a key tool in multi-organ support strategies when liver dysfunction becomes a central driver of shock physiology [73, 74].

8.6.5 Why Other Liver Support Technologies Cannot Be Used with ECMO

Several extracorporeal liver support modalities beyond SPAD and MARS have been developed, including fractionated plasma separation systems such as Prometheus, high-volume plasma exchange (HVPE), and bioartificial liver devices incorporating hepatocytes [61, 75]. Although each has a physiological rationale in isolated liver failure, they are poorly suited technically and clinically for integration into a multi-organ support strategy that already includes ECMO and CRRT. Prometheus and other fractionated plasma separation and adsorption (FPSA) systems require stable, low-pressure, low-shear flow conditions to maintain the integrity of the albumin-permeable fractionator [76, 77]. These devices are vulnerable to pressure oscillations and high blood flows, which are intrinsic to ECMO circuits. Because ECMO operates at 3–5 L/min with highly variable inlet pressures, coupling Prometheus to an ECMO circuit risks membrane collapse, failure of the FPSA fractionator, and hemodynamic instability [76, 78]. Clinical experience with simultaneous ECMO + Prometheus is virtually nonexistent, and technical concerns make the combination impractical in real-world settings. The interaction between HVPE and ECMO depends heavily on the choice of replacement fluid. When albumin is used as the replacement solution, HVPE causes marked depletion of coagulation factors (II, V, VII, IX, X) and fibrinogen, leading to significant coagulopathy that is incompatible with the systemic anticoagulation mandatory in ECMO [79]. In this configuration, HVPE is essentially contraindicated during ECMO. When fresh frozen plasma (FFP) is used instead, HVPE replenishes rather than depletes coagulation factors, theoretically allowing coexistence with ECMO. However, the technique still presents major limitations. The large exchange volumes required (8–12 L per session) can cause hemodynamic instability, disrupt fluid management goals during CRRT, and introduce abrupt shifts in plasma viscosity and oncotic pressure that may compromise ECMO circuit stability [79, 80]. Plasma transfusion also carries risks of TRALI, complement activation, and immunological reactions, which are particularly hazardous in patients already receiving ECMO [79, 81]. For these reasons, although HVPE with plasma is not formally contraindicated, its risk–benefit profile is generally unfavorable within an integrated ECOS strategy [16, 79]. Bioartificial liver systems face even greater obstacles. These devices require strict control of shear stress, complement activation, inflammatory mediators, and flow stability, conditions fundamentally incompatible with ECMO physiology [77, 78]. Hepatocytes used in these systems are extremely vulnerable to complement activation, cytokine surges, and anticoagulation-related perturbations, all of which are amplified during ECMO [16, 80]. Consequently, bioartificial liver systems have remained confined to research environments, with no meaningful clinical application alongside ECMO [77, 78]. Taken together, these physiological and technical limitations explain why SPAD and MARS remain the only liver support modalities realistically compatible with ECMO and CRRT. They specifically target albumin-bound toxin clearance, can be integrated safely into extracorporeal strategies, and do not impose hemodynamic or immunological constraints incompatible with high-flow extracorporeal support [62, 64, 79].

8.6.6 Integrating ECMO, CRRT, and Albumin Dialysis (SPAD/MARS)

The need to integrate ECMO, CRRT, and albumin dialysis arises when the internal environment collapses simultaneously along several axes: oxygen transport, perfusion, solute composition, fluid distribution, and toxin clearance. No single modality can correct all of these dimensions. ECMO restores gas exchange and circulatory support, CRRT stabilizes solute and fluid balance, and albumin dialysis removes protein-bound toxins that neither ECMO nor CRRT can access [16, 79]. When multi-organ failure progresses despite conventional therapy, these modalities must be combined in a way that is physiologically coherent and technically safe.

8.6.7 Physiological Logic of Integration

From a physiological perspective, ECMO, CRRT, and liver support act on different but interconnected domains of the same system: the bloodstream. ECMO supports the macrocirculation and gas exchange by ensuring adequate oxygen delivery and carbon dioxide removal even when the native lung or heart fails. CRRT stabilizes the chemical and volumetric environment by correcting acidemia, hyperkalemia, uremia, and fluid overload, thereby relieving right ventricular strain, improving pulmonary mechanics, and reducing hepatic congestion [16, 82]. Albumin dialysis with SPAD or MARS addresses a third layer of derangement: the accumulation of bilirubin, bile acids, aromatic amino acids, ammonia, and other albumin-bound toxins that depress myocardial contractility, worsen vasoplegia, impair mitochondrial respiration, and aggravate encephalopathy [60, 61, 63]. In clinical practice, the benefits of integration become evident in patients with severe ARDS on VV-ECMO who develop AKI and fluid overload requiring CRRT, followed by progressive cholestasis or ALF requiring albumin dialysis [60, 69, 73]. A similar sequence occurs in VA-ECMO–supported cardiogenic shock complicated by ischemic hepatitis or ACLF. In these scenarios, ECMO alone cannot reverse multi-organ failure if the biochemical environment remains hostile; CRRT alone cannot compensate for profound gas-exchange or circulatory failure; and detoxification alone is ineffective if oxygen delivery and perfusion are inadequate. Only the combined use of ECMO, CRRT, and SPAD or MARS can reconstitute a milieu in which organ recovery becomes physiologically possible [16, 77].

8.6.8 Connecting CRRT to ECMO

Technically, CRRT is most often integrated with ECMO by connecting the CRRT circuit directly to the ECMO circuit rather than inserting a separate dialysis catheter (Fig. 8.2). This approach reduces the number of vascular accesses, simplifies line management, and ensures stable blood flows [18, 26]. In a typical configuration:

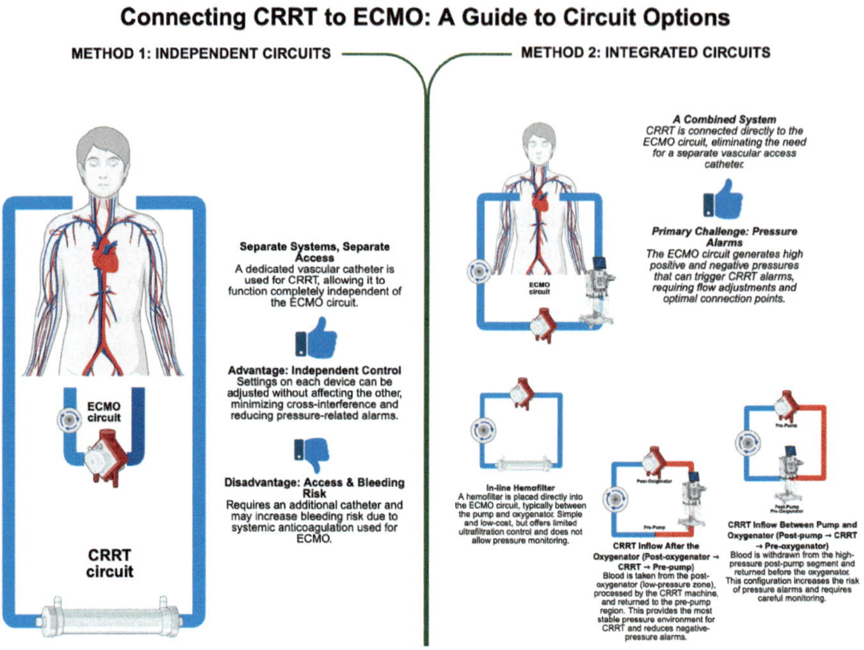

Fig. 8.2 CRRT–ECMO connection options. Created in BioRender. Romero-González, G. (2026) https://BioRender.com/d8w8t4xSummary of independent and integrated strategies for connecting CRRT to an ECMO circuit, including in-line hemofilter configurations and pre-/post-oxygenator access points. *CRRT* continuous renal replacement therapy, *ECMO* extracorporeal membrane oxygenation, *UF* ultrafiltration

- *CRRT withdrawal port*: pre-oxygenator (negative-pressure, stable segment)
- *CRRT return port*: post-oxygenator (positive-pressure, nonpulsatile segment) [27, 28]

This configuration allows the CRRT machine to operate within its usual pressure ranges while preserving alarms, ultrafiltration precision, and solute control. Observational data demonstrate that this arrangement is safe and effective in most ECMO patients with AKI [18, 27].

A parallel approach uses a separate dual-lumen catheter, typically in the right internal jugular vein, to run CRRT independently [27]. This is advantageous when:

- ECMO circuit pressures fluctuate excessively
- Hemolysis or suction events interfere with CRRT performance
- Regional citrate anticoagulation is preferred for CRRT

The cost is additional vascular access and more complex line management. The historical practice of inserting an in-line hemofilter directly into the ECMO tubing without a full CRRT machine is now considered suboptimal. This method lacks precise ultrafiltration control, provides limited solute clearance, and offers no reliable alarm system for clotting or pressure excursions. In the era of sophisticated multi-organ support, this approach is rarely justified [26, 28].

8.6.9 Anticoagulation in the Combined ECMO–CRRT Setting

When CRRT is integrated with ECMO, anticoagulation must be managed as a unified problem rather than as two independent protocols. In most centers, UFH remains the cornerstone of anticoagulation for ECMO and, by extension, for CRRT connected to the ECMO circuit [56]. Systemic UFH targets are set primarily to protect the oxygenator; the CRRT filter benefits from the same anticoagulant milieu [18, 27].

- *Monitoring*: anti-Xa levels and ACT/aPTT trends
- *Decision-making*: guided by circuit performance, bleeding, and evolving physiology

Regional citrate anticoagulation (RCA) introduces complexity. When CRRT is run independently via a separate catheter, RCA can safely prolong filter life and reduce bleeding risk, provided hepatic metabolism is adequate [32, 36]. However, when CRRT is directly connected to the ECMO circuit, the systemic impact of citrate becomes more unpredictable, especially in ALF, ACLF, or profound shock [27, 28]. In these cases, many centers prefer to maintain UFH for both circuits, accepting a higher bleeding risk in exchange for predictability [18, 27]. Ultimately, anticoagulation in the ECMO–CRRT combination is a dynamic process [26]. Every drop in hemoglobin, new circuit alarm, rise in oxygenator pressure gradient, or change in lactate may signal the need to adjust anticoagulation targets or circuit configuration.

8.6.10 Adding SPAD to ECMO–CRRT

SPAD is uniquely suited to integration with ECMO and CRRT because it does not require a separate extracorporeal circuit [60]. It builds directly upon the CRRT platform already in use [67]. Once CRRT is established, SPAD is implemented by replacing the standard dialysate with albumin-enriched dialysate (2–4% HSA), prepared through careful pre-mixing [60].

The CRRT machine then operates in CVVHD or CVVHDF mode:

- *Blood flow*: 120–200 mL/min
- *Dialysate flow*: 1–2 L/h
- *Duration*: 6–12 h

In ECMO patients, blood entering the CRRT circuit has already passed through the ECMO pump and oxygenator, but the principles of albumin dialysis remain unchanged: albumin-bound toxins dissociate from plasma albumin and diffuse into the albumin-rich dialysate.

Key advantages of SPAD in this context:

- No additional vascular access
- Precise ultrafiltration control through CRRT
- Physiological compatibility with ECMO flows and pressures
- Flexibility for repeated or prolonged sessions

Observational studies and controlled comparisons demonstrate meaningful reductions in bilirubin, bile acids, and ammonia, with clinically relevant improvements in hepatic encephalopathy even in highly unstable patients [83, 84].

8.6.11 Adding MARS to ECMO–CRRT

MARS, unlike SPAD, requires its own dedicated extracorporeal circuit and cannot be connected directly to ECMO limbs [67, 68] (Fig. 8.3). The reasons are primarily technical: ECMO operates at flows of 3–5 L/min, far exceeding the tolerances of MARS pumps and membranes; albumin-containing extracorporeal lines risk fouling or coating of the ECMO oxygenator; and the pressure oscillations generated by ECMO may impair the function of the charcoal and anion-exchange columns that regenerate albumin [43, 85]. For these reasons, MARS must be delivered through a separate double-lumen catheter, most commonly in the right internal jugular vein, allowing it to run independently of the ECMO circuit [49, 68]. Once established, the MARS system circulates blood through an albumin-containing compartment where bilirubin, bile acids, and other protein-bound toxins dissociate and are captured [68, 72]. The albumin solution is continuously regenerated by charcoal and anion-exchange resins, preserving its binding capacity, while a secondary hemodialysis or hemofiltration circuit clears water-soluble toxins and maintains electrolyte balance [75, 76]. When ECMO, CRRT, and MARS are all active, the total extracorporeal volume increases substantially, and careful attention must be paid to vascular access, anticoagulation, hemodynamic tolerance, and fluid balance [16, 82]. Even modest ultrafiltration or albumin loss can provoke intravascular depletion, particularly in patients whose circulatory reserve is already limited by shock or hepatic dysfunction [74, 81]. Despite these complexities, MARS can produce clinically significant improvements in bilirubin, bile acids, ammonia, and encephalopathy in selected patients with ALF or ACLF, particularly when the objective is stabilization while awaiting transplantation [69, 73]. Although not universally beneficial, it remains the most potent form of albumin-based detoxification available and a valuable adjunct when liver dysfunction becomes a dominant driver of multi-organ instability.

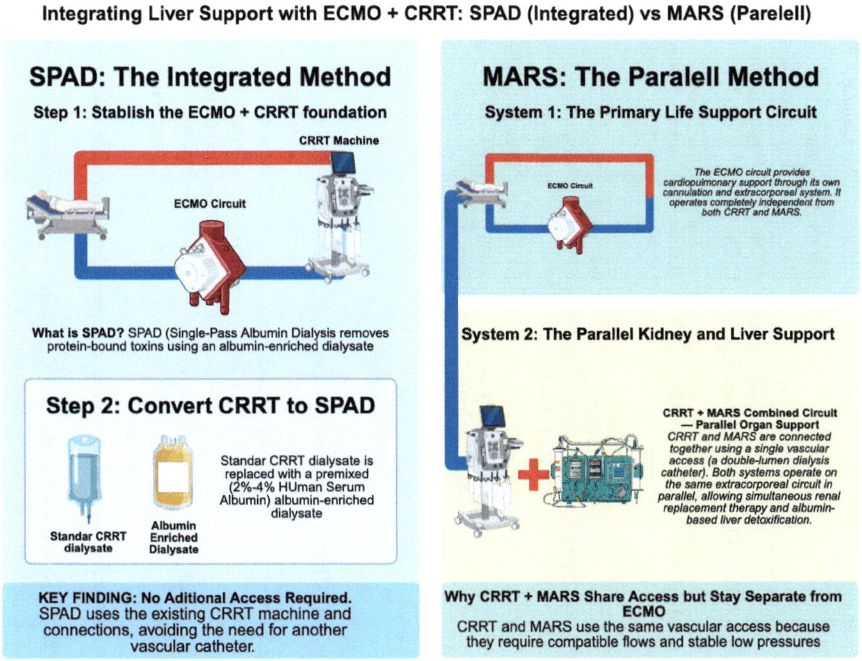

Fig. 8.3 Integration of Liver Support With ECMO + CRRT (SPAD vs. MARS). Created in BioRender. Romero-González, G. (2026) https://BioRender.com/d8w8t4xComparison between SPAD, delivered through the CRRT platform using albumin-enriched dialysate, and MARS, which runs as an independent detoxification circuit, while ECMO remains the primary extracorporeal support. *SPAD* single-pass albumin dialysis, *MARS* molecular adsorbent recirculating system, *ECMO* extracorporeal membrane oxygenation, *CRRT* continuous renal replacement therapy, *HSA* human serum albumin

8.6.12 Clinical Sequencing and Load Management

In clinical practice, ECMO, CRRT, and albumin dialysis are seldom initiated at the same time. Their introduction follows the physiological priorities imposed by the patient's evolving state. ECMO is typically established first when oxygen delivery or perfusion can no longer be maintained by conventional means. As AKI, acidosis, or fluid overload emerge (often within the initial 24–48 h), CRRT is added to stabilize the biochemical and volumetric environment. Albumin dialysis with SPAD or MARS is introduced later, once it becomes clear that liver dysfunction is contributing significantly to hemodynamic instability, encephalopathy, or systemic inflammation (Table 8.2). This sequence reflects the natural hierarchy of physiological needs. Oxygen delivery and perfusion must be secured before meaningful metabolic correction is possible. Solute and fluid homeostasis must then be restored to prevent further organ injury. Only after these two foundations are stabilized can albumin-bound toxins be effectively cleared [85–90]. Attempting to reverse hepatic toxin accumulation before correcting oxygen debt, acidosis, or venous congestion is

Table 8.2 Summary of published cases and series reporting the use of albumin-based liver support (SPAD/MARS) in combination with ECMO and/or CRRT

Authors	Year	Study design	Patient cohort	Primary therapy	Key outcomes	Survival rate	Major complications
Hui WF et al. [84]	2024	Case series	2 pediatric (16 years) amlodipine OD	SPAD (3–4%) + CytoSorb + VA-ECMO	VIS ↓240→0; lactate 10.6→1 mmol/L	100% (2/2)	Hypokalemia
Essink J et al. [83]	2022	Case report	1 adolescent (17 years, 103 kg) amlodipine	SPAD (1.25–2.5%) + VA-ECMO	117 h SPAD; ECMO wean d11	100% (1/1)	Fluid overload (>10 L); stroke
Villarreal-Ondarza I et al. [89]	2023	Case report	1 adult (60 years) COVID-19 ARDS	MARS (2 × 12 h) + VV-ECMO + CRRT	Bilirubin ↓18.5→3.8 mg/dL; CRP ↓166→50	0% (died m^2)	Sepsis (Klebsiella/Candida)
Sparks BE et al. [85].	2017	Retrospective	14 ECMO+ALF vs. 14 controls	MARS (8 ± 9 days) + VA/VV-ECMO	Bilirubin ↓7.9 mg/dL; ECMO wean 64% vs. 21% ($p = 0.02$)	64% wean (9/14)	Bleeding 79%; DIC 14%
Pinto VL et al. [88]	2019	Case report	1 pediatric (14 years) amlodipine	MARS (11+8+26 h) + VA-ECMO	Amlodipine ↓340→90 ng/mL	100% (1/1)	Circuit clotting (2/3)
Peerapornratana S et al. [91]	2025	Case series	ECMO + multi-organ failure	Combined ECOS (ECMO/CRRT/MARS)	Improved organ recovery rates	Not specified	Technical complexity
Tiruvoipati R et al. [87]	2007	Case series	6 pediatric MOF	MARS + VV/VA-ECMO	Bilirubin clearance; 3/6 ECMO wean	50% (3/6)	Circuit thrombosis; hemorrhage
Peek GJ et al. [86]	2002	Case series	5 MOF + ECMO-ALF	MARS (bilirubin > 17 mg/dL)	2/5 survived vs. predicted 100% mortality	40% (2/5)	MOF progression

The table includes patient characteristics, primary extracorporeal modality, key biochemical or hemodynamic outcomes, survival data, and major complications

ECMO extracorporeal membrane oxygenation, *VA-ECMO* veno-arterial ECMO, *VV-ECMO* veno-venous ECMO, *CRRT* continuous renal replacement therapy, *SPAD* single-pass albumin dialysis, *MARS* molecular adsorbent recirculating system, *ALF* acute liver failure, *MOF* multi-organ failure, *VIS* vasoactive-inotropic score, *CRP* C-reactive protein rarely successful. Managing the total extracorporeal load requires a dynamic, rather than procedural, approach. Excessive ultrafiltration may precipitate hypotension in a patient whose circulatory reserve is marginal. Conversely, insufficient fluid removal may perpetuate pulmonary edema or right ventricular failure. Albumin dialysis must be dosed carefully to avoid destabilizing protein-bound drug levels or provoking intravascular shifts. Each therapy influences the others: ECMO performance improves when acidosis is corrected by CRRT; CRRT is more effective when perfusion is stabilized by ECMO; SPAD or MARS exert their maximal benefit only once oxygenation, perfusion, and solute balance have been restored. Integration, therefore, is not the act of connecting devices but of continuously recalibrating a multi-circuit system to meet the changing physiology of the patient. The clinician's task is to navigate this interplay in real time, guided by hemodynamics, biochemical trends, neurological status, and circuit behavior—to create and maintain a biochemical and hemodynamic environment in which organ recovery remains possible.

8.7 Conclusion

Multi-organ failure is not the collapse of individual organs but the breakdown of the internal environment that sustains them. ECMO, CRRT, and albumin-based liver support act on distinct yet interdependent physiological domains: oxygenation and perfusion, metabolic and volumetric stability, and the clearance of protein-bound toxins. When applied coherently, these therapies enable the reconstruction of an internal milieu compatible with recovery in advanced shock. In practice, their integration should follow the sequence imposed by physiology: stabilizing circulation, reestablishing metabolic continuity, and then addressing the toxin burden. This alignment between the patient's evolving internal environment and the timing of each modality is central to the success of multi-organ support. Ultimately, the purpose of extracorporeal therapies is not to replace life but to create the physiological conditions in which recovery remains possible, offering a realistic chance of survival in one of the most fragile scenarios in critical care medicine.

References

1. Levy MM, Fink MP, Marshall JC, Abraham E, Angus D, Cook D, et al. SCCM/ESICM/ACCP/ATS/SIS international sepsis definitions conference. Crit Care Med [Internet]. Crit Care Med; 2003 [cited 2025 Nov 30];31:1250–6. 2001; https://doi.org/10.1097/01.CCM.0000050454.01978.3B.
2. Angus DC, van der Poll T. Severe sepsis and septic shock. N Engl J Med [Internet]. N Engl J Med; 2013 [cited 2025 Nov 30];369:840–851. https://doi.org/10.1056/NEJMRA1208623.
3. Rudd KE, Johnson SC, Agesa KM, Shackelford KA, Tsoi D, Kievlan DR, et al. Global, regional, and national sepsis incidence and mortality, 1990–2017: analysis for the Global Burden of Disease Study. The Lancet [Internet]. Lancet Publishing Group; 2020 [cited 2025 Nov 30];395:200–211. https://doi.org/10.1016/S0140-6736(19)32989-7.
4. Vincent JL, De Mendonça A, Cantraine F, Moreno R, Takala J, Suter PM, et al. Use of the SOFA score to assess the incidence of organ dysfunction/failure in intensive care units:

results of a multicenter, prospective study. Working group on "sepsis-related problems" of the European Society of Intensive Care Medicine. Crit Care Med [Internet]. Crit Care Med; 1998 [cited 2025 Nov 30];26:1793–800. https://doi.org/10.1097/00003246-199811000-00016.

5. Lopes Ferreira F, Peres Bota D, Bross A, Mélot C, Vincent JL. Serial evaluation of the SOFA score to predict outcome in critically ill patients. JAMA [Internet]. JAMA; 2001 [cited 2025 Nov 30];286:1754–1758. https://doi.org/10.1001/JAMA.286.14.1754.
6. Marshall JC, Cook DJ, Christou N V., Bernard GR, Sprung CL, Sibbald WJ. Multiple organ dysfunction score: a reliable descriptor of a complex clinical outcome. Crit Care Med [Internet]. Crit Care Med; 1995 [cited 2025 Nov 30];23:1638–52. https://doi.org/10.1097/00003246-199510000-00007.
7. Paoli CJ, Reynolds MA, Sinha M, Gitlin M, Crouser E. Epidemiology and costs of sepsis in the United States-an analysis based on timing of diagnosis and severity level. Crit Care Med [Internet]. Lippincott Williams and Wilkins; 2018 [cited 2025 Nov 30];46:1889–1897. https://doi.org/10.1097/CCM.0000000000003342.
8. Torio CM, Moore BJ. National inpatient hospital costs: the most expensive conditions by Payer, 2013. Healthcare Cost and Utilization Project (HCUP) Statistical Briefs [Internet]. 2006 [cited 2025 Nov 30]; http://www.ncbi.nlm.nih.gov/pubmed/27359025. Accessed 30 Nov 2025.
9. van den Berg M, van Beuningen FE, ter Maaten JC, Bouma HR. Hospital-related costs of sepsis around the world: a systematic review exploring the economic burden of sepsis. J Crit Care [Internet]. W.B. Saunders; 2022 [cited 2025 Nov 30];71:154096. https://doi.org/10.1016/J.JCRC.2022.154096.
10. Burchardi H, Schneider H. Economic aspects of severe sepsis: a review of intensive care unit costs, cost of illness and cost effectiveness of therapy. Pharmacoeconomics [Internet]. Pharmacoeconomics; 2004 [cited 2025 Nov 30];22:793–813. https://doi.org/10.2165/00019053-200422120-00003.
11. Bellumkonda L, Gul B, Masri SC. Evolving concepts in diagnosis and management of cardiogenic shock. Am J Cardiol [Internet]. Elsevier Inc.; 2018 [cited 2025 Nov 30];122:1104–10. https://doi.org/10.1016/j.amjcard.2018.05.040.
12. Finfer SR, Vincent J-L, De D. Circulatory shock. Finfer SR, Vincent J-L, editors. New England Journal of Medicine [Internet]. Massachusetts Medical Society; 2013 [cited 2025 Nov 30];369:1726–34. https://doi.org/10.1056/NEJMRA1208943.
13. Meyer NJ, Prescott HC. Sepsis and septic shock. Hardin CC, editor. New England Journal of Medicine [Internet]. Massachusetts Medical Society; 2024 [cited 2025 Nov 30];391:2133–46. https://doi.org/10.1056/NEJMRA2403213.
14. Ronco C, Ricci Z, Husain-Syed F. From multiple organ support therapy to extracorporeal organ support in critically ill patients. Blood Purif [Internet]. Blood Purif; 2019 [cited 2025 Nov 30];48:99–105. https://doi.org/10.1159/000490694.
15. Husain-Syed F, Ricci Z, Brodie D, Vincent JL, Ranieri VM, Slutsky AS, et al. Extracorporeal organ support (ECOS) in critical illness and acute kidney injury: from native to artificial organ crosstalk. Intens Care Med 2018 44:9 [Internet]. Springer; 2018 [cited 2025 Nov 30];44:1447–1459. https://doi.org/10.1007/S00134-018-5329-Z.
16. Papamichalis P, Oikonomou KG, Xanthoudaki M, Valsamaki A, Skoura A-L, Papathanasiou SK, et al. Extracorporeal organ support for critically ill patients: overcoming the past, achieving the maximum at present, and redefining the future. World J Crit Care Med [Internet]. Baishideng Publishing Group Inc.; 2024 [cited 2025 Nov 30];13:92458. https://doi.org/10.5492/wjccm.v13.i2.92458.
17. Ostermann M, Lumlertgul N, Jeong R, See E, Joannidis M, James M. Acute kidney injury. The Lancet [Internet]. Elsevier; 2025 [cited 2025 Dec 1];405:241–256. https://doi.org/10.1016/S0140-6736(24)02385-7.
18. Selewski DT, Wille KM. Continuous renal replacement therapy in patients treated with extracorporeal membrane oxygenation. Semin Dial [Internet]. Semin Dial; 2021 [cited 2025 Dec 1];34:537–49. https://doi.org/10.1111/SDI.12965.

19. Ostermann M, Liu K, Kashani K. Fluid management in acute kidney injury. Chest [Internet]. Elsevier Inc; 2019 [cited 2025 Dec 1];156:594–603. https://doi.org/10.1016/j.chest.2019.04.004.
20. Hayashi Y, Shimazui T, Tomita K, Shimada T, Miura RE, Taka-Aki Nakada & Associations between fluid overload and outcomes in critically ill patients with acute kidney injury: a retrospective observational study. Scientific Reports | [Internet]. 123AD [cited 2025 Dec 1];13:17410. https://doi.org/10.1038/s41598-023-44778-0.
21. Tolwani A. Continuous renal-replacement therapy for acute kidney injury. N Engl J Med [Internet]. Massachussetts Medical Society; 2012 [cited 2020 Mar 17];367:2505–2514. https://doi.org/10.1056/NEJMct1206045.
22. Teixeira JP, Hiremath S, Kabli AO, Rewa OG, Clark EG. Continuous kidney replacement therapies: core curriculum 2025. Am J Kidney Dis [Internet]. W.B. Saunders; 2025 [cited 2025 Dec 1];85:767–786. https://doi.org/10.1053/j.ajkd.2024.09.015.
23. Wald R, Gaudry S, da Costa BR, Adhikari NKJ, Bellomo R, Du B, et al. Initiation of continuous renal replacement therapy versus intermittent hemodialysis in critically ill patients with severe acute kidney injury: a secondary analysis of STARRT-AKI trial. Inten Care Med 2023 49:11 [Internet]. Springer; 2023 [cited 2025 Dec 1];49:1305–1316. https://doi.org/10.1007/S00134-023-07211-8.
24. Barbar SD, Wald R, Quenot JP. Acute kidney injury: when and how to start renal replacement therapy. Intens Care Med 2025 51:6 [Internet]. Springer; 2025 [cited 2025 Dec 1];51:1172–1175. https://doi.org/10.1007/S00134-025-07933-X.
25. Cardoso FS, Gottfried M, Tujios S, Olson JC, Karvellas CJ; US Acute Liver Failure Study Group. Continuous renal replacement therapy is associated with reduced serum ammonia levels and mortality in acute liver failure. Hepatology. 2018 Feb;67(2):711–720. https://doi.org/10.1002/hep.29488.
26. Chen H, Yu RG, Yin NN, Zhou JX. Combination of extracorporeal membrane oxygenation and continuous renal replacement therapy in critically ill patients: a systematic review. Crit Care [Internet]. Crit Care; 2014 [cited 2025 Dec 1];18. https://doi.org/10.1186/S13054-014-0675-X.
27. Karakala N, Juncos LA. Providing continuous renal replacement therapy in patients on extracorporeal membrane oxygenation. Clin J Am Soc Nephrol [Internet]. American Society of Nephrology; 2020 [cited 2025 Dec 1];15:704. https://doi.org/10.2215/CJN.11220919.
28. Ostermann M, Connor M, Kashani K. Continuous renal replacement therapy during extracorporeal membrane oxygenation: why, when and how? Curr Opin Crit Care [Internet]. Curr Opin Crit Care; 2018 [cited 2025 Dec 1];24:493–503. https://doi.org/10.1097/MCC.0000000000000559.
29. Oudemans-van Straaten HM, Kellum JA, Bellomo R. Clinical review: anticoagulation for continuous renal replacement therapy – heparin or citrate? Crit Care [Internet]. Crit Care; 2011 [cited 2025 Dec 1];15. https://doi.org/10.1186/CC9358.
30. Doidge JC, Gould DW, Sadique Z, Borthwick M, Hatch RA, Caskey FJ, et al. Regional citrate anticoagulation versus systemic heparin anticoagulation for continuous kidney replacement therapy in intensive care. J Crit Care [Internet]. W.B. Saunders; 2023 [cited 2025 Dec 1];74:154218. https://doi.org/10.1016/J.JCRC.2022.154218.
31. Section 5: Dialysis Interventions for Treatment of AKI. Kidney Int Suppl (2011) [Internet]. Elsevier; 2012 [cited 2025 Dec 1];2:89–115. https://doi.org/10.1038/KISUP.2011.35.
32. Morabito S, Pistolesi V, Tritapepe L, Fiaccadori E. Regional citrate anticoagulation for RRTs in critically ill patients with AKI. Clin J Am Soc Nephrol [Internet]. Clin J Am Soc Nephrol; 2014 [cited 2025 Dec 1];9:2173–88. https://doi.org/10.2215/CJN.01280214.
33. Schilder L, Nurmohamed SA, Bosch FH, Purmer IM, den Boer SS, Kleppe CG, et al. Citrate anticoagulation versus systemic heparinisation in continuous venovenous hemofiltration in critically ill patients with acute kidney injury: a multi-center randomized clinical trial. Crit Care [Internet]. Crit Care; 2014 [cited 2025 Dec 1];18. https://doi.org/10.1186/S13054-014-0472-6.
34. Peng B, Lu J, Guo H, Liu J, Li A. Regional citrate anticoagulation for replacement therapy in patients with liver failure: a systematic review and meta-analysis. Front Nutr [Internet].

Frontiers Media S.A.; 2023 [cited 2025 Dec 1];10:1031796. https://doi.org/10.3389/FNUT.2023.1031796/BIBTEX.
35. Patel S, Wendon J. Regional citrate anticoagulation in patients with liver failure – time for a rethink? Crit Care 2012 16:5 [Internet]. BioMed Central; 2012 [cited 2025 Dec 1];16:153. https://doi.org/10.1186/CC11492.
36. Honoré PM, Rimmelé T, Joannes-Boyau O. Citrate anticoagulation for continuous renal replacement therapy. Intens Care Med 2024 50:9 [Internet]. Springer; 2024 [cited 2025 Dec 1];50:1553–1556. https://doi.org/10.1007/S00134-024-07531-3.
37. Liu C, Fan S, Yang L, Wei W, Huang Y, Chen Z, et al. Higher blood flow rates in anticoagulation free CRRT improve circuit survival and clinical outcomes. Clin Kidney J [Internet]. 2025 [cited 2025 Dec 1]; https://doi.org/10.1093/CKJ/SFAF360.
38. Gajkowski EF, Herrera G, Hatton L, Velia Antonini M, Vercaemst L, Cooley E. ELSO guidelines for adult and pediatric extracorporeal membrane oxygenation circuits. ASAIO J [Internet]. ASAIO J; 2022 [cited 2025 Dec 1];68:133–152. https://doi.org/10.1097/MAT.0000000000001630.
39. Bartos JA, Grunau B, Carlson C, Duval S, Ripeckyj A, Kalra R, et al. Improved survival with extracorporeal cardiopulmonary resuscitation despite progressive metabolic derangement associated with prolonged resuscitation. Circulation [Internet]. Circulation; 2020 [cited 2025 Dec 1];141:877–886. https://doi.org/10.1161/CIRCULATIONAHA.119.042173.
40. Combes A, Hajage D, Capellier G, Demoule A, Lavoué S, Guervilly C, et al. Extracorporeal membrane oxygenation for severe acute respiratory distress syndrome. N Engl J Med [Internet]. Massachusetts Medical Society; 2018 [cited 2025 Dec 1];378:1965–1975. https://doi.org/10.1056/NEJMOA1800385;CTYPE:STRING:JOURNAL.
41. Rochwerg B, Brochard L, Elliott MW, Hess D, Hill NS, Nava S, et al. Official ERS/ATS clinical practice guidelines: noninvasive ventilation for acute respiratory failure. Eur Respir J [Internet]. Eur Respir J; 2017 [cited 2025 Dec 1];50. https://doi.org/10.1183/13993003.02426-2016.
42. Wieruszewski PM, Ortoleva JP, Cormican DS, Seelhammer TG. Extracorporeal membrane oxygenation in acute respiratory failure. Pulm Ther [Internet]. Adis; 2023 [cited 2025 Dec 1];9:109. https://doi.org/10.1007/S41030-023-00214-2.
43. Guglin M, Zucker MJ, Bazan VM, Bozkurt B, El Banayosy A, Estep JD, et al. Venoarterial ECMO for adults: JACC scientific expert panel. J Am Coll Cardiol [Internet]. Elsevier USA; 2019 [cited 2025 Dec 1];73:698–716. https://doi.org/10.1016/J.JACC.2018.11.038;TAXONOMY:TAXONOMY:CME;PAGEGROUP:STRING:PUBLICATION.
44. Sun T, Guy A, Sidhu A, Finlayson G, Grunau B, Ding L, et al. Veno-arterial extracorporeal membrane oxygenation (VA-ECMO) for emergency cardiac support. J Crit Care [Internet]. W.B. Saunders; 2018 [cited 2025 Dec 1];44:31–38. https://doi.org/10.1016/J.JCRC.2017.10.011.
45. ELSO Adult Cardiac Failure Supplement to the ELSO General Guidelines Extracorporeal Life Support Organization (ELSO) Guidelines for Adult Cardiac Failure. 2013.
46. Fernández-Mondéjar E, Fuset-Cabanes MP, Grau-Carmona T, López-Sánchez M, Peñuelas Ó, Pérez-Vela JL, et al. The use of ECMO in ICU. Recommendations of the Spanish Society of Critical Care Medicine and Coronary Units. Medicina Intensiva (English Edition) [Internet]. Elsevier; 2019 [cited 2025 Dec 1];43:108–120. https://doi.org/10.1016/J.MEDINE.2018.12.002.
47. Bohman JK, Radosevich M, Sugeir S. Extracorporeal membrane oxygenation contraindications. Cardiopulmonary bypass: advances in extracorporeal life support [Internet]. Academic; 2023 [cited 2025 Dec 1];835–45. https://doi.org/10.1016/B978-0-443-18918-0.00053-X.
48. Javidfar J, Brodie D, Wang D, Ibrahimiye AN, Yang J, Zwischenberger JB, et al. Use of bicaval dual-lumen catheter for adult venovenous extracorporeal membrane oxygenation. Annals of Thoracic Surgery [Internet]. Elsevier USA; 2011 [cited 2025 Dec 1];91:1763–1769. https://doi.org/10.1016/j.athoracsur.2011.03.002.

49. Pappalardo F, Ruggeri L, Pieri M, Maj G, de Bonis M, Zangrillo A. Dual lumen catheter cannulation for venovenous ECMO. Intens Care Med 2015 41:5 [Internet]. Springer; 2015 [cited 2025 Dec 1];41:941–942. https://doi.org/10.1007/S00134-015-3740-2.
50. Banfi C, Pozzi M, Siegenthaler N, Brunner ME, Tassaux D, Obadia JF, et al. Veno-venous extracorporeal membrane oxygenation: cannulation techniques. J Thorac Dis [Internet]. AME Publishing Company; 2016 [cited 2025 Dec 1];8:3762–3773. https://doi.org/10.21037/JTD.2016.12.88.
51. Parker LP, Svensson Marcial A, Brismar TB, Broman LM, Prahl Wittberg L. Hemodynamic and recirculation performance of dual lumen cannulas for venovenous extracorporeal membrane oxygenation. Sci Rep [Internet]. Sci Rep; 2023 [cited 2025 Dec 1];13. https://doi.org/10.1038/S41598-023-34655-1.
52. Cheng R, Hachamovitch R, Kittleson M, Patel J, Arabia F, Moriguchi J, et al. Complications of extracorporeal membrane oxygenation for treatment of cardiogenic shock and cardiac arrest: a meta-analysis of 1,866 adult patients. Annals of Thoracic Surgery [Internet]. Ann Thorac Surg; 2014 [cited 2025 Dec 1];97:610–616. https://doi.org/10.1016/j.athoracsur.2013.09.008.
53. Pisani A, Braham W, Brega C, Lajmi M, Provenchere S, Danial P, et al. Right axillary artery cannulation for venoarterial extracorporeal membrane oxygenation: a retrospective single centre observational study. Eur J Cardiothorac Surg [Internet]. Eur J Cardiothorac Surg; 2021 [cited 2025 Dec 1];59:601–609. https://doi.org/10.1093/EJCTS/EZAA397.
54. Raffa GM, Kowalewski M, Brodie D, Ogino M, Whitman G, Meani P, et al. Meta-analysis of peripheral or central extracorporeal membrane oxygenation in postcardiotomy and non-postcardiotomy shock. Ann Thorac Surg [Internet]. Elsevier USA; 2019 [cited 2025 Dec 1];107:311–321. https://doi.org/10.1016/j.athoracsur.2018.05.063.
55. McMichael ABV, Ryerson LM, Ratano D, Fan E, Faraoni D, Annich GM. ELSO adult and pediatric anticoagulation guidelines. ASAIO J [Internet]. ASAIO J; 2022 [cited 2025 Dec 1];68:303–10. 2021; https://doi.org/10.1097/MAT.0000000000001652.
56. Vajter J, Volod O. Anticoagulation management during ECMO: narrative review. JHLT Open [Internet]. Elsevier; 2025 [cited 2025 Dec 1];8:100216. https://doi.org/10.1016/J.JHLTO.2025.100216.
57. Zhong H, Zhu ML, Yu YT, Li W, Xing SP, Zhao XY, et al. Management of bivalirudin anticoagulation therapy for extracorporeal membrane oxygenation in heparin-induced thrombocytopenia: a case report and a systematic review. Front Pharmacol [Internet]. Front Pharmacol; 2020 [cited 2025 Dec 1];11. https://doi.org/10.3389/FPHAR.2020.565013.
58. Wendon J, Cordoba J, Dhawan A, Larsen FS, Manns M, Nevens F, et al. EASL Clinical Practical Guidelines on the management of acute (fulminant) liver failure. J Hepatol [Internet]. Elsevier; 2017 [cited 2025 Dec 2];66:1047–1081. https://doi.org/10.1016/J.JHEP.2016.12.003.
59. Shingina A, Mukhtar N, Wakim-Fleming J, Alqahtani S, Wong RJ, Limketkai BN, et al. Acute liver failure guidelines. Am J Gastroenterol [Internet]. Wolters Kluwer Health; 2023 [cited 2025 Dec 2];118:1128–1153. https://doi.org/10.14309/AJG.0000000000002340.
60. Hernández DR, Valdez-Gaona A, García-Velasco LA, Lemus JS, Herrera OG, Membrila GC. Single-Pass Albumin Dialysis (SPAD) as a therapeutic extracorporeal liver support in a low-resource setting: case report and literature review. Cureus [Internet]. Springer Science and Business Media LLC; 2025 [cited 2025 Dec 2];17:e85782. https://doi.org/10.7759/CUREUS.85782.
61. Tandon R, Froghi S. Artificial liver support systems. J Gastroenterol Hepatol [Internet]. J Gastroenterol Hepatol; 2021 [cited 2025 Dec 2];36:1164–1179. https://doi.org/10.1111/JGH.15255.
62. Piechota M, Piechota A. An evaluation of the usefulness of single pass albumin dialysis: key role of dialysate flow rate. Crit Care [Internet]. BioMed Central Ltd.; 2016 [cited 2025 Dec 2];20:156. https://doi.org/10.1186/S13054-016-1287-4.
63. Gadour E, Kaballo MA, Shrwani K, Hassan Z, Kotb A, Aljuraysan A, et al. Safety and efficacy of Single-Pass Albumin Dialysis (SPAD), Prometheus, and Molecular Adsorbent Recycling System (MARS) liver haemodialysis vs. Standard Medical Therapy (SMT): meta-analysis and

systematic review. Prz Gastroenterol [Internet]. Termedia Publishing House Ltd.; 2024 [cited 2025 Dec 2];19:101. https://doi.org/10.5114/PG.2024.139297.
64. Schmuck RB, Nawrot GH, Fikatas P, Reutzel-Selke A, Pratschke J, Sauer IM. Single pass albumin dialysis – a dose-finding study to define optimal albumin concentration and dialysate flow. Artif Organs [Internet]. Wiley; 2017 [cited 2025 Dec 2];41:153–161. https://doi.org/10.1111/AOR.12736;WGROUP:STRING:PUBLICATION.
65. Hutapea TPH, Madurani KA, Syahputra MY, Hudha MN, Asriana AN, Suprapto, et al. Albumin: source, preparation, determination, applications, and prospects. J Sci Adv Mater Dev [Internet]. Elsevier; 2023 [cited 2025 Dec 2];8:100549. https://doi.org/10.1016/J.JSAMD.2023.100549.
66. Silvariño R, San Román S, Peluffo L, Opertti A, Grecco G, Noboa O, et al. Extended online hemodiafiltration associated with single-pass albumin dialysis, a feasible alternative for patients with hepatorenal insufficiency. Nefrología (English Edition) [Internet]. Elsevier; 2023 [cited 2025 Dec 2];43:801–3. https://doi.org/10.1016/J.NEFROE.2024.01.003.
67. Wallon G, Guth C, Guichon C, Thevenon S, Gazon M, Viale JP, et al. Extracorporeal albumin dialysis in liver failure with MARS and SPAD: a randomized crossover trial. Blood Purif [Internet]. Blood Purif; 2022 [cited 2025 Dec 2];51:243–250. https://doi.org/10.1159/000515825.
68. Boyle M, Kurtovic J, Bihari D, Riordan S, Steiner C. Equipment review: the molecular adsorbents recirculating system (MARS®). Crit Care [Internet]. 2004 [cited 2025 Dec 2];8:280. https://doi.org/10.1186/CC2895.
69. Mielnicki W, Dyla A, Karczewski M. Clinical effectiveness of MARS treatment – multidirectional analysis of positive clinical response to treatment. Clin Exp Hepatol [Internet]. Termedia Publishing House Ltd.; 2019 [cited 2025 Dec 2];5:271. https://doi.org/10.5114/CEH.2019.89163.
70. Kapoor D. Molecular adsorbent recirculating system: albumin dialysis-based extracorporeal liver assist device. J Gastroenterol Hepatol (Australia) [Internet]. Blackwell Publishing; 2002 [cited 2025 Dec 2];17:S280–S286. https://doi.org/10.1046/J.1440-1746.17.S3.14.X;ISSUE:ISSUE:DOI.
71. He GL, Feng L, Duan CY, Hu X, Zhou CJ, Cheng Y, et al. Meta-analysis of survival with the molecular adsorbent recirculating system for liver failure. Int J Clin Exp Med [Internet]. E-Century Publishing Corporation; 2015 [cited 2025 Dec 2];8:17046. https://pmc.ncbi.nlm.nih.gov/articles/PMC4694195/. Accessed 2 Dec 2025.
72. Sen S, Mookerjee RP, Davies NA, Williams R, Jalan R. Review article: the molecular adsorbents recirculating system (MARS) in liver failure. Aliment Pharmacol Ther [Internet]. Aliment Pharmacol Ther; 2002 [cited 2025 Dec 2];16 Suppl 5:32–38. https://doi.org/10.1046/J.1365-2036.16.S5.5.X.
73. Bañares R, Nevens F, Larsen FS, Jalan R, Albillos A, Dollinger M, et al. Extracorporeal albumin dialysis with the molecular adsorbent recirculating system in acute-on-chronic liver failure: the RELIEF trial. Hepatology [Internet]. Hepatology; 2013 [cited 2025 Dec 2];57:1153–1162. https://doi.org/10.1002/HEP.26185.
74. Ballester MP, Elshabrawi A, Jalan R. Extracorporeal liver support and liver transplantation for acute-on-chronic liver failure. Liver Int [Internet]. Wiley; 2023 [cited 2025 Dec 2];45:e15647. https://doi.org/10.1111/LIV.15647.
75. Karvellas CJ, Gibney N, Kutsogiannis D, Wendon J, Bain VG. Bench-to-bedside review: current evidence for extracorporeal albumin dialysis systems in liver failure. Crit Care [Internet]. 2007 [cited 2025 Dec 2];11:215. https://doi.org/10.1186/CC5922.
76. Evenepoel P, Laleman W, Wilmer A, Claes K, Maes B, Kuypers D, et al. Detoxifying capacity and kinetics of prometheus – a new extracorporeal system for the treatment of liver failure. Blood Purif [Internet]. Blood Purif; 2005 [cited 2025 Dec 2];23:349–358. https://doi.org/10.1159/000086885.
77. van Hoek B. Defining the value of extracorporeal liver support in acute and acute-on-chronic liver failure. J Clin Transl Hepatol [Internet]. Xia and He Publishing Inc.; 2023 [cited 2025 Dec 2];11:517. https://doi.org/10.14218/JCTH.2022.00025.

78. Matar AJ, Subramanian R. Extracorporeal liver support: a bridge to somewhere. Clin Liver Dis (Hoboken) [Internet]. Wiley; 2021 [cited 2025 Dec 2];18:274. https://doi.org/10.1002/CLD.1140.
79. Sanchez AP, Ward DM, Cunard R. Therapeutic plasma exchange in the intensive care unit: rationale, special considerations, and techniques for combined circuits. Therapeutic Apheresis and Dialysis. Wiley; 2022;26:41–52. https://doi.org/10.1111/1744-9987.13814.
80. Kanjo A, Ocskay K, Gede N, Kiss S, Szakács Z, Párniczky A, et al. Efficacy and safety of liver support devices in acute and hyperacute liver failure: a systematic review and network meta-analysis. Scientific Reports 2021 11:1 [Internet]. Nature Publishing Group; 2021 [cited 2025 Dec 2];11:4189. https://doi.org/10.1038/s41598-021-83292-z.
81. Angeli P, Bernardi M, Villanueva C, Francoz C, Mookerjee RP, Trebicka J, et al. EASL Clinical Practice Guidelines for the management of patients with decompensated cirrhosis. J Hepatol [Internet]. Elsevier B.V.; 2018 [cited 2025 Dec 2];69:406–460. https://doi.org/10.1016/j.jhep.2018.03.024.
82. Samoni S, Husain-syed F, Villa G, Ronco C. Continuous renal replacement therapy in the critically ill patient: from garage technology to artificial intelligence. J Clin Med [Internet]. MDPI; 2021 [cited 2025 Dec 2];11:172. https://doi.org/10.3390/JCM11010172.
83. Essink J, Berg S, Montange J, Sankey A, Taylor V, Salomon J. Single-pass albumin dialysis as rescue therapy for pediatric calcium channel blocker overdose. J Investig Med High Impact Case Rep [Internet]. J Investig Med High Impact Case Rep; 2022 [cited 2025 Dec 2];10. https://doi.org/10.1177/23247096221105251.
84. Hui WF, Choi AWM, Cheung WL, Hon KL, Ku SW. The use of single pass albumin dialysis and hemoadsorption in management of life-threatening amlodipine overdose. Semin Dial [Internet]. Semin Dial; 2025 [cited 2025 Dec 2];38:146–151. https://doi.org/10.1111/SDI.13236.
85. Sparks BE, Cavarocchi NC, Hirose H. Extracorporeal membrane oxygenation with multiple-organ failure: can molecular adsorbent recirculating system therapy improve survival? J Heart Lung Transp [Internet]. Elsevier USA; 2017 [cited 2025 Dec 2];36:71–76. https://doi.org/10.1016/j.healun.2016.09.014.
86. Peek GJ, Killer HM, Sosnowski MA, Firmin RK. Modular extracorporeal life support for multiorgan failure patients. Liver [Internet]. Wiley; 2002 [cited 2025 Dec 2];22:69–71. https://doi.org/10.1034/J.1600-0676.2002.00014.X;WGROUP:STRING:PUBLICATION.
87. Tiruvoipati R, Moorthy T, Balasubramanian SK, Platt V, Peek GJ. Extracorporeal membrane oxygenation and extracorporeal albumin dialysis in pediatric patients with sepsis and multi-organ dysfunction syndrome. Int J Artif Organs [Internet]. Int J Artif Organs; 2007 [cited 2025 Dec 2];30:227–234. https://doi.org/10.1177/039139880703000308.
88. Pinto VL, Wenderfer SE, Morris J, Akcan-Arikan A. Treatment of severe amlodipine toxicity with molecular adsorbent recirculating system. Kidney Int Rep [Internet]. Elsevier; 2019 [cited 2025 Dec 2];4:346–349. https://doi.org/10.1016/J.EKIR.2018.09.017.
89. Villarreal-Ondarza I, Rodríguez-Salinas CA, Gómez-Gutierrez R, Guerrero-Izaguirre I, Rizo-Topete LM. Use of hepatic support with MARS in a patient with SARS-CoV-2 Pneumonia, in treatment with ECMO and CRRT therapies: case report. J Extra Corpor Technol [Internet]. J Extra Corpor Technol; 2023 [cited 2025 Dec 2];55:130–133. https://doi.org/10.1051/JECT/2023025.
90. Sparks B, Hirose H, Cavarocchi N. ECMO with multiple-organ failure: can liver dialysis improve survival? J Heart Lung Transp [Internet]. Elsevier BV; 2016 [cited 2025 Dec 2];35:S152. https://doi.org/10.1016/j.healun.2016.01.421.
91. Peerapornratana S, Manrique-Caballero CL, Gómez H, Kellum JA. Acute kidney injury from sepsis: current concepts, epidemiology, pathophysiology, prevention and treatment. Kidney Int [Internet]. Elsevier; 2019 [cited 2022 May 12];96:1083–1099. https://doi.org/10.1016/J.KINT.2019.05.026.

Blood Purification in Cardiac Surgery and Transplantation

9

Martin H. Bernardi

9.1 Introduction

Cardiac surgery and heart transplantation are among the most physiologically demanding interventions, frequently complicated by profound inflammatory and immunologic disturbances causing a systemic inflammatory response syndrome (SIRS) [1, 2]. In contrast to general intensive care medicine, SIRS in cardiac surgery is usually directly related to the procedure and not to inflammation caused by sepsis [3]. This makes blood purification particularly interesting in this field, as it could be able to proactively mitigate procedure-specific inflammatory responses.

Additionally, in heart transplantation, the persistent risk of acute cellular and antibody-mediated rejection (ACR, AMR) and the high early mortality associated with primary graft dysfunction (PGD) may necessitate extracorporeal strategies such as plasma exchange or immunoadsorption to remove isoagglutinins or donor-specific antibodies (DSA) [4, 5].

9.1.1 Pathophysiology

Massive cytokine release, whether triggered by infection, cardiopulmonary bypass (CPB), ischemia/reperfusion (I/R) injury, or allograft-directed immune responses, can lead to vasodilation, capillary leak, coagulopathy, and immune suppression, ultimately progressing to multiorgan failure [6–8]. CPB plays a central role but also initiates a SIRS through blood contact with artificial surfaces, elevated free hemoglobin, activation of complement and coagulation pathways, oxidative stress, and

M. H. Bernardi (✉)
Medical University of Vienna, Division of Cardiac Thoracic Vascular Anaesthesia and Intensive Care Medicine, Vienna, Austria
e-mail: martin.bernardi@meduniwien.ac.at

S. De Rosa, S. Lassola (eds.), *Next-Gen Blood Purification*,
https://doi.org/10.1007/978-3-032-27033-7_9

the release of endotoxins, free radicals, and cytokines [2] [9–12]. This inflammatory cascade impairs organ perfusion and increases postoperative complications. Modulating cytokines is therefore a key therapeutic target, as SIRS is closely linked to microcirculatory dysfunction, endothelial injury, and coagulopathy, as well as hemodilution, capillary leak, vasoplegia, and postoperative organ dysfunction [13–15].

9.1.2 Therapeutic Rationale of Blood Purification

To counteract these processes, several extracorporeal blood purification techniques have been adopted from nephrology and critical care, aiming to non-selectively reduce inflammatory mediators and restore homeostasis [6, 7, 16, 17]. These modalities operate via diffusion, convection, combined diffusive–convective clearance, or solute adsorption using sorbent materials [6, 7, 18–20].

Across these settings, extracorporeal blood purification techniques offer targeted or broad removal of inflammatory mediators, endotoxins, or pathological antibodies; support fluid and electrolyte balance; improve coagulopathy; and promote organ recovery [21]. Their integration into cardiac surgery and transplantation has expanded considerably, prompting the need for a comprehensive evaluation of their mechanisms, indications, limitations, and clinical outcomes [2, 12].

This chapter synthesizes contemporary evidence on conventional ultrafiltration, modified ultrafiltration, zero-balance ultrafiltration, continuous renal replacement therapy, and emerging adsorptive techniques, alongside blood purification strategies used in heart transplantation, such as plasma exchange, immunoadsorption, and extracorporeal photopheresis.

9.2 Ultrafiltration

An ultrafiltration is used during CPB to remove excess fluid and circulating aggregates. Particles smaller than the semipermeable membrane's pore size pass through under a transmembrane pressure gradient, allowing plasma water and aggregates to be removed in proportion to their concentrations in the blood (Table 9.1) [16, 22].

9.2.1 Conventional Ultrafiltration (CUF)

Conventional ultrafiltration (CUF) is a standard blood purification technique during CPB, using a semipermeable membrane to remove plasma water and small solutes while returning concentrated blood to the circuit [17, 23]. It counteracts CPB-induced hemodilution, supports electrolyte and coagulation balance, and modestly reduces inflammatory mediators [17]. Because cardiac surgery uses an estimated 10–15% of the national blood supply, patient blood management programs increasingly emphasize strategies to reduce transfusions [24]. CUF has been incorporated

Table 9.1 Ultrafiltration techniques

Technique	Indication	Timing	Effects	Strengths	Limitations
Conventional ultrafiltration (CUF)	Hemoconcentration; optimize electrolytes	During CPB	Hemoconcentration; modest reduction of small soluble molecules; improved metabolic balance	Simple to integrate into CPB; widely familiar; may reduce transfusion need	Outcome benefits inconsistent; excessive volume removal may precipitate hypotension or AKI
Modified ultrafiltration (MUF)	Hemoconcentration; removal of inflammatory molecules	After CPB	Hemoconcentration; less tissue edema; reduced chest drainage and transfusion need	More efficient hemoconcentration than CUF	Requires stable hemodynamic and additional time; adult RCT data limited
Zero-balance ultrafiltration (ZBUF)	Removal of inflammatory molecules; optimize electrolytes without changing volume	During CPB	Washout of cytokines/activated proteins; correction of electrolytes	Maintains intravascular volume; electrolyte control; reduced inflammatory mediators	Limited evidence for hard outcome improvement; no blood-conservation

to increase hemoglobin concentration and potentially decrease blood product use [17, 23, 25, 26]. Over the past 25 years, multiple studies have evaluated these techniques, showing possible reductions in transfusion but also raising concerns about organ injury, particularly acute kidney injury when large ultrafiltrate volumes are removed [26, 27]. Consequently, guideline recommendations vary, prompting renewed interest in clarifying the impact of CUF on postoperative transfusion and requirements outcomes [28–30].

9.2.2 Modified Ultrafiltration (MUF)

Compared to CUF, which is typically performed during the rewarming stage of CPB, modified ultrafiltration (MUF) is used most often in pediatric cardiac surgery to concentrate the patient's blood volume after termination from CPB and provides greater efficiency in filtration and hemoconcentration [31–33]. In adult cardiac patients, a prior meta-analysis [34] of combined ultrafiltration techniques showed reduced postoperative bleeding, though MUF-specific data remain limited. As older, multimorbid patients increasingly undergo cardiac surgery [35] and face higher postoperative risk [36], MUF may offer particular benefit after CPB and has proven to be safe and feasible in adults, improving postoperative hematocrit, reducing chest tube bleeding, transfusion requirements, and intensive care unit (ICU) stay [31].

9.2.3 Zero-Balance Ultrafiltration

Zero-balanced ultrafiltration (ZBUF) replaces the filtered fluid with an equal volume of balanced crystalloid, providing no net fluid removal. Its benefits stem from clearing circulating aggregates and inflammatory by-products rather than hemoconcentration [37]. During CPB, ZBUF is used to reduce inflammatory mediators and correct electrolyte disturbances, particularly those arising from cardioplegic solutions; its use is comparatively of lesser importance [33, 38, 39].

9.3 Adsorptive Blood Purification Techniques

Adsorptive blood purification is an emerging extracorporeal approach that uses specialized membranes or coated systems to selectively bind inflammatory mediators, endotoxins, and other pathogenic substances directly to membrane surfaces, rather than relying on ultrafiltration or diffusion. In contrast, hemoadsorption uses sorbent particles packed into cartridges to create a tortuous sorbent bed. As blood or plasma flows through, solutes are selectively adsorbed onto the bead surfaces. Molecules physically adhere to the surface of the sorbent, allowing removal of medium-to-high-molecular-weight and protein-bound toxins [18, 20, 40].

In cardiac surgery, adsorptive blood purification techniques such as CytoSorb, Jafron, polymyxin B hemoperfusion (PMX-HP), and AN69-Oxiris are increasingly used to mitigate CPB-induced SIRS. CytoSorb and Jafron remove circulating cytokines, PMX-HP targets endotoxin, and AN69-Oxiris provides combined cytokine and endotoxin clearance [40]. Currently, evidence and clinical benefits are unclear, because patient populations and inflammatory responses are heterogeneous, unclear timing of intervention, and the non-selective nature of the devices (Table 9.2) [41–43].

Table 9.2 Hemoadsorption devices during cardiopulmonary bypass

Device	Indication	Technique	Target molecules	Evidence status
CytoSorb®	Complex/ high-risk cardiac surgery	Cross-linked divinylbenzene polymer beads	Broad-spectrum adsorption of cytokines; various hydrophobic molecules <55 kDa; drugs (e.g., ticagrelor)	No outcome benefit in routine clinical cardiac surgery; removal of DOACs reduced perioperative bleeding complications
Jafron HA380	Complex/ high-risk cardiac surgery	Cross-linked styrene–divinylbenzene copolymer beads	Broad-spectrum adsorption of cytokines; various molecules	Robust evidence in cardiac surgery is limited. Larger trials are ongoing to confirm impact on clinical outcomes.
Polymyxin B hemoperfusion	Endotoxin removal in gram-negative sepsis; adult cardiac surgical patients with suspected endotoxemia	Polymyxin B–immobilized fiber column	Endotoxin binding (highly specific to gram-negative bacterial endotoxins)	No robust clinical trial evidence in adult cardiac surgery
AN69-Oxiris	Complex/ high-risk cardiac surgery	Three-layered hollow-fiber membrane (AN69 copolymer hydrogel; polyethyleneimine layer; heparin-treated surface)	Combined cytokine and endotoxin adsorption	No robust clinical trial evidence in adult cardiac surgery

9.3.1 CytoSorb®

CytoSorb® (CytoSorbents Inc., Princeton, NJ) effectively adsorbs hydrophobic molecules up to 55 kDa, including cytokines, bile acids, and myoglobin, using cross-linked divinylbenzene polymer beads [44]. Its use has been reported in conditions marked by severe inflammation, such as sepsis, acute respiratory distress syndrome related to SARS-CoV-2, and liver failure, and for the removal of direct oral anticoagulants (DOACs) and certain toxins [45]. However, a recent systematic review and meta-analysis [43] found no clinical benefit of CytoSorb® in cardiac surgery. Treatment was not associated with reduced mortality, and subgroup analyses similarly showed no positive effect, with study heterogeneity limiting firm conclusions. In patients on DOACs undergoing cardiac surgery, intraoperative hemadsorption has been associated with reduced perioperative bleeding complications [46–49].

9.3.2 Jafron HA380

The Jafron HA380 device (Jafron Biomedical Co., Ltd., Zhuhai, China) uses a neutral macroporous resin composed of cross-linked styrene–divinylbenzene copolymers designed to remove circulating cytokines [50]. Compared with CytoSorb®, differences in material composition, pore size distribution, surface characteristics, adsorption kinetics, sorbent capacity, and recommended treatment duration result in distinct technical and clinical performance [51, 52]. Although both devices target cytokine removal in sepsis and other hyperinflammatory states, their adsorption behavior is not comparable [52]. Consequently, clinical outcomes and safety data from CytoSorb® cannot be extrapolated to Jafron HA380, and dedicated studies in cardiac surgery and on DOAC adsorption for Jafron are lacking.

9.3.3 Polymyxin B Hemoperfusion

PMX-HP (Toraymyxin, Toray Industries, Tokyo, Japan) is primarily used in Gram-negative sepsis and refractory septic shock, where endotoxemia plays a central pathogenic role. It employs a polymyxin B–immobilized fiber column that selectively binds the lipid A component of lipopolysaccharide (LPS) as blood passes through the cartridge. Because polymyxin B is covalently fixed to the fibers, endotoxin is removed without exerting an antibiotic effect. By clearing circulating endotoxin, PMX-HP interrupts TLR-4–mediated inflammatory signaling, reduces proinflammatory cytokine production, stabilizes vascular tone, and lowers vasopressor requirements. These effects may also help preserve endothelial integrity and mitigate organ injury [40].

Clinical evidence in septic patients is mixed [53, 54], but several potential benefits of PMX-HP have been reported in the cardiac surgical setting. PMX-HP has been shown to reduce the inflammatory response induced by CPB [55], improve outcomes in patients who develop postoperative sepsis [56, 57], and, in active infective endocarditis, markedly reduce inotropic requirements and shorten mechanical ventilation times [58].

9.3.4 AN69-Oxiris

The hollow-fiber AN69 membrane used in the AN69-Oxiris device (Gambro Industries, Meyzieu Cedex, France) has a distinctive three-layer structure: an AN69 copolymer hydrogel for cytokine adsorption, a positively charged polyethyleneimine layer for effective endotoxin binding, and a heparin-treated surface to reduce thrombosis risk and extend filter lifespan, supporting efficient continuous renal replacement therapy performance. This configuration enables broad, nonselective adsorption of both pro- and anti-inflammatory mediators [12, 40]. However, despite its theoretical advantages, the clinical benefit of AN69-Oxiris in cardiac surgery remains uncertain [12].

9.4 Blood Purification in Heart Transplantation

In cardiac surgery, blood purification aims to mitigate acute inflammatory disturbances caused by CPB. In heart transplantation, additional extracorporeal therapies are used to control alloimmune responses, donor-specific antibodies, and rejection.

Heart transplantation is the gold-standard treatment for selected patients with end-stage heart failure. Unfortunately, long-term success can be hindered by immune-mediated rejection of the cardiac allograft, particularly acute cellular rejection, antibody-mediated rejection, and cardiac allograft vasculopathy [59]. According to the 2019 annual report of the International Society for Heart and Lung Transplantation, over 5500 heart transplants were performed worldwide in 2017, with median post-transplant survival currently approaching 13 years [60, 61]. Despite significant advances in surgical techniques and immunosuppressive therapy, allograft rejection remains a persistent clinical challenge [4, 5].

Since the first heart transplant in 1967, improvements in immunosuppression have helped reduce rejection rates. Standard first-year triple therapy includes calcineurin inhibitors, antimetabolites, and glucocorticoids. ACR and AMR are managed with high-dose steroids and intensified immunosuppression; severe episodes may require antithymocyte globulin, while AMR treatment often includes intravenous immunoglobulins (IVIG), plasma exchange, or B-cell–targeted therapies. Nevertheless, recurrent rejection can occur despite aggressive management. Moreover, newer targeted agents are associated with substantial adverse effects, such as nephrotoxicity, increased malignancy risk, and opportunistic infections, and still fail to fully prevent the immune responses driving long-term graft failure. Over the past two decades, however, several studies have demonstrated that extracorporeal photopheresis (ECP) offers immunomodulatory benefits with a favorable side-effect profile in selected heart transplant recipients [59, 62, 63].

9.4.1 Immunoadsorption and Plasma Exchange

DSAs play a key role in AMR, which is associated with high mortality and increased risk of cardiac allograft vasculopathy. Anti-HLA antibodies are present in up to 11% of patients at heart transplantation, and de novo DSAs develop in up to one third post-transplant, reducing graft and patient survival. As no consensus exists on how best to eliminate HLA antibodies, most centers rely on plasmapheresis or immunoadsorption in combination with rituximab and/or IVIG for DSA reduction and AMR treatment [64].

Immunoadsorption is an advanced form of plasma exchange in which plasma is removed and passed over ligand-containing columns (e.g., Protein A) to selectively eliminate immunoglobulins, after which the purified plasma is reinfused. Unlike plasma exchange, immunoadsorption preserves other plasma components such as fibrinogen and coagulation factors, reducing adverse effects [65, 66].

9.4.2 Extracorporeal Photopheresis

ECP is a leukapheresis-based therapy approved for T-cell–mediated disorders such as cutaneous T-cell lymphoma, autoimmune diseases, and graft-versus-host disease after hematopoietic stem cell transplantation [67, 68]. Evidence also supports its use as prophylaxis or treatment for solid organ allograft rejection and as an immunosuppression-modifying therapy in solid organ transplant recipients [63, 67–69].

ECP is typically performed using a single integrated system [67]. Leukocytes are collected, treated with 8-methoxypsoralen, exposed to UVA light, and reinfused [67, 68]. The treated leukocytes undergo apoptosis and are phagocytosed by immature dendritic cells, resulting in immunomodulatory effects [68, 70]. Although the exact mechanism is not fully defined, ECP appears to act through dendritic cell activation, cytokine modulation, and T-cell regulation [68]. Apoptosis induction and monocyte activation initiate these processes, contributing to anti-tumor immunity as well [71–74]. Crucially, ECP promotes immune tolerance primarily through Treg induction and increased anti-inflammatory cytokines such as IL-10 and TGF-β [68, 71, 75]. Thus, unlike conventional immunosuppressive therapies, ECP modulates immune responses without causing global immunosuppression [67, 69, 70].

Disclosure of Interest Martin Bernardi received travel funding and research grants from CytoSorbents Europe GmbH.

References

1. Tomic V, Russwurm S, Moller E, Claus RA, Blaess M, Brunkhorst F, et al. Transcriptomic and proteomic patterns of systemic inflammation in on-pump and off-pump coronary artery bypass grafting. Circulation. 2005;112(19):2912–20.
2. Bernardi MH, Rinoesl H, Dragosits K, Ristl R, Hoffelner F, Opfermann P, et al. Effect of hemoadsorption during cardiopulmonary bypass surgery – a blinded, randomized, controlled pilot study using a novel adsorbent. Crit Care. 2016;20:96.
3. Viikinkoski E, Aittokallio J, Lehto J, Ollila H, Relander A, Vasankari T, et al. Prolonged systemic inflammatory response syndrome after cardiac surgery. J Cardiothorac Vasc Anesth. 2024;38(3):709–16.
4. Lund LH, Edwards LB, Kucheryavaya AY, Benden C, Christie JD, Dipchand AI, et al. The registry of the International Society for Heart and Lung Transplantation: thirty-first official adult heart transplant report–2014; focus theme: retransplantation. J Heart Lung Transplant. 2014;33(10):996–1008.
5. Augusto JF, Benden C, Diekmann F, Zuckermann A. The value of extracorporeal photopheresis as an immunosuppression-modifying approach in solid organ transplantation: a potential solution to an unmet medical need. Front Immunol. 2024;15:1371554.
6. Zhou F, Peng Z, Murugan R, Kellum JA. Blood purification and mortality in sepsis: a meta-analysis of randomized trials. Crit Care Med. 2013;41(9):2209–20.
7. Jarczak D, Nierhaus A. Cytokine storm-definition, causes, and implications. Int J Mol Sci. 2022;23(19)
8. Liu Z, Zhai Q. Inflammatory biomarkers to predict clinical outcomes in adults after cardiac surgery in China: a prospective observational trial. Cytokine. 2025;193:156987.
9. Laffey JG, Boylan JF, Cheng DC. The systemic inflammatory response to cardiac surgery: implications for the anesthesiologist. Anesthesiology. 2002;97(1):215–52.
10. Wan IY, Arifi AA, Wan S, Yip JH, Sihoe AD, Thung KH, et al. Beating heart revascularization with or without cardiopulmonary bypass: evaluation of inflammatory response in a prospective randomized study. J Thorac Cardiovasc Surg. 2004;127(6):1624–31.
11. Klein DJ, Briet F, Nisenbaum R, Romaschin AD, Mazer CD. Endotoxemia related to cardiopulmonary bypass is associated with increased risk of infection after cardiac surgery: a prospective observational study. Crit Care. 2011;15(1):R69.
12. Abou-Arab O, Huette P, Ibrahima A, Beyls C, Bayart G, Guilbart M, et al. Cytokine Hemoadsorption versus standard Care in Cardiac Surgery Using the Oxiris membrane: the OXICARD single-center randomized trial. Anesthesiology. 2025;142(5):874–84.
13. Hall R. Identification of inflammatory mediators and their modulation by strategies for the management of the systemic inflammatory response during cardiac surgery. J Cardiothorac Vasc Anesth. 2013;27(5):983–1033.
14. Koning NJ, Overmars MA, van den Brom CE, van Bezu J, Simon LE, Vonk AB, et al. Endothelial hyperpermeability after cardiac surgery with cardiopulmonary bypass as assessed using an in vitro bioassay for endothelial barrier function. Br J Anaesth. 2016;116(2):223–32.
15. den Os MM, van den Brom CE, van Leeuwen ALI, Dekker NAM. Microcirculatory perfusion disturbances following cardiopulmonary bypass: a systematic review. Crit Care. 2020;24(1):218.
16. Clar A, Larson DF. Hemofiltration: determinants of drug loss and concentration. J Extra Corpor Technol. 1995;27(3):158–63.
17. Hensley NB, Colao JA, Zorrilla-Vaca A, Nanavati J, Lawton JS, Raphael J, et al. Ultrafiltration in cardiac surgery: results of a systematic review and meta-analysis. Perfusion. 2024;39(4):743–51.
18. Ankawi G, Neri M, Zhang J, Breglia A, Ricci Z, Ronco C. Extracorporeal techniques for the treatment of critically ill patients with sepsis beyond conventional blood purification therapy: the promises and the pitfalls. Crit Care. 2018;22(1):262.

19. Ronco C, Ricci Z, Husain-Syed F. From multiple organ support therapy to extracorporeal organ support in critically ill patients. Blood Purif. 2019;48(2):99–105.
20. Clark WR, Ferrari F, La Manna G, Ronco C. Extracorporeal sorbent technologies: basic concepts and clinical application. Contrib Nephrol. 2017;190:43–57.
21. Malard B, Lambert C, Kellum JA. In vitro comparison of the adsorption of inflammatory mediators by blood purification devices. Intensive Care Med Exp. 2018;6(1):12.
22. Naik SK, Elliott MJ. Ultrafiltration and paediatric cardiopulmonary bypass. Perfusion. 1993;8(1):101–12.
23. Boodhwani M, Hamilton A, de Varennes B, Mesana T, Williams K, Wells GA, et al. A multicenter randomized controlled trial to assess the feasibility of testing modified ultrafiltration as a blood conservation technology in cardiac surgery. J Thorac Cardiovasc Surg. 2010;139(3):701–6.
24. Warner MA, Schulte PJ, Hanson AC, Madde NR, Burt JM, Higgins AA, et al. Implementation of a comprehensive patient blood management program for hospitalized patients at a large United States medical center. Mayo Clin Proc. 2021;96(12):2980–90.
25. Sniecinski RM, Chandler WL. Activation of the hemostatic system during cardiopulmonary bypass. Anesth Analg. 2011;113(6):1319–33.
26. Manning MW, Li YJ, Linder D, Haney JC, Wu YH, Podgoreanu MV, et al. Conventional ultrafiltration during elective cardiac surgery and postoperative acute kidney injury. J Cardiothorac Vasc Anesth. 2021;35(5):1310–8.
27. Paugh TA, Dickinson TA, Martin JR, Hanson EC, Fuller J, Heung M, et al. Impact of ultrafiltration on kidney injury after cardiac surgery: the Michigan experience. Ann Thorac Surg. 2015;100(5):1683–8.
28. Raphael J, Mazer CD, Subramani S, Schroeder A, Abdalla M, Ferreira R, et al. Society of Cardiovascular Anesthesiologists Clinical Practice Improvement Advisory for Management of Perioperative Bleeding and Hemostasis in cardiac surgery patients. Anesth Analg. 2019;129(5):1209–21.
29. Tibi P, McClure RS, Huang J, Baker RA, Fitzgerald D, Mazer CD, et al. STS/SCA/AmSECT/SABM update to the clinical practice guidelines on patient blood management. J Cardiothorac Vasc Anesth. 2021;35(9):2569–91.
30. Casselman FPA, Lance MD, Ahmed A, Ascari A, Blanco-Morillo J, Bolliger D, et al. 2024 EACTS/EACTAIC guidelines on patient blood Management in Adult Cardiac Surgery in collaboration with EBCP. J Cardiothorac Vasc Anesth. 2025;39(8):1964–2018.
31. Low ZK, Gao F, Sin KYK, Yap KH. Modified ultrafiltration reduces postoperative blood loss and transfusions in adult cardiac surgery: a meta-analysis of randomized controlled trials. Interact Cardiovasc Thorac Surg. 2021;32(5):671–82.
32. Williams GD, Ramamoorthy C, Chu L, Hammer GB, Kamra K, Boltz MG, et al. Modified and conventional ultrafiltration during pediatric cardiac surgery: clinical outcomes compared. J Thorac Cardiovasc Surg. 2006;132(6):1291–8.
33. Stammers AH, Tesdahl EA, Mongero LB, Patel KP, Petersen CC, Vucovich JA, et al. Zero-balance ultrafiltration during cardiopulmonary bypass is associated with decreased urine output. J Extra Corpor Technol. 2021;53(1):27–37.
34. Boodhwani M, Williams K, Babaev A, Gill G, Saleem N, Rubens FD. Ultrafiltration reduces blood transfusions following cardiac surgery: a meta-analysis. Eur J Cardiothorac Surg. 2006;30(6):892–7.
35. Nicolini F, Agostinelli A, Vezzani A, Manca T, Benassi F, Molardi A, et al. The evolution of cardiovascular surgery in elderly patient: a review of current options and outcomes. Biomed Res Int. 2014;2014:736298.
36. Alexander KP, Anstrom KJ, Muhlbaier LH, Grosswald RD, Smith PK, Jones RH, et al. Outcomes of cardiac surgery in patients > or = 80 years: results from the National Cardiovascular Network. J Am Coll Cardiol. 2000;35(3):731–8.
37. Matata BM, Scawn N, Morgan M, Shirley S, Kemp I, Richards S, et al. A single-center randomized trial of intraoperative zero-balanced ultrafiltration during cardiopulmonary bypass

for patients with impaired kidney function undergoing cardiac surgery. J Cardiothorac Vasc Anesth. 2015;29(5):1236–47.
38. Journois D, Israel-Biet D, Pouard P, Rolland B, Silvester W, Vouhe P, et al. High-volume, zero-balanced hemofiltration to reduce delayed inflammatory response to cardiopulmonary bypass in children. Anesthesiology. 1996;85(5):965–76.
39. Tallman RD, Dumond M, Brown D. Inflammatory mediator removal by zero-balance ultrafiltration during cardiopulmonary bypass. Perfusion. 2002;17(2):111–5.
40. Kim EY. Extracorporeal blood purification treatments for refractory septic shock following surgery. J Acute Care Surg. 2025;5(1):5–12.
41. Matejic-Spasic M, Lindstedt S, Lebreton G, Dzemali O, Suwalski P, Folliguet T, et al. The role of hemoadsorption in cardiac surgery – a systematic review. BMC Cardiovasc Disord. 2024;24(1):258.
42. Diab M, Lehmann T, Bothe W, Akhyari P, Platzer S, Wendt D, et al. Cytokine Hemoadsorption during cardiac surgery versus standard surgical Care for Infective Endocarditis (REMOVE): results from a multicenter randomized controlled trial. Circulation. 2022;145(13):959–68.
43. Becker S, Lang H, Vollmer Barbosa C, Tian Z, Melk A, Schmidt BMW. Efficacy of CytoSorb(R): a systematic review and meta-analysis. Crit Care. 2023;27(1):215.
44. Scharf C, Liebchen U, Paal M, Irlbeck M, Zoller M, Schroeder I. Blood purification with a cytokine adsorber for the elimination of myoglobin in critically ill patients with severe rhabdomyolysis. Crit Care. 2021;25(1):41.
45. Kohler T, Schwier E, Praxenthaler J, Kirchner C, Henzler D, Eickmeyer C. Therapeutic modulation of the host defense by Hemoadsorption with CytoSorb((R))-basics, indications and perspectives-a scoping review. Int J Mol Sci. 2021;22(23)
46. Schmoeckel M, Thielmann M, Vitanova K, Eberle T, Marczin N, Hassan K, et al. Direct-acting oral anticoagulant removal by intraoperative hemoadsorption in CABG and/or single valve surgery: interim analysis of the international safe and timely antithrombotic removal (STAR) registry. J Cardiothorac Surg. 2025;20(1):74.
47. Hassan K, Thielmann M, Easo J, Kamler M, Wendt D, Haidari Z, et al. Removal of Apixaban during emergency cardiac surgery using Hemoadsorption with a porous polymer bead sorbent. J Clin Med. 2022;11(19)
48. Hassan K, Kannmacher J, Wohlmuth P, Budde U, Schmoeckel M, Geidel S. Cytosorb adsorption during emergency cardiac operations in patients at high risk of bleeding. Ann Thorac Surg. 2019;108(1):45–51.
49. Mair H, Ulrich S, Rosenzweig D, Goeppl J, Jurma C, Vogt F, et al. Antithrombotic drug removal with hemoadsorption during off-pump coronary artery bypass grafting. J Cardiothorac Surg. 2024;19(1):246.
50. Chen J, Han W, Chen J, Zong W, Wang W, Wang Y, et al. High performance of a unique mesoporous polystyrene-based adsorbent for blood purification. Regener Biomater. 2017;4(1):31–7.
51. Schildboeck C, Harm S, Hartmann J. In vitro removal of protein-bound retention solutes by extracorporeal blood purification procedures. Blood Purif. 2024;53(4):231–42.
52. Nierhaus A, Morales J, Wendt D, Scheier J, Gutzler D, Jarczak D, et al. Comparison of the CytoSorb((R)) 300 mL and Jafron HA380 hemoadsorption devices: an in vitro study. Minim Invasive Ther Allied Technol. 2022;31(7):1058–65.
53. Garcia-Ramos S, Caamano E, Rodriguez Benitez P, Benito P, Calvo A, Ramos S, et al. Mortality risk prediction in abdominal septic shock treated with Polymyxin-B Hemoperfusion: a retrospective cohort study. J Pers Med. 2023;13(7)
54. Dellinger RP, Bagshaw SM, Antonelli M, Foster DM, Klein DJ, Marshall JC, et al. Effect of targeted Polymyxin B Hemoperfusion on 28-day mortality in patients with septic shock and elevated endotoxin level: the EUPHRATES randomized clinical trial. JAMA. 2018;320(14):1455–63.
55. Ohki S, Oshima K, Takeyoshi I, Matsumoto K, Morishita Y. Endotoxin removal with a polymyxin B-immobilized hemoperfusion cartridge improves cardiopulmonary function after cardiopulmonary bypass. J Surg Res. 2008;145(1):74–9.

56. Yaroustovsky M, Abramyan M, Komardina E, Nazarova H, Popov D, Plyushch M, et al. Selective LPS adsorption using Polymyxin B-immobilized fiber cartridges in sepsis patients following cardiac surgery. Shock. 2018;49(6):658–66.
57. Murakami M, Miyauchi Y, Nishida M, Okada H, Hamano K. Direct hemoperfusion using polymyxin-B immobilized fiber for septic shock after cardiac surgery. Circ J. 2009;73(4):658–61.
58. Totsugawa T, Kuinose M, Yoshitaka H, Tsushima Y, Ishida A, Chikazawa G, et al. Intraoperative direct hemoperfusion with a polymyxin-B immobilized fiber column for treatment of infective endocarditis. Gen Thorac Cardiovasc Surg. 2011;59(2):98–104.
59. Slomovich S, Bell J, Clerkin KJ, Habal MV, Griffin JM, Raikhelkar JK, et al. Extracorporeal photopheresis and its role in heart transplant rejection: prophylaxis and treatment. Clin Transpl. 2021;35(7):e14333.
60. Khush KK, Cherikh WS, Chambers DC, Harhay MO, Hayes D Jr, Hsich E, et al. The international thoracic organ transplant registry of the International Society for Heart and Lung Transplantation: thirty-sixth adult heart transplantation report – 2019; focus theme: donor and recipient size match. J Heart Lung Transplant. 2019;38(10):1056–66.
61. Chambers DC, Cherikh WS, Harhay MO, Hayes D Jr, Hsich E, Khush KK, et al. The International Thoracic Organ Transplant Registry of the International Society for Heart and Lung Transplantation: thirty-sixth adult lung and heart-lung transplantation report-2019; focus theme: donor and recipient size match. J Heart Lung Transplant. 2019;38(10):1042–55.
62. Padmanabhan A, Connelly-Smith L, Aqui N, Balogun RA, Klingel R, Meyer E, et al. Guidelines on the use of therapeutic apheresis in clinical practice – evidence-based approach from the Writing Committee of the American Society for apheresis: the eighth special issue. J Clin Apher. 2019;34(3):171–354.
63. Jaksch P, Knobler R. ECP and solid organ transplantation. Transfus Apher Sci. 2014;50(3):358–62.
64. Barten MJ, Schulz U, Beiras-Fernandez A, Berchtold-Herz M, Boeken U, Garbade J, et al. The clinical impact of donor-specific antibodies in heart transplantation. Transplant Rev (Orlando). 2018;32(4):207–17.
65. Marco I, Lopez-Azor Garcia JC, Gonzalez Martin J, Severo Sanchez A, Garcia-Cosio Carmena MD, Mancebo Sierra E, et al. De novo donor-specific antibodies after heart transplantation: a comprehensive guide for clinicians. J Clin Med. 2023;12(23)
66. Dandel M. Autoimmunity in cardiomyopathy-induced heart failure and cardiac autoantibody removal by Immunoadsorption. J Clin Med. 2025;14(3)
67. Arora S, Setia R. Extracorporeal photopheresis: review of technical aspects. Asian J Transfus Sci. 2017;11(2):81–6.
68. Cho A, Jantschitsch C, Knobler R. Extracorporeal Photopheresis-an overview. Front Med (Lausanne). 2018;5:236.
69. Knobler R, Berlin G, Calzavara-Pinton P, Greinix H, Jaksch P, Laroche L, et al. Guidelines on the use of extracorporeal photopheresis. J Eur Acad Dermatol Venereol. 2014;28 Suppl 1(Suppl 1):1–37.
70. Hachem R, Corris P. Extracorporeal Photopheresis for bronchiolitis obliterans syndrome after lung transplantation. Transplantation. 2018;102(7):1059–65.
71. Akilov OE. What does the future hold for biomarkers of response to extracorporeal Photopheresis for mycosis Fungoides and Sezary syndrome? Cells. 2023;12(18)
72. Edelson RL. Mechanistic insights into extracorporeal photochemotherapy: efficient induction of monocyte-to-dendritic cell maturation. Transfus Apher Sci. 2014;50(3):322–9.
73. Heshmati F. Updating ECP action mechanisms. Transfus Apher Sci. 2014;50(3):330–9.
74. Han P, Hanlon D, Arshad N, Lee JS, Tatsuno K, Robinson E, et al. Platelet P-selectin initiates cross-presentation and dendritic cell differentiation in blood monocytes. Sci Adv. 2020;6(11):eaaz1580.
75. Bladon J, Taylor PC. Extracorporeal photopheresis: a focus on apoptosis and cytokines. J Dermatol Sci. 2006;43(2):85–94.

Extracorporeal Liver Support (ECLS) Systems

10

Federico Nalesso, Rime Kalf, Martina Cacciapuoti, Leda Cattarin, Ruggero Zanella, Giuseppe Scaparrotta, Francesca K. Martino, and Lucia Federica Stefanelli

10.1 Introduction

Acute liver failure (ALF) and acute-on-chronic liver failure (ACLF) remain among the most lethal conditions in critical care, with mortality rates that have not substantially declined despite advances in intensive care and transplantation [1, 2]. The two most common causes of death in patients with ALF are cerebral edema and multiorgan system failure, with a mortality rate of 25–50% [3]. In this type of patient, it is necessary to establish a series of specific medical therapies in order to achieve clinical recovery or stabilization. When this fails, one option is to apply a series of blood purification methods aimed at ensuring a bridge to recovery or liver transplantation. ALF is less frequent in developed countries, where vaccination

F. Nalesso (✉) · R. Kalf · L. Cattarin · R. Zanella · G. Scaparrotta · F. K. Martino · L. F. Stefanelli
Department of Medicine, University of Padua, Nephrology, Dialysis and Transplant Unit, Padua, Italy
e-mail: rime.khalf@studenti.unipd.it; LEDA.CATTARIN@AOPD.VENETO.IT; RUGGERO.ZANELLA@AOPD.VENETO.IT; GIUSEPPE.SCAPARROTTA@AOPD.VENETO.IT; francescakatiana.martino@aopd.veneto.it; luciafederica.stefanelli@unipd.it

M. Cacciapuoti
Department of Medicine (DIMED), University of Padua, Nephrology, Dialysis and Transplant Unit, Padua, Italy
e-mail: martina.cacciapuoti@studenti.unipd.it

S. De Rosa, S. Lassola (eds.), *Next-Gen Blood Purification*,
https://doi.org/10.1007/978-3-032-27033-7_10

and sanitation have reduced viral hepatitis. As a result, drug-induced liver injury now represents the most frequent cause of ALF in these settings, accounting for approximately 50% of the cases in the United States [4], especially caused by paracetamol (acetaminophen) overdose [5]. During this type of poisoning, medical therapy may not be effective in restoring organ function, and blood purification may be a valid option for supporting patients awaiting urgent liver transplants or for improving the liver's response to medical therapies. Although liver transplantation remains the definitive therapy, donor organ scarcity and contraindications necessitate alternative strategies [6]. From this perspective, blood purification has evolved in this field, providing clinicians with a range of purification treatments, from simple dialysis with albumin-rich dialysate to the development of complex methods for adsorbing the patient's albumin on resin devices specifically designed for the adsorption of hepatic toxins [7]. In summary, Extracorporeal Liver Support (ECLS) systems, both biological and non-biological, have emerged as adjunctive therapies designed to stabilize patients, mitigate toxin burden, and bridge them to recovery or transplantation. The challenge of these methods is to remove both water-soluble toxins that are easily removed by diffusion and convection processes (typically dialysis and hemofiltration) and hydrophobic molecules bound to albumin that cannot be physically removed by diffusion and convection processes, but with the use of specific resins inserted into devices with reduced hemocompatibility requiring mandatory plasma perfusion [8, 9]. Often, the hardware complexity of these methods limits their use in common clinical practice, while simplifying them reduces their purifying effectiveness, providing clinicians with methods that are sufficiently useful to ensure a bridge to transplantation or recovery of liver function in selected patient cases. Overall, ECLS aims to replace or augment the liver's detoxification, synthetic, immunomodulatory, and metabolic functions [7]. Contemporary systems vary widely in design and mechanism, ranging from albumin-based detoxification platforms to bioreactors containing living hepatocytes. This chapter reviews the principles, classifications, mechanisms, evidence base, and clinical applications of ECLS systems.

10.2 Pathophysiological Rationale for ECLS

ECLS systems in common clinical practice must ensure the removal of hepatic toxins and, ideally, should also be equipped with a synthetic capacity to compensate for the reduced metabolic functions of the liver. This does not involve the simple removal of "hepatic toxins," but rather the more complex support of hepatic functions, which, in the most advanced systems, requires a bioreactor capable of synthesizing all those proteins that the insufficient liver does not produce or produces in lower concentrations, such as coagulation factors and albumin. This crucial point is more evident when considering the liver's physiology.

10.2.1 Key Functions Lost in Liver Failure

Hepatic insufficiency, regardless of the cause that led to its onset, results in:

- *Accumulation of toxins* (bilirubin, bile acids, aromatic amino acids, ammonia, cytokines).
- *Loss of synthetic capacity* (coagulation factors, albumin).
- *Impaired metabolic and regulatory functions* (glucose homeostasis, hormone metabolism).
- *Systemic inflammatory activation* leading to endothelial dysfunction and multi-organ failure.

10.2.2 Target Functions for ECLS

ECLS systems are designed to address:

- *Detoxification* (removal of albumin-bound and water-soluble toxins).
- *Metabolic support* (urea cycle activity, lactate clearance, energy substrate processing).
- *Synthetic functions* (production of proteins and coagulation factors—only possible in bioartificial systems).
- *Hemodynamic and immunological modulation* through reduction of inflammatory mediators.

To address these pathophysiological derangements, ECLS systems rely on fundamental principles of solute transport and mass transfer. These principles can be used individually in the most basic "liver function support" technologies or combined in complex ways in systems that seek to ensure "liver function replacement." However, each technology has clear and easily identifiable purification limitations linked to multiple factors, which will be analyzed in detail in this chapter and are summarized in Table 10.1.

Table 10.1 Comparison of extracorporeal liver support systems

System	Type	Main mechanism(s)	What removes/provides	Advantages	Limitations	Clinical status
MARS (molecular adsorbent recirculating system)	Artificial	Albumin dialysis + diffusion + adsorption	Albumin-bound toxins (bilirubin, bile acids), ammonia (via diffusion only), aromatic amino acids	Well-studied; good bilirubin clearance; improves encephalopathy; widely available	Cost; intermittent therapy; modest effect on ammonia; unclear survival benefit	Used clinically as bridge to transplant or decision; no proven mortality benefit
Prometheus/FPSA	Artificial	Fractionated plasma separation + adsorption + high-flux dialysis	Strong removal of albumin-bound toxins; water-soluble toxins (via dialysis)	Higher bilirubin/bile acid clearance vs. MARS; simultaneous renal support	Hemodynamic demands; complex system; mixed survival results	Used clinically; no clear survival advantage in large trials
SPAD (single-pass albumin dialysis)	Artificial	Diffusion using albumin-enriched dialysate (single-pass)	Bilirubin and some albumin-bound toxins	Simple; low-cost; usable where MARS absent	Less effective; high albumin consumption; intermittent	Limited to specific ICU uses; not standard for ALF/ACLF
TPE (therapeutic plasma exchange)	Artificial	Bulk plasma removal and replacement	Broad removal of toxins, cytokines, autoantibodies; replenishes clotting factors	Strong evidence of survival benefit in hyperacute ALF (high-volume TPE); improves coagulopathy	Requires large plasma volumes; risk of reactions, bleeding	Widely used; strongest evidence for transplant-free survival in ALF
CytoSorb/HA330 (Hemoadsorption cartridges)	Artificial	Adsorption of inflammatory mediators and some bilirubin	Cytokines, myoglobin, some albumin-bound toxins	Useful adjunct to CKRT; reduces inflammatory burden	Non-selective adsorption (removes antibiotics); variable toxin clearance	Common adjunct in sepsis-associated ACLF; emerging evidence
CKRT (with liver support intent)	Artificial	Diffusion + convection (hemodialysis + hemofiltration)	Ammonia, lactate, water-soluble toxins	Useful for hepatorenal failure; stabilizes electrolytes and pH	Does not remove albumin-bound toxins	Standard in ACLF with kidney failure; supportive measure only

ELAD	Bioartificial	Human hepatocyte-like C3A cell bioreactors; metabolic & synthetic support	Limited ammonia metabolism; albumin/transferrin secretion; cytokine modulation	Human cells; metabolic & synthetic function; unique immunomodulation	Lower detox capacity than artificial systems; high cost; mixed trial results	Not FDA/EMA approved; experimental; possible benefit in select alcoholic hepatitis subgroups
BAL-AMC	Bioartificial	Porcine hepatocyte bioreactor + adsorption + dialysis	Detoxification and metabolic activity	Higher metabolic potential; hepatocyte-like function	Xenogeneic risks; logistical complexity; trials did not show long-term survival benefit	Experimental; no longer commercialized
Hybrid BAL systems (experimental)	Bioartificial/ hybrid	Combination of adsorption + albumin dialysis + hepatocyte modules	Mixed detox + metabolic support	Potential to combine best features of both worlds	Still developmental; engineering challenges; no clinical approval	Preclinical or early-phase research

ALF acute liver failure (insufficienza epatica acuta), *ACLF* acute-on-chronic liver failure, *ICU* intensive care unit, *MARS*: molecular adsorbent recirculating system (Recirculating circuit albumin dialysis for extracorporeal liver support), *Prometheus/FPSA* fractionated plasma separation and adsorption (Fractionated plasma separation and adsorption (Prometheus system)), *SPAD* single-pass albumin dialysis single-pass (albumin dialysis using an albumin-containing dialysate), *TPE* therapeutic plasma exchange (therapeutic plasmapheresis), *CytoSorb* hemoadsorption cartridge for the removal of inflammatory mediators and selected toxins, *HA330* Hemoadsorption cartridge (a family of sorbent devices, often described as providing "non-selective" adsorption of inflammatory mediators), *CKRT* continuous kidney replacement therapy (Continuous renal replacement therapy: continuous hemodialysis and/or hemofiltration), *pH* hydrogen potential (pH), an index of acidity/alkalinity, *ELAD* extracorporeal liver assist device (bioartificial/experimental extracorporeal liver support device), *C3A* cell line derived from human hepatoma, used in selected bioartificial liver bioreactors, *FDA* Food and Drug Administration, *EMA* European Medicines Agency, *BAL* Bioartificial liver, *BAL-AMC* Bioartificial liver–AMC (Bioartificial system developed at the Academic Medical Center, Amsterdam), *Hybrid BAL Systems* Hybrid bioartificial liver systems (combining adsorption/dialysis with cellular modules)

10.3 Fundamental Principles of Mass Transfer in Extracorporeal Liver Support

Extracorporeal Liver Support (ECLS) systems rely on physical and chemical mechanisms that govern the movement and removal of solutes from blood or plasma. Three foundational mass-transfer principles, diffusion, convection, and adsorption, form the basis for detoxification in all artificial liver support technologies. Understanding these mechanisms is essential when evaluating device performance, toxin clearance capacity, clinical indications, and the possible limitations due to the technology used [10].

10.3.1 Diffusion

Diffusion is the movement of solutes from an area of higher concentration to an area of lower concentration across a semipermeable membrane. It is governed by Fick's Law, where solute flux is proportional to the concentration gradient and membrane characteristics.

Key Determinants

- Concentration gradient between blood and dialysate
- Membrane surface area and thickness, structural and functional characteristics of the membrane
- Solute molecular size and charge, solute-membrane interaction based on the elements described in the previous points
- Temperature and physicochemical properties of the solute under purification conditions

Role in ECLS

- Removes small, water-soluble molecules such as ammonia, urea, lactate, and electrolytes.
- Central to hemodialysis and the small-solute clearance component of MARS (Molecular Adsorbent Recirculating System), Prometheus, SPAD (Single Pass Albumin Dialysis), and CKRT (Continuous Kidney Replacement Therapy).

Limitations

- Ineffective for albumin-bound toxins (e.g., bilirubin, bile acids), which require albumin-binding dynamics or adsorptive processes. Since the diffusion process is based on the spontaneous movement of molecules induced by a concentration gradient and operated by the interaction between the characteristics of the molecule and the membrane, it is clear that large molecules or molecules with poor positive interaction with the membrane cannot be removed from the blood through the diffusion process alone. To increase the purification capabilities of this method, it is necessary to introduce the possibility of dragging these molecules and "forcing" their interaction with the membrane through a process of convection.

10.3.2 Convection

Convection refers to solute movement driven by solvent drag, where water transport across a membrane carries dissolved solutes with it. This process depends on hydrostatic pressure gradients, as described by Starling forces.

Key Determinants

- Transmembrane pressure
- Membrane permeability to water (ultrafiltration coefficient)
- Solute sieving coefficient (the fraction of solute passing with water). This becomes the fundamental point of interaction between molecule and membrane, as molecules capable of crossing the membrane will be removed with varying degrees of efficiency, while molecules that cannot be transported across the membrane will be retained, as is typically the case with albumin. However, this limitation is protective, as the elimination of useful molecules due to "excess permeability" of the membrane would cause harm to the patient
- Flow rate of ultrafiltration

Role in ECLS

- Clearance of middle-molecular-weight solutes such as cytokines, vasoactive substances, and some metabolites.
- Critical for hemofiltration, high-volume hemofiltration (HVHF), and the convective component of CKRT integrated with liver support.

Limitations

- Still limited for large, albumin-bound toxins unless combined with albumin-containing fluids or secondary adsorptive stages. This method also does not allow the removal of molecules bound to albumin, as it is not possible to remove albumin directly from the patient's blood without causing damage. Although membranes capable of removing albumin and higher molecular weight proteins are available (hollow fiber plasma separators), these devices cannot be used to indirectly remove albumin-bound hepatic toxins without also removing albumin itself, which is a protein essential for organic homeostasis, determining not only the oncotic force of the blood but also the transport of nutrients, catabolites, nutrients and drugs to various parts of the body for their actions or catabolism.

10.3.3 Adsorption

Adsorption is the binding of solutes to the surface of a solid matrix through physical (van der Waals forces, hydrophobic interactions) or chemical (ionic, covalent) interactions. It does not require a membrane or concentration gradient. Very often, the surface characteristics of the resins used in such devices do not allow their use on whole blood (hemoperfusion, HP) due to the possible activation of platelets, leukocytes, and complement. The solution is found in their use to adsorb plasma or albumin solutions from the patient (plasma perfusion, PP, or plasma adsorption, PA) or in completely covering the structure of the resin spheres with more compatible materials such as those used in membranes for kidney replacement therapy (KRT), but this process inevitably results in the loss of part of the device's purifying effectiveness due to the limitations of toxic-resin interactions.

Key Determinants

- Sorbent material (charcoal, resins, polymer beads)
- Surface area and pore size
- Binding affinities for specific toxins
- Flow rates and contact time

Role in ECLS

- Essential for removing protein-bound and albumin-bound toxins, including bilirubin, bile acids, aromatic amino acids, and various inflammatory mediators.
- Found in MARS detoxification columns, Prometheus adsorption cartridges, CytoSorb, HA330, and other hemoadsorption devices.
  Strengths:
- Highly effective for substances that cannot be removed via diffusion or convection.

Limitations

- Saturation of adsorbent materials requires cartridge changes. Reduced purification efficacy when used on whole blood in hemoperfusion to cover the resin with specific membranes to increase its biocompatibility. Reduced purification efficacy for treating reduced plasma volumes, as plasma production from whole blood provides the device with a much lower plasma flow rate in mL/min than the blood flow rate in mL/min obtainable through the common catheters used for extracorporeal circulation in KRT.
- Non-selective adsorption can remove therapeutically important molecules (e.g., antibiotics). These adsorbent devices are not generally tested for the removal of all drugs used in common clinical practice. Only case reports exist in the literature, and there is no robust literature available in this regard, leading to doubts and uncertainties about the removal of very useful molecules such as antibiotics, which play a fundamental role in this type of patient as part of medical therapy that could also be used during the liver transplant period.

10.4 Major Artificial ECLS Systems

10.4.1 Therapeutic Plasma Exchange (TPE)

Therapeutic plasma exchange is an extracorporeal blood purification technique performed using either centrifugation or membrane filtration. Substances most effectively removed by TPE are typically characterized by large molecular weight, with a predominant intravascular distribution and a prolonged half-life [11, 12]. The procedure relies on extracorporeal separation of plasma from cellular blood components in either continuous or intermittent flow modalities, with comparable therapeutic efficacy assumed between techniques [13, 14]. The cellular components are subsequently reinfused together with replacement fluid, resulting in effective removal of circulating toxins, immune complexes, cytokines, and other pathogenic macromolecules [12]. The technical description shows that this method does not use any principles of diffusion, convection, or adsorption to determine purification. In summary, the purification mechanism involves removing plasma from the patient and replacing it with donor plasma. In practice, the patient is purified by diluting the toxins present in the plasma. The process is similar, but not technically identical, to hemofiltration, with which it shares the principle of removing toxins by dilution. In ALF, TPE corrects hemostatic derangements by supplying coagulation factors while avoiding the volume overload associated with large-volume plasma infusion [15]. The choice of the anticoagulation strategy depends on the apheresis platform, with citrate anticoagulation being most commonly used [13]. Although the American Society for Apheresis classifies TPE in liver failure as a therapy requiring individualized consideration, it is widely recognized as a valuable intervention in ALF. In this setting, high-volume plasma exchange (8–12 L per session, performed daily for up to 3 days) improves transplant-free survival, as demonstrated in a randomized controlled trial by Larsen et al., and is associated with reductions in circulating toxins and inflammatory mediators (more effective removal of damage-associated molecular patterns (DAMPs), cytokines, ammonia), correction of coagulopathy, and improvement in hemodynamic stability (reduced vasopressor requirement, improved mean arterial pressure), particularly in patients not immediately eligible for liver transplantation [15].

In ACLF, TPE consistently improves biochemical parameters and systemic inflammation; however, a definitive survival benefit has not been demonstrated. This likely reflects the complex pathophysiology of ACLF, including underlying cirrhosis, immune dysregulation, and multiorgan dysfunction. Consequently, in ACLF, TPE is primarily employed as a supportive or bridging therapy, often integrated with other extracorporeal support modalities [16].

Advantages

- Provides rapid extracorporeal removal of circulating toxins, cytokines, and immune mediators
- Demonstrates documented transplant-free survival benefit in acute liver failure, particularly with high-volume exchange
- Improves coagulation abnormalities through plasma replacement
- Exerts a systemic immunomodulatory effect, attenuating inflammatory responses
- Technically established and widely available in tertiary care settings
- Serves as an effective bridge to transplantation, liver recovery, or clinical decision-making

Limitations

- Non-selective depletion of beneficial plasma components, including immunoglobulins and protein-bound drugs.
- Temporary physiological support, with potential rebound of toxins.
- Large volumes of replacement fluid, increasing resource utilization, and cost.
- Another limitation of the method, as a relative risk, is the anticoagulation of the circuit required by the devices used. Any underuse of anticoagulation could lead to a reduction in the efficiency of the method, with the achievement of partial purification objectives and a consequent reduction in patient outcomes (Table 10.1).

10.4.2 Single-Pass Albumin Dialysis (SPAD)

Single-pass albumin dialysis (SPAD) is a simpler and more cost-effective method of albumin dialysis that uses a CKRT platform modified by the addition of albumin to the dialysate, enabling the removal of albumin-bound toxins such as bilirubin and bile acids. Unlike MARS or Prometheus, the albumin solution is not recirculated but discarded after a single pass, which makes the technique technically simple but less efficient and more albumin-consuming [17, 18]. The clearance of albumin-bound solutes occurs through diffusion of toxins across the dialysis membrane into the albumin-containing dialysate, followed by their elimination in the effluent. SPAD has been used in a variety of clinical contexts, including adult and pediatric acute liver failure, cholestatic disorders, and drug-induced liver injury, and may be particularly useful in centers where MARS or Prometheus are unavailable or when rapid implementation is required. It has shown meaningful reductions in bilirubin, bile acids, and, to a lesser extent, ammonia, with case series describing clinical improvement, including encephalopathy reduction and hemodynamic stabilization. Thanks to its simplicity in terms of hardware and execution, this method is particularly useful in all healthcare contexts where experience in the field of CKRT is basic and more complex methods, such as HP, PP, and PA, are not available. SPAD provides a pragmatic, low-complexity option in settings where more advanced systems are unavailable.

Characteristics

- Used primarily in ICUs where MARS is not available.
- Lower efficacy due to reduced dialysate reuse. Specifically, the method is characterized as "single pass," meaning that the spent dialysate cannot be regenerated by any device and is therefore discarded. This affects the production costs of a high-volume albumin-enriched dialysate.
- Useful for refractory cholestasis and specific toxin ingestions.

It should be emphasized that CKRT primarily provides metabolic and ammonia control but does not address the accumulation of albumin-bound toxins, which requires albumin-based or adsorptive technologies.

10.4.3 Molecular Adsorbent Recirculating System (MARS)

MARS is the most widely studied artificial liver support system. It uses albumin dialysis to remove albumin-bound toxins. It is a high-cost intermittent method, whose effectiveness decreases over time, that also combines renal purification. Specifically, the patient's blood is interfaced through a specific membrane against a dialysate containing donor albumin. From this interaction, the toxins bound to the patient's albumin are transferred to the dialysate albumin, which recirculates in a closed circuit where it undergoes adsorption processes. The albumin solvent in this circuit consists of plasma water, which balances with the patient's plasma water through the membrane, ensuring the diffusion of small molecules and electrolytes. The closed donor albumin circuit also interfaces with a standard dialysate for CRT through a high-flow membrane, thus making it possible to dialysate the plasma water in the circuit and ensure renal purification of hydrophilic toxins for the patient. In a nutshell, hepatic toxins are removed by adsorption, while water-soluble molecules, including ammonium, pass sequentially from the patient's plasma water to the plasma water of the closed-loop recirculating donor albumin circuit and finally to the KRT dialysate [19–22].

Mechanism

- Patient blood circulates through a high-flux dialyzer against albumin-enriched dialysate (20% of albumin in the dialysate).
- The dialysate is cleaned by activated charcoal and anion-exchange resin columns and recirculated.

Clearance Targets

- Bilirubin (adsorption)
- Bile acids (adsorption)
- Aromatic amino acids (adsorption and diffusion)
- Ammonia (diffusion)
- Cytokines and nitric oxide derivatives (adsorption)

Evidence

- Improves biochemical parameters and encephalopathy.
- Mortality benefit remains controversial, though some survival advantages are seen in ACLF subsets. The method acts as a bridge to transplantation or recovery of organ function and can be implemented for a limited period of time due to its costs [19].

10.4.4 Fractionated Plasma Separation and Adsorption (FPSA) and Prometheus

Prometheus is the system that implements a combination of fractionated plasma separation with high-flux hemodialysis, aiming to combine the strengths of albumin dialysis with direct albumin purification. This method is unique because it treats the patient's own albumin, rather than relying on exogenous albumin dialysate (as MARS and SPAD) [23]. Specifically, this method consists of two steps in series. In the first step, a hollow fiber plasma separator produces albumin, which is adsorbed onto two specific cartridges. Once the albumin has been purified, it is returned to the bloodstream, and the blood undergoes a high-flow hemodialysis process (internal hemodiafiltration). In the first step, the hepatic toxins bound to the patient's albumin are removed by two adsorbent devices. In the second step, all water-soluble hepatic toxins, including ammonium, are removed by diffusion and convection. In the case of coexisting AKI (acute kidney injury) or AKI on CKD (chronic kidney disease), the second step is able to provide renal metabolic support to restore water-electrolyte and acid-base balance. This renal purification is also feasible in SPAD and MARS processes with varying degrees of efficiency depending on the treatment setting, but in all cases, these methods can achieve and maintain clinically relevant renal compensation in addition to removing water-soluble hepatic toxins, including ammonium.

Mechanism

The Prometheus system combines three sequential processes:

- *Fractionated Plasma Separation*: Blood enters a special high-permeability filter that allows albumin (66 kDa) to pass through, together with small and middle molecules, but retains larger proteins (immunoglobulins, clotting factors). This creates albumin-rich plasma filtrate, which is the focus of treatment. This solution is essentially an albuminate, i.e., it contains high concentrations of the patient's albumin dissolved in plasma water.
- *Adsorption (Detoxification of Albumin)*: The albumin-rich filtrate then passes through two adsorption columns: anion-exchange resin and neutral resin, allowing the removal of several toxins (bilirubin, bile acids, aromatic amino acids, fatty acids, phenols and phenol conjugates, medium-sized inflammatory mediators, endogenous benzodiazepine-like substances). This direct albumin purification results in higher clearance of bilirubin and bile acids than MARS in comparative studies [24, 25]. Unlike MARS, Prometheus directly purifies the patient's own albumin, which is purified directly by two devices in an extracorporeal circuit.

- *Conventional Hemodialysis/Hemofiltration*: The blood passes through a high-flux dialysis filter to remove water-soluble toxins. This integrates renal support with liver detoxification, which is beneficial because ACLF patients often develop hepatorenal dysfunction simultaneously (AKI or AKI/CKD).

Advantages vs MARS

- Greater clearance of bilirubin and bile acids.
- Higher mass transfer efficiency.

Limitations

- Less global survival improvement in large trials [18, 23]
- Another limitation of the method, as a relative risk, is the anticoagulation of the circuit required by the devices used. Any underuse of anticoagulation could lead to a reduction in the efficiency of the method, with the achievement of partial purification objectives and a consequent reduction in patient outcomes. This becomes particularly evident when adsorbent devices are used that have a marked activation of the coagulation cascade (Table 10.1)

10.4.5 Adsorption Technologies (CytoSorb, HA330, Resin Cartridges)

Hemoadsorption systems are increasingly used in combined liver-kidney failure or sepsis-associated ACLF. This technology involves adsorbing the patient's whole blood onto specific devices that have been made more hemocompatible by coating the resin spheres with a specially designed dialysis membrane. This process greatly increases hemocompatibility but reduces adsorbent capacity, as it introduces an additional interaction, namely the toxin-membrane interaction followed by the toxin-resin interaction. Technically, this increase in hemocompatibility can simplify the hardware of the method, as it no longer requires the production of plasma in order to perfuse a less hemocompatible device. This type of treatment also raises the issue of the non-specific removal of substances that may be beneficial, such as antibiotics or other drugs administered to the patient for specific intercurrent conditions. The possibility of hemoperfusion with these devices further simplifies the purification method, allowing this technology to be used in single hemoperfusion or in combination with CKRT.

Targets

- Cytokines (IL-6, TNF-α)
- Bilirubin (CytoSorb)
- Myoglobin

Often used as an adjunct to CKRT or MARS to modulate systemic inflammation.

10.5 Bioartificial Liver Support Systems (BALSS)

Bioartificial Liver Support Systems aim to temporarily replace both detoxification and true metabolic/synthetic functions of the liver. Unlike purely artificial devices (MARS, Prometheus, SPAD), which exclusively rely on physicochemical toxin removal, BALSS incorporate living hepatocytes within bioreactors, enabling partial replication of the liver's essential cellular activities [26]. These systems are designed to serve as a bridge to recovery or a bridge to transplantation, stabilizing patients with ALF or ACLF during the critical window before either liver regeneration or organ replacement occurs. BALSS use primary hepatocytes (porcine or human) or hepatocyte-like cell lines, seeded on hollow-fiber scaffolds or other three-dimensional matrices [27]. These cells aim to mimic the liver (the human liver performs more than 500 functions). By integrating hepatocyte bioreactors, BLASS theoretically offer detoxification, synthetic activity, metabolic regulation, and immunomodulation, although metabolic efficiency varies widely across systems [28]. Early clinical trials demonstrated biochemical improvements, particularly in ammonia and encephalopathy, but no consistent survival benefit has been established [26, 29].

10.5.1 Cell Sources

10.5.1.1 Primary Porcine Hepatocytes

Historically, it has been the most common source.

Advantages

- Abundant, metabolically active
- Good cytochrome activity

Limitations

- Immunologic concerns (xenoantigens)
- Risk of porcine endogenous retroviruses transmission (zoonoses)
- Short viability in culture
- Ethical and regulatory concerns
- When using cells from immortalized cell lines (hepatoblastoma), additional devices are required to protect against the release of cells from the bioreactor into the patient's systemic circulation during treatment.

10.5.1.2 Human Hepatocytes

Used less often due to limited availability and poor expansion in vitro.

10.5.1.3 Human Hepatoblastoma/Hepatocyte Cell Lines

Example: C3A cell line, used in the ELAD system.

Pros: Continuous expansion, stable phenotype.
Cons: Lower metabolic activity vs. primary hepatocytes.

10.5.1.4 Stem-Cell-Derived Hepatocyte-Like Cells

Highly promising but still experimental:

- Induced Pluripotent Stem Cells (iPSCs)
- Mesenchymal Stem Cells (MSCs)
- 3D liver organoids

These may overcome supply shortages and reduce zoonotic risks.

10.5.2 The Extracorporeal Liver Assist Device (ELAD) System

ELAD uses a large mass of viable human hepatocyte-like cells (C3A cells) in hollow-fiber bioreactors to perform functions the failing liver can no longer sustain. Patient plasma circulates through four hollow-fiber cartridges containing approximately 200–400 grams of live cells, allowing controlled exchange of solutes, nutrients, and hepatocyte-produced factors [30].

The patient's blood is withdrawn and passes through a plasma separator. Then the plasma goes through the hollow fiber bioreactors, a semipermeable membrane ($\approx$70 kDa cutoff) that allows diffusion of solutes (ammonia, bilirubin metabolites, small proteins) but retains cells on both sides [31]. The structure mimics a 3D microenvironment. Oxygenation and nutrient flow support cell viability, metabolic, and synthetic activity. After exposure to the bioreactors, the "treated" plasma is filtered again, combined with the cellular blood fraction, and finally returned to the patient's circulation [30].

Advantages of ELAD

- Human cell source (C3A): avoids xenogeneic risks associated with porcine hepatocytes
- Metabolic and synthetic capabilities beyond artificial detox systems
- Potential immunomodulatory effect, which may benefit inflammatory liver failure states
- Prolonged cell viability, allowing continuous therapy for 3–10 days
- No need for exogenous albumin, unlike MARS/SPAD

Limitations

- Lower albumin-bound toxin clearance vs. MARS or Prometheus
- Limited cytochrome P450 activity and incomplete replication of hepatocyte function
- High complexity and cost of bioreactor manufacturing and ICU operation
- Large, randomized trials have not shown a consistent survival benefit
- Most effective only in narrow patient subgroups (e.g., select alcoholic hepatitis phenotypes)

- Device logistics (transport, storage, priming, sterility) limit broad implementation

Despite encouraging biochemical and mechanistic data [32, 33], ELAD has produced mixed results in clinical trials:

- ALF: Some early stabilization observed, but no significant improvement in overall survival in large multicenter trials.
- Alcoholic Hepatitis (AH): A subgroup (younger patients, lower MELD, preserved renal function) showed potential benefit, but results were insufficient for regulatory approval.
- ACLF and post-transplant dysfunction: Limited evidence and no consistent outcome advantages (Table 10.1).

Currently, this method is not FDA-approved or EMA-approved and is considered experimental, with ongoing research focused on refining indications and improving cell and bioreactor performance.

10.5.3 BAL-AMC (Bioartificial Liver-Amsterdam Medical Center)

The BAL-AMC is a second-generation bioartificial liver support system developed at the Amsterdam Medical Center, designed to provide both detoxification and true metabolic support through the use of viable primary porcine hepatocytes cultured within a highly oxygenated hollow-fiber bioreactor. Unlike artificial systems that rely on physicochemical principles, the AMC-BAL delivers active hepatic functions such as urea cycle activity, ammonia detoxification, albumin synthesis, gluconeogenesis, and phase I/II detoxification. The system operates in a plasma-only circuit, preventing direct immune contact with xenogeneic cells while allowing bidirectional exchange of metabolites across semipermeable membranes. A defining feature of the AMC-BAL is its high-density hepatocyte culture supported by an optimized oxygenation system, enabling sustained metabolic performance during several hours of treatment. Early clinical studies in ALF demonstrated improvements in ammonia levels, hemodynamic stability, and hepatic encephalopathy, with a favorable safety profile and no evidence of porcine viral transmission. While the AMC-BAL showed promising biological activity, its use remains experimental, and further large-scale trials are required to confirm survival benefits and clinical applicability [33]. Current guidelines do not recommend their use in patients with liver failure [16, 34].

10.6 Clinical Indications and Device Selection

Selection of an extracorporeal liver support modality should be guided by the dominant pathophysiological abnormality, clinical context, and therapeutic goals. The decision algorithm presented in this chapter provides a structured approach to device selection in acute liver failure, acute-on-chronic liver failure, and related conditions (Fig. 10.1).

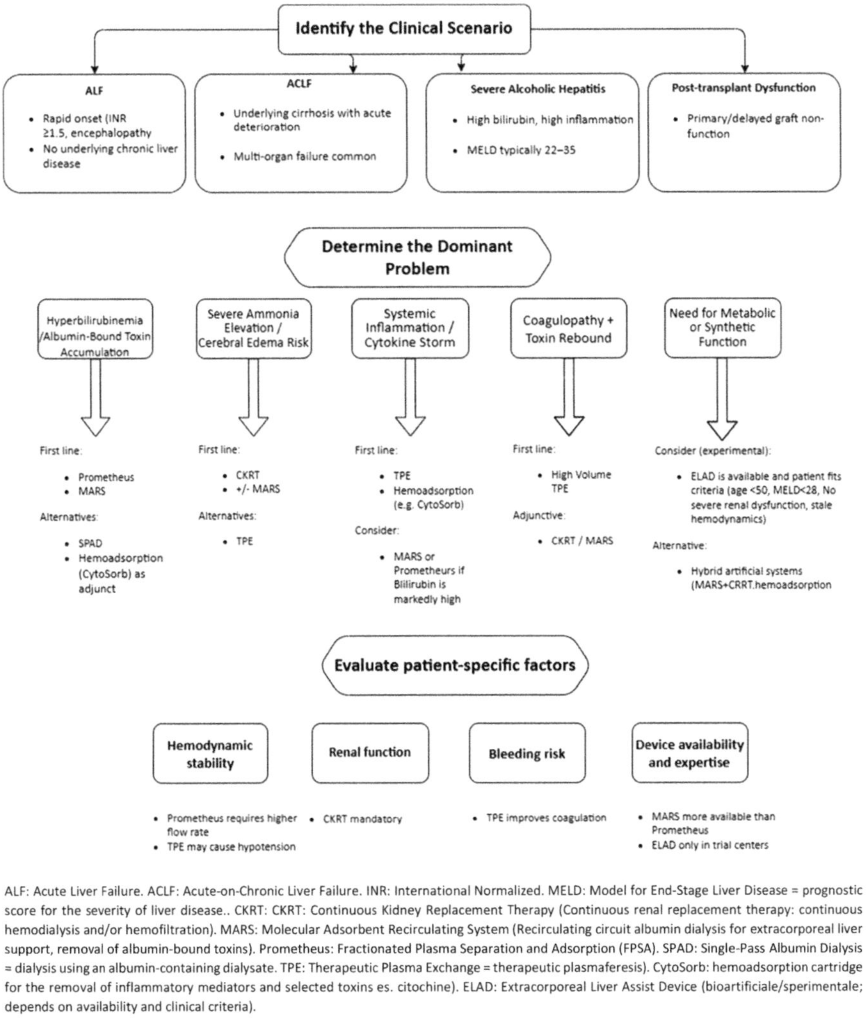

Fig. 10.1 Algorithm for selecting an extracorporeal liver support system. ALF: Acute Liver Failure. ACLF: Acute-on-Chronic Liver Failure. INR: International Normalized. MELD: Model for End-Stage Liver Disease = prognostic score for the severity of liver disease. CKRT: Continuous Kidney Replacement Therapy (Continuous renal replacement therapy: continuous hemodialysis and/or hemofiltration). MARS: Molecular Adsorbent Recirculating System (Recirculating circuit albumin dialysis for extracorporeal liver support, removal of albumin-bound toxins). Prometheus: Fractionated Plasma Separation and Adsorption (FPSA). SPAD: Single-Pass Albumin Dialysis = dialysis using an albumin-containing dialysate. TPE: Therapeutic Plasma Exchange = therapeutic plasmapheresis. CytoSorb: hemoadsorption cartridge for the removal of inflammatory mediators and selected toxins (es. citochine). ELAD: Extracorporeal Liver Assist Device (bioartificiale/sperimentale; depends on availability and clinical criteria)

10.7 Conclusion

ECLS systems represent an essential therapeutic bridge in the management of ALF, ACLF, and other severe hepatic dysfunctions where native liver recovery or transplantation is still possible. Artificial and bioartificial liver support has been studied for more than three decades; however, clinical results are far from comparable to those of whole liver transplantation. Considering that the purification by non-selective adsorption of blood components (bound to albumin) by artificial devices seems to be insufficient to support a sophisticated process such as the regeneration of a diseased liver, the clinical impact of bioartificial devices is mainly limited by a conceptual issue: their membranes. At the end of the last century, several artificial liver devices began to be developed for use as supportive therapy until liver transplantation (bridge-to-transplant) or liver regeneration (bridge-to-recovery). Modern artificial systems such as MARS, Prometheus/FPSA, SPAD, hemoadsorption cartridges, and therapeutic plasma exchange have demonstrated meaningful biochemical improvements and clinical stabilization, although robust survival benefits remain limited to specific scenarios, most notably high-volume TPE in ALF.

In the years that followed, experimental work and initial clinical applications were reported, and to date, many thousands of patients have already been treated with these devices [35].

MARS has proven to be a safe method with rare adverse events; its use leads to an improvement in encephalopathy without, however, having demonstrated a definite effect on the survival of treated patients [36–39].

Bioartificial liver systems, exemplified by ELAD and AMC-BAL, attempt to overcome the limitations of purely physicochemical detoxification by incorporating viable hepatocytes within engineered bioreactors. These systems offer the theoretical advantage of providing metabolic, synthetic, and immunomodulatory functions, yet challenges related to cell sourcing, bioreactor design, regulatory approval, and consistent clinical efficacy have thus far limited widespread adoption. Nevertheless, they remain a critical avenue of research, as true hepatic replacement therapy will ultimately require functional restoration and not detoxification alone. Given the diversity of underlying mechanisms in liver failure, no single ECLS modality is optimal for all patients. Instead, therapy must be tailored to the dominant pathophysiological problem and integrated with the patient's broader clinical context, including organ support requirements and transplant eligibility. Looking ahead, advances in stem cell–derived hepatocytes, 3D bioprinting, xeno-safe porcine lines, and microfluidic bioreactor engineering hold the potential to transform bioartificial liver therapy. Likewise, hybrid systems that combine adsorption, albumin dialysis, and biologic modules may offer more comprehensive support. Until then, current ECLS systems play a critical role as bridges to recovery, transplantation, or clinical decision, expanding therapeutic possibilities in what remains one of the most challenging areas of acute and critical care medicine.

Until true biological liver replacement becomes feasible, ECLS will remain a critical bridge that expands survival and therapeutic opportunity in patients with otherwise fatal liver failure.

Key Points

- ECLS systems are essential bridge therapies in ALF and ACLF, providing time for liver regeneration or transplantation.
- Artificial systems rely on diffusion, convection, and adsorption to remove toxins; TPE has the strongest evidence for survival benefit in ALF.
- MARS and Prometheus effectively clear albumin-bound toxins, while CKRT addresses ammonia and metabolic derangements.
- Bioartificial systems (ELAD, AMC-BAL) provide partial metabolic and synthetic support but remain experimental due to limited efficacy and logistical challenges.
- Device choice should be guided by the dominant clinical problem: bilirubin, ammonia, inflammation, or synthetic dysfunction.
- No current technology replaces full liver function; advances in stem-cell hepatocytes, organoids, and hybrid bioreactors may enable true functional liver replacement in the future.

References

1. Girish V, Royer A, John S. Acute liver failure.
2. Reuben A, Tillman H, Fontana RJ, Davern T, McGuire B, Stravitz RT, et al. Outcomes in adults with acute liver failure between 1998 and 2013: an observational cohort study. Ann Intern Med. 2016;164(11):724–32.
3. Bernal W, Wendon J. Acute liver failure. N Engl J Med. 2013;369(26):2525–34.
4. Reuben A, Koch DG, Lee WM. Drug-induced acute liver failure: results of a US multicenter, prospective study. Hepatology. 2010;52(6):2065–76.
5. Angeli P, Bernardi M, Villanueva C, Francoz C, Mookerjee RP, Trebicka J, et al. EASL Clinical Practice Guidelines for the management of patients with decompensated cirrhosis. J Hepatol. 2018;69(2):406–60.
6. Krisper P, Stauber RE. Technology Insight: artificial extracorporeal liver support—how does Prometheus® compare with MARS®? Nat Clin Pract Nephrol. 2007;3(5):267–76.
7. Nalesso F. L'evoluzione dei Trattamenti Combinati. Dalla Mars Alla PFAD: IL Plasma Come Mezzo Di Purificazione
8. Nalesso F, Brendolan A, Crepaldi C, Cruz D, De Cal M, Bellomo R, et al. Albumin dialysis and plasma filtration adsorption dialysis system. Contrib Nephrol. 2007;156(R):411.
9. Nalesso F. Plasma filtration adsorption dialysis (PFAD): a new technology for blood purification. Int J Artif Organs. 2005;28(7):731–8.
10. Hanish SI, Stein DM, Scalea JR, Essien E-o, Thurman P, Hutson WR, et al. Molecular adsorbent recirculating system effectively replaces hepatic function in severe acute liver failure. Ann Surg. 2017;266(4):677–84.
11. Fernández-Zarzoso M, Gómez-Seguí I, de la Rubia J. Therapeutic plasma exchange: review of current indications. Transfus Apher Sci. 2019;58(3):247–53.
12. Reeves HM, Winters JL. The mechanisms of action of plasma exchange. Br J Haematol. 2014;164(3):342–51.
13. Ward DM. Conventional apheresis therapies: a review. J Clin Apher. 2011;26(5):230–8.
14. Island T. StatPearls Publishing; 2022 Jan. PMID[Google Scholar]. 2023.
15. Larsen FS, Schmidt LE, Bernsmeier C, Rasmussen A, Isoniemi H, Patel VC, et al. High-volume plasma exchange in patients with acute liver failure: an open randomised controlled trial. J Hepatol. 2016;64(1):69–78.

16. Moreau R, Tonon M, Krag A, Angeli P, Berenguer M, Berzigotti A, et al. EASL Clinical Practice Guidelines on acute-on-chronic liver failure. J Hepatol. 2023;79(2):461–91.
17. Karvellas CJ, Gibney N, Kutsogiannis D, Wendon J, Bain VG. Bench-to-bedside review: current evidence for extracorporeal albumin dialysis systems in liver failure. Crit Care. 2007;11(3):215.
18. Stadlbauer V, Krisper P, Aigner R, Haditsch B, Jung A, Lackner C, et al. Effect of extracorporeal liver support by MARS and Prometheus on serum cytokines in acute-on-chronic liver failure. Crit Care. 2006;10(6):R169.
19. Gerth HU, Pohlen M, Thölking G, Pavenstädt H, Brand M, Hüsing-Kabar A, et al. Molecular adsorbent recirculating system can reduce short-term mortality among patients with acute-on-chronic liver failure—a retrospective analysis. Crit Care Med. 2017;45(10):1616–24.
20. Mitzner SR. Extracorporeal liver support-albumin dialysis with the Molecular Adsorbent Recirculating System (MARS). Ann Hepatol. 2016;10(S1):21–8.
21. Nguyen A, Mirza S, Javed N, Hanif H, Ryu M, Mirza RT, et al. Extracorporeal liver support: an updated review of mechanisms and current literature. Journal of Community Hospital Internal Medicine Perspectives. 2022;12(4):43.
22. Hernández DR, Valdez-Gaona A, García-Velasco LA, Lemus JS, Herrera OG, Membrila GC, et al. Single-Pass Albumin Dialysis (SPAD) as a Therapeutic Extracorporeal Liver Support in a Low-Resource Setting. Case Report and Literature Review Cureus. 2025;17(6)
23. Kribben A, Gerken G, Haag S, Herget-Rosenthal S, Treichel U, Betz C, et al. Effects of fractionated plasma separation and adsorption on survival in patients with acute-on-chronic liver failure. Gastroenterology. 2012;142(4):782–9. e3
24. Stadlbauer V, Krisper P, Beuers U, Haditsch B, Schneditz D, Jung A, et al. Removal of bile acids by two different extracorporeal liver support systems in acute-on-chronic liver failure. ASAIO J. 2007;53(2):187–93.
25. Evenepoel P, Laleman W, Wilmer A, Claes K, Kuypers D, Bammens B, et al. Prometheus versus molecular adsorbents recirculating system: comparison of efficiency in two different liver detoxification devices. Artif Organs. 2006;30(4):276–84.
26. Struecker B, Raschzok N, Sauer IM. Liver support strategies: cutting-edge technologies. Nat Rev Gastroenterol Hepatol. 2014;11(3):166–76.
27. He Y-T, Qi Y-N, Zhang B-Q, Li J-B, Bao J. Bioartificial liver support systems for acute liver failure: a systematic review and meta-analysis of the clinical and preclinical literature. World J Gastroenterol. 2019;25(27):3634.
28. Demetriou AA, Brown RS Jr, Busuttil RW, Fair J, McGuire BM, Rosenthal P, et al. Prospective, randomized, multicenter, controlled trial of a bioartificial liver in treating acute liver failure. Ann Surg. 2004;239(5):660–70.
29. Thompson J, Jones N, Al-Khafaji A, Malik S, Reich D, Munoz S, et al. Extracorporeal cellular therapy (ELAD) in severe alcoholic hepatitis: a multinational, prospective, controlled, randomized trial. Liver Transpl. 2018;24(3):380–93.
30. Pless G. Artificial and bioartificial liver support. Organogenesis. 2007;3(1):20–4.
31. Duan Z, Xin S, Zhang J, You S, Chen Y, Liu H, et al. Comparison of extracorporeal cellular therapy (ELAD®) vs standard of care in a randomized controlled clinical trial in treating Chinese subjects with acute-on-chronic liver failure. Hepatic Med Evid Res. 2018:139–52.
32. van Wenum M, Adam AA, Hakvoort TB, Hendriks EJ, Shevchenko V, van Gulik TM, et al. Selecting cells for bioartificial liver devices and the importance of a 3D culture environment: a functional comparison between the HepaRG and C3A cell lines. Int J Biol Sci. 2016;12(8):964.
33. Van de Kerkhove M, Poyck P, Deurholt T, Hoekstra R, Chamuleau R, Van Gulik T. Liver support therapy: an overview of the AMC-bioartificial liver research. Dig Surg. 2005;22(4):254–64.
34. Alexandra S, Nizar M, Jamilé W-F, Saleh A, Wong RJ, Limketkai BN, et al. Acute Liver Failure Guidelines. Am J Gastroenterol. 2023;118(7):1128–53.
35. García Martínez JJ, Bendjelid K. Artificial liver support systems: what is new over the last decade? Ann Intensive Care. 2018;8(1):109.

36. Mitzner SR, Stange J, Klammt S, Risler T, Erley CM, Bader BD, et al. Improvement of hepatorenal syndrome with extracorporeal albumin dialysis MARS: results of a prospective, randomized, controlled clinical trial. Liver Transpl. 2000;6(3):277–86.
37. Heemann U, Treichel U, Loock J, Philipp T, Gerken G, Malago M, et al. Albumin dialysis in cirrhosis with superimposed acute liver injury: a prospective, controlled study. Hepatology. 2002;36(4):949–58.
38. Sen S, Davies NA, Mookerjee RP, Cheshire LM, Hodges SJ, Williams R, et al. Pathophysiological effects of albumin dialysis in acute-on-chronic liver failure: a randomized controlled study. Liver Transpl. 2004;10(9):1109–19.
39. Hassanein TI, Tofteng F, Brown RS Jr, McGuire B, Lynch P, Mehta R, et al. Randomized controlled study of extracorporeal albumin dialysis for hepatic encephalopathy in advanced cirrhosis. Hepatology. 2007;46(6):1853–62.

Extracorporeal CO_2 Removal: Techniques and Clinical Applications

11

Vlad Cristian Sanda, Sergio Lassola, and Francesco Alessandri

11.1 Physiopathology of CO_2

Carbon dioxide (CO_2) is a waste molecule produced during the citric acid cycle (Krebs cycle) in the cytoplasm and mitochondria. CO_2 production at rest is approximately 250 mL/min, and 1 liter of blood carries approximately 500 mL of CO_2. It is transported to the lungs via hemoglobin, in the form of HCO_3−, or dissolved in plasma. In the lungs, at the interface between blood and air, the partial pressure gradient of CO_2 ($PaCO_2$) and the alveolar partial pressure of CO_2 ($PACO_2$) is close to zero. The diffusion coefficient of CO_2 is 20 times higher than that of O_2, which speeds up the elimination of CO_2 [1]. Considering this mechanism, the ratio between ventilated areas and perfused areas has a central role. The ventilation/perfusion (V/Q) ratio is a validated index showing how gas exchange is optimized when this ratio is close to 1. In healthy lungs, the ventilated areas are also well perfused so the gas exchange is guaranteed by the gradient formed by the different partial pressures of CO_2. In pathological situations in which there is an alteration of this gradient with

V. C. Sanda
Rianimazione Polivalente Azienda Ospedaliero-Universitaria Policlinico Umberto I di Roma, Rome, Italy
e-mail: V.Sanda@policlinicoumberto1.it

S. Lassola
Anestesia e Rianimazione 1, Ospedale Santa Chiara, Trento, Italy
e-mail: sergio.lassola@apss.tn.it

F. Alessandri (✉)
Rianimazione Polivalente Azienda Ospedaliero-Universitaria Policlinico Umberto I di Roma, Rome, Italy

Dipartimento Chirurgia Generale, Specialistica e Anestesiologia, Università Sapienza di Roma, Rome, Italy
e-mail: francesco.alessandri@uniroma1.it

S. De Rosa, S. Lassola (eds.), *Next-Gen Blood Purification*,
https://doi.org/10.1007/978-3-032-27033-7_11

a decrease in CO_2 exchange, hypercapnia occurs. Hypercapnia increases mortality, and it may have deleterious effects on different systems and functions: respiratory, cardiovascular, neurologic, and metabolic. On the respiratory system, hypercapnia induces tachypnea, air hunger, and general patient discomfort. On the cardiovascular side induces tachycardia, increases cardiac output, pulmonary and systemic resistance, leading to pulmonary hypertension. Severe hypercapnia may lead to myocardial depression and arrhythmias. It increases cerebral blood flow and intracranial pressure. Hypercapnia induces the release of endogenous catecholamines and corticosteroids, but it reduces the effects of exogenous vasopressors, particularly when acidosis occurs [2–4].

11.2 $ECCO_2$ Removal

Extracorporeal CO_2 removal ($ECCO_2R$) has been discussed since the late 1970s, when Kobolov and Gattinoni hypothesized that lung rest with near-apneic ventilation could improve outcomes in patients with acute respiratory failure. When the lungs are at rest, the problem is increased CO_2 levels, so the use of an $ECCO_2R$ system could solve the problem, with particular attention to anticoagulation monitoring [5, 6]. Several studies were conducted in the following years with increasing attractiveness toward extracorporeal therapy, although Morris et al. in 1994 published a randomized clinical trial that was unable to assess improvement in mortality rate among patients treated with $ECCO_2R$. On the contrary, it reported an augmented risk of adverse events such as bleeding [7]. In 2009, Terragni et al. published a study on the application of an ultraprotective 4 mL/Kg of predicted body weight (PBW) in moderate ARDS patients along with $ECCO_2R$ in order to compensate for the iatrogenic hypercapnia caused by the reduction in tidal volume. A low-flow (500 mL/min) $ECCO_2R$ normalized pH while maintaining ultraprotective ventilation, suggesting the use of this strategy in the rescue therapy of ARDS patients [8].

11.2.1 $ECCO_2R$ System

$ECCO_2R$ is a system consisting of a cannula that drains venous blood from a large caliber vein (usually the femoral, internal jugular, or subclavian vein) and a roller, centrifugal, or magnetic levitation pump at the air-blood interface inside a membrane (Fig. 11.1). The reoxygenated and decarbonated blood returns to the venous circulation through the same double-lumen inlet cannula (low-flow systems) or through a separate cannula (usually in high-flow systems). This veno-venous $ECCO_2R$ configuration is now the most common. In the past, arterio-venous $ECCO_2R$ was also used: these systems do not require a pump. A cannula placed in the femoral artery drains blood, which, under the pressure of the patient's cardiac output, reaches the membrane. The treated blood then returned to the patient through the femoral vein. This system was dependent on the patient's cardiac output (cardiac

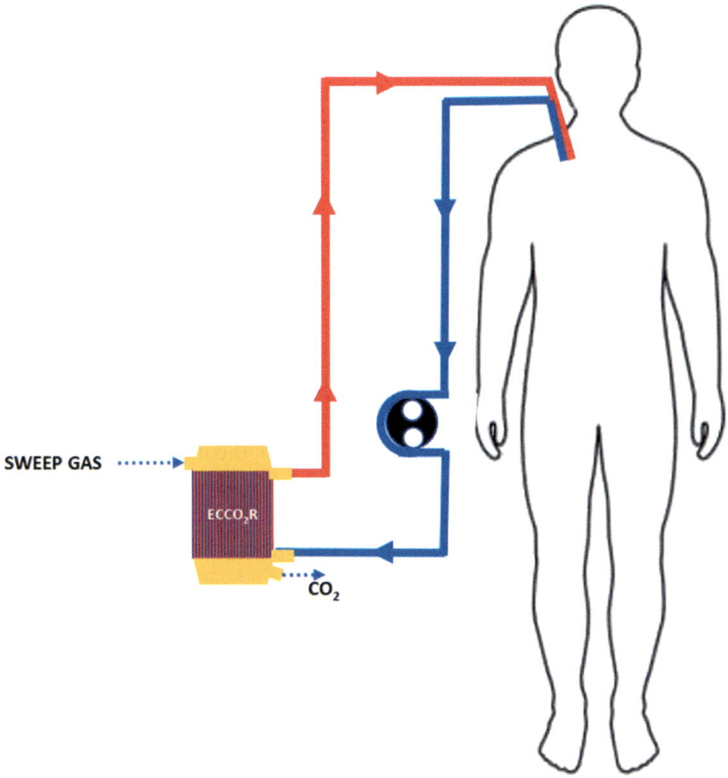

Fig. 11.1 Low-flow $ECCO_2R$ system

index of at least 3 L/min/m^2), which had to maintain an average arterial pressure of at least 70 mmHg. The high risk of serious complications (limb ischemia, vascular damage) led to the discontinuation of the arteriovenous system in favor of the veno-venous system. The veno-venous (VV) $ECCO_2R$ is more feasible for critically ill patients, particularly in case of heart failure or acute hemodynamic instability [9–12]. Based on the type of technology capable of developing a different blood flow, we distinguish between high-flow VV $ECCO_2R$ (blood flow 500–1000 mL/min) and low-flow VV $ECCO_2R$ (blood flow 200–500 mL/min). The first comes from VV ECMO technology, which is very efficient in removing CO_2, but usually requires two cannulas of at least 18–19 Fr. This system guarantees full control of CO_2 removal, but results in a higher risk of complications for the patient. It requires two cannulas, with an increased risk of bleeding and thrombosis. Otherwise, the low-flow $ECCO_2R$ comes from continuous renal replacement therapy (CRRT) technology; it is less invasive and requires a smaller double-lumen cannula (13–15 Fr). This system removes about 33% of the CO_2 produced with a lower risk of patient complications [13]. Among the variables involved in CO_2 reduction, in addition to blood flow, we must include the sweep gas flow and the specific characteristics of the artificial membrane, as well as its surface area. Artificial lung membranes designed specifically for CO_2 removal are made of non-porous polymethylpentene with a surface area ranging from 0.32 m^2 to 1.8 m^2. Another important component of $ECCO_2R$ systems is the pump, which is essential for creating blood flow in veno-venous systems. There are several types: roller, centrifugal, or diagonal, electric, or electromagnetic. Roller pumps are most commonly used in low-flow systems; other types of pumps generate higher flows (Table 11.1).

VV $ECCO_2R$ circuits are the most widely used and include the following:

- A drainage and reinfusion cannula, placed in a central vein (14–15Fr double-lumen catheter in low-flow circuits or two separate cannulas in high-flow systems).
- A pump that ensures negative pressure on the drainage side and positive pressure on the reinfusion side of the circuit.
- A membrane lung with a sweep gas flow (O_2 or medical air), which, according to the laws of diffusion, ensures the washing out of CO_2.

Normally, the amount of CO_2 in the blood is approximately 500 mL/L of blood. Ideally, a flow rate of 500 mL/min, as in low-flow $ECCO_2R$, should be sufficient to remove all the CO_2 produced. Unfortunately, in clinical practice, CO_2 removal depends on several other factors, such as the efficiency and duration of the membrane lung, constant blood flow (i.e., circulating blood volume), cardiac preload, pump efficiency, and the amount of blood recirculating in the system [14] (Fig. 11.1).

11.2.2 Anticoagulation

Anticoagulation is a main topic required; hence, blood flows through a non-physiological system. At this time, there is no gold standard of anticoagulation systems in $ECCO_2R$. Heparin is the most used systemic anticoagulation. Activated clotting time (ACT) and activated partial thromboplastin time (aPTT) are the main tests used to monitor the effectiveness of the anticoagulant system when unfractionated heparin or direct thrombin inhibitors (DTIs) are used. The most widely accepted target is 1.5–2.0 times the normal value for aPTT; this value is derived from ECMO

Table 11.1 Different characteristics of the low- and high-flow $ECCO_2R$

	Low-flow $ECCO_2R$	High-flow $ECCO_2R$
Blood flow mL/min	300–500	500–1000
Vascular access	VV	VV
Cannula size (Fr)	14–15	18–21
Cannula configuration	Double-lumen cannula	Arterial and venous cannulas
Membrane surface m^2	0.32–1.8	>4
Pumps	Roller	Centrifugal
CO_2 extraction (% of initial value)	50%	>50%

Table 11.2 Anticoagulation management

Anticoagulant agent	
Unfractionated heparin (UFH);	Standard anticoagulant for extracorporeal circuits given its reversibility
Direct thrombin inhibitors (i.e., bivalirudin, argatroban)	Especially in heparin-induced thrombocytopenia (HIT) scenarios
Monitoring tools	
Activated partial thromboplastin time (aPTT)	50–70 s, equivalent to 1.5–2.5× baseline; 40–60 s in low-flow $ECCO_2R$ settings. Monitoring frequency: Every 2–4 h initially;
Activated clotting time (ACT)	ACT >200 s: Unchanged ACT ≥180 ≤ 200 s increase infusion rate by 50% ACT <180 s: Intravenous heparin bolus (12.5 IU/kg) + increase infusion rate by 50% Generally, poor correlation with UFH levels;
Anti-Xa assays	0.3–0.5 IU/mL (some centers may use lower range 0.2–0.3 IU/mL in low-flow circuits) More specificity for heparin activity and stability in the presence of confounding factors (e.g., low antithrombin, hemolysis) Monitoring frequency: Anti-Xa once daily or in first 24 h if used
Viscoelastic assays (TEG/ROTEM)	Provide real-time insight into coagulation dynamics and help guide component transfusion or adjustment of anticoagulation therapy Monitoring frequency: Recommended early (first 24 h) to assess hemostatic profile; repeated as needed for bleeding or clot events

$ECCO_2R$ extracorporeal CO_2 removal, *TEG* thromboelastography, *ROTEM* rotational thromboelastometry

practice, and there is no $ECCO_2R$-specific consensus. ACT is less reliable and influenced by lots of variables, such as platelet count, hemodilution, or recent transfusions, and should not be used alone for anticoagulation monitoring (Table 11.2). During anticoagulation with heparin, considering its pharmacodynamics, it is necessary to constantly monitor the concentration of antithrombin III (ATIII) [15].

11.2.3 Complications

Adverse events are common during these therapies. They can be classified according to their correlation with the patient, with cannulation, or with the device. Among those related to the patient, the most important are worsening hypoxemia, bleeding, and hemolysis. During cannulation, the most common complications are bleeding from the insertion site, thrombosis, cannula twisting, cannula displacement, or aneurysm formation. Finally, possible complications of the device are mainly due to its malfunction, such as pump failure, air in the circuit, circuit clotting, oxygenator or heat exchanger failure [13].

11.3 Evidences

11.3.1 ARDS

Mortality in ARDS is about 40%. ARDSnet in the 2000s demonstrated the benefit of a protective ventilation strategy in reducing mortality, despite the fact that in one-third of patients, mechanical stress and hyperinflation persist, causing worsening inflammation. Further reduction of tidal volume to 4 mL/kg PBW inevitably causes iatrogenic hypercapnia, which $ECCO_2R$ can compensate for by maintaining normal pH. Several studies have been conducted in order to validate the use of this technique that at least theoretically permits to limit the lung damage induced by mechanical ventilation. According to the SUPERNOVA trial conducted by Combes et al., ultraprotective ventilation—facilitated by $ECCO_2R$—is a technically viable strategy for patients with moderate ARDS [16]. While the study reported a 28-day survival rate of 73%, the high incidence of complications (39%), including intracranial hemorrhage, suggests that the safety profile remains a concern. Notably, the data suggests that clinical benefit is most pronounced in patients with significant alveolar dead space or reduced lung compliance [16]. Conversely, the subsequent REST trial—a large-scale randomized controlled trial—failed to show a mortality benefit. Enrolling 405 patients, the study was prematurely terminated for futility after finding no significant difference in 90-day mortality between the $ECCO_2R$ group (41.5%) and the standard care group (39.5%) [17]. Furthermore, the intervention group saw fewer ventilator-free days and a higher incidence of serious complications, particularly bleeding and intracranial hemorrhage [17]. Several factors may have contributed to the REST trial's neutral findings: first, patient selection; the inclusion criteria focused primarily on oxygenation deficits rather than the severe acidosis or ventilatory failure that $ECCO_2R$ is specifically designed to treat. Second, equipment limitations, the use of centrifugal pumps may have reduced hydraulic efficiency at low flow rates, potentially increasing shear stress and blood component damage. Third, procedural risks, the combination of 15.5 Fr catheters and aggressive anticoagulation protocols (aPTT 45–90 s) likely exacerbated the observed bleeding risks [17]. Finally, institutional experience, a lack of standardized expertise across the participating centers, may have influenced the outcomes. However, due to several limitations, the conclusions remain uncertain, and ARDS guidelines restrict its use in this type of patient to clinical trials only [18]. Further studies are needed to validate its use as an adjunct to conventional therapy.

11.3.2 COPD

In patients suffering from COPD, the reduction in the lung surface area dedicated to gas exchange, associated with edema, inflammation, and bronchial secretions, causes prolonged expiratory time and air trapping. The residual expiratory lung volume exerts a certain intrinsic end-expiratory pressure ($PEEP_i$). The patient normally tries to compensate for gas exchange with rapid and frequent but inefficient breathing, which leads to compensated respiratory acidosis. CO_2 reaches a higher-than-normal baseline level as a result of renal compensation. When an acute exacerbation occurs, the pH becomes unbalanced, and respiratory acidosis develops. Non-invasive mechanical ventilation (NIV) is the gold standard for treating acute exacerbations of COPD, but in severe cases where there is no clinical improvement, the patient is intubated and invasively ventilated, with a worsening of the outcome. In this context, the use of $ECCO_2R$ could prevent orotracheal intubation in cases of NIV failure.

Del Sorbo et al. [19] investigated the potential of combining NIV with $ECCO_2R$ to prevent intubation in COPD patients at high risk of treatment failure. The study compared 25 patients against historical controls, defining "high risk" based on severe acidosis and significant tachypnea. While the addition of appeared to drastically reduce the risk of being intubated, the absolute difference in intubation rates (12% vs. 33%) did not reach statistical significance. Furthermore, the intervention carried a high complication rate; over half of the group experienced adverse events, including system malfunctions and rare but serious vascular injuries like vein perforation.

In the multicentric case-control ECLAIR study, 25 patients, treated with $ECCO_2R$ when NIV failed, were matched with 25 controls. Intubation was avoided in 14 patients (56%) in the $ECCO_2R$ group [20]. However, adverse events associated with $ECCO_2R$, such as bleeding, were observed in 11 patients, of whom major bleeding was observed in 9 patients (36%). The use of VV $ECCO_2R$ to avoid invasive mechanical ventilation was successful in just over half of the cases. However, relevant $ECCO_2R$-associated complications occurred in over one-third of cases. Despite the shorter period of IMV in the $ECCO_2R$ group, there were no significant differences in length of stay or in 28- and 90-day mortality rates between the two groups [20].

In the VENT-AVOID trial, researchers evaluated the impact of $ECCO_2R$ on ventilator-free days for COPD exacerbations. Enrolling 113 patients before being halted early due to slow recruitment, the study compared $ECCO_2R$ plus standard care against standard care alone across NIV and invasive mechanical ventilation (IMV) strata [21]. The primary endpoint, ventilator-free days, showed no significant improvement with $ECCO_2R$. Furthermore, a safety signal emerged in the NIV subgroup, where $ECCO_2R$ was associated with a 22% mortality rate compared to 0% in the control arm. The study concluded that $ECCO_2R$ does not provide a benefit for early ventilator independence in these patients [21].

Pisani et al. [22] reported that in COPD patients who are not yet ready to be weaned, the addition of $ECCO_2R$ during unsupported breathing avoids the increase in $PaCO_2$ and inspiratory effort. Among the participants who finished the full 24-hour protocol [22], Pisani et al. observed a significant reduction in $PaCO_2$, with decreases ranging from 23% to 47%. Notably, the effects persisted beyond the treatment period; it took between 2 and 4 days for CO_2 levels to revert to baseline once the extracorporeal support was removed [22].

$ECCO_2R$ can be applied in weaning from mechanical ventilation. There is no universal consensus in using $ECCO_2R$ as an adjuvant support to reduce fatigue of respiratory muscles in COPD exacerbation, but the perspective can be interesting. Numerous ongoing randomized studies are required to determine the efficacy of $ECCO_2R$ in patients with acute hypercapnic respiratory failure because there is insufficient evidence that it can reduce the rate of NIV failure and wean hypercapnic patients from IMV.

11.3.3 Bridge to Lung Transplant

Patients waiting for a lung transplant are often in respiratory failure due to the basal pathology. Extracorporeal devices in support of these patients can be required. The most common support in hypoxemia is ECMO, although in selected patients with respiratory acidosis but with sufficient oxygenation, $ECCO_2R$ can be an adequate option. In these patients, $ECCO_2R$ avoids intubation in the preoperative period. It can facilitate weaning from mechanical ventilation after surgery. The use of $ECCO_2R$ is less invasive than ECMO, and intraoperative control of gas exchange could be feasible [23]. A retrospective study by Ruberto et al. investigated whether using intraoperative $ECCO_2R$ could prevent the need for emergency ECMO in lung transplant patients exhibiting “intermediate” respiratory distress (characterized by severe acidosis but stable oxygenation). $ECCO_2R$ reduces ECMO reliance: patients receiving $ECCO_2R$ plus standard care required emergency ECMO significantly less frequently than those receiving standard care alone [24]. The use of $ECCO_2R$ successfully lowered mean pulmonary artery pressure (mPAP) while improving pH levels [24]. While $ECCO_2R$ appears to be an effective bridge that avoids more invasive ECMO in these specific cases, the authors emphasize that current evidence for this application is still limited.

11.3.4 Other Indications

Asthma is defined by persistent airway inflammation and bronchial hyperresponsiveness, often requiring ventilatory assistance when standard medical therapies fail during acute exacerbations. In cases of life-threatening respiratory failure, extracorporeal techniques such as ECMO and $ECCO_2R$ serve as vital adjuncts to manage gas exchange by ensuring adequate oxygenation or decarboxylation. A narrative review examining five studies—four focusing on VV ECMO and one on $ECCO_2R$—suggested that these supports may offer a survival benefit for mechanically ventilated patients with severe asthma compared to conventional ventilation alone [25]. However, the current body of evidence remains insufficient to recommend $ECCO_2R$ as a routine intervention for asthma exacerbations. Otherwise, it is viewed as a “rescue” therapy for refractory cases.

11.4 $ECCO_2R$ Plus CRRT

In a patient with acute kidney injury (AKI), lung function can be impaired, and vice versa, an acute lung injury can affect kidney function. It depends on a network of inflammatory mediators known as the kidney-lung crosstalk. During AKI, tubular epithelial cells release high amounts of pro-inflammatory molecules locally but also into the bloodstream, reaching distant organs. Interleukin 1 (IL-1), interleukin 6 (IL-6), interleukin 8 (IL-8), TNF-α, tumor necrosis factor receptor 1, caspase-3, T cells, nitric oxide, and others increase vascular permeability, inflammation, cellular apoptosis, and oxidative stress. Considering its high capillary system, the lung is one of the most important targets of these inflammatory mediators, making the lung highly related to the kidney. Moreover, during AKI, patients are treated with high amounts of fluids that can affect the lung by accumulating in the interstitial space or worsening gas exchange. These are only some of the mechanisms that lead to lung injury during AKI. CRRT plus $ECCO_2R$ may be useful to treat patients suffering from acute hypoxic respiratory failure who develop AKI requiring CRRT. The rationale is to support both the respiratory system, allowing an ultraprotective ventilation strategy 4 mL/Kg of PBW, and avoiding fluid overload and worsening of renal function in patients that have already shown renal impairment [26]. The combined approach allows for better fluid management. Several studies on CRRT plus $ECCO_2R$ approach have hypothesized early recovery of renal function and a synergistic effect of the combination on reducing inflammation. The use of such platforms, capable of treating multiple organs simultaneously, could become increasingly widespread in the future to treat the trigger of inflammation that links various disorders in critically ill patients.

While $ECCO_2R$ is highly effective at clearing and allowing for "ultra-protective" lung ventilation (reducing tidal volumes to <4 mL/Kg PBW), this physiological success has not consistently translated into better long-term survival. According to current guideline positions, $ECCO_2R$ use is restricted to selected patients, specialized centers, and predominantly research settings.

References

1. Doyle J, Cooper JS. Physiology, carbon dioxide transport [Updated 2023 Jul 4]. In: StatPearls [Internet]. Treasure Island (FL): StatPearls Publishing; 2025. Available from: https://www.ncbi.nlm.nih.gov/books/NBK532988/
2. Bigatello LM, Patroniti N, Sangalli F. Permissive hypercapnia. Curr Opin Crit Care. 2001;7(1):34–40.
3. Nassar B. Should we be permissive with hypercapnia? Ann Am Thorac Soc. 2022;19(2):165–6.
4. Baumgardner JE, Hedenstierna G. Ventilation/perfusion distributions revisited. Curr Opin Anaesthesiol. 2016;29(1):2–7.
5. Scaramuzzo G, Ottaviani I, Volta CA, Spadaro S. Mechanical ventilation and COPD: from pathophysiology to ventilatory management. Minerva Med. 2022;113(3):460–70.
6. Kolobow T, Gattinoni L, Tomlinson TA, Pierce JE. Control of breathing using an extracorporeal membrane lung. Anesthesiology. 1977;46(2):138–41.

7. Morris AH, Wallace CJ, Menlove RL, Clemmer TP, Orme JF Jr, Weaver LK, Dean NC, Thomas F, East TD, Pace NL, Suchyta MR, Beck E, Bombino M, Sittig DF, Böhm S, Hoffmann B, Becks H, Butler S, Pearl J, Rasmusson B. Randomized clinical trial of pressure-controlled inverse ratio ventilation and extracorporeal CO2 removal for adult respiratory distress syndrome. Am J Respir Crit Care Med. 1994;149(2 Pt 1):295–305. Erratum in: Am J Respir Crit Care Med 1994;149(3 Pt 1):838
8. Terragni PP, Birocco A, Faggiano C, Ranieri VM. Extracorporeal CO2 removal. Contrib Nephrol. 2010;165:185–96.
9. Taccone FS, Malfertheiner MV, Ferrari F, Di Nardo M, Swol J, Broman LM, Vercaemst L, Barrett N, Pappalardo F, Belohlavek J, Mueller T, Lorusso R, Belliato M, EuroELSO Workgroup "Innovation on ECMO and ECLS". Extracorporeal CO2 removal in critically ill patients: a systematic review. Minerva Anestesiol. 2017;83(7):762–72.
10. Karagiannidis C, Kampe KA, Sipmann FS, Larsson A, Hedenstierna G, Windisch W, Mueller T. Veno-venous extracorporeal CO2 removal for the treatment of severe respiratory acidosis: pathophysiological and technical considerations. Crit Care. 2014;18(3):R124.
11. Morimont P, Batchinsky A, Lambermont B. Update on the role of extracorporeal CO_2 removal as an adjunct to mechanical ventilation in ARDS. Crit Care. 2015;19(1):117.
12. Camporota L, Barrett N. Current applications for the use of extracorporeal carbon dioxide removal in critically ill patients. Biomed Res Int. 2016:9781695.
13. Morelli A, Del Sorbo L, Pesenti A, Ranieri VM, Fan E. Extracorporeal carbon dioxide removal ($ECCO_2R$) in patients with acute respiratory failure. Intensive Care Med. 2017;43(4):519–30.
14. Tonetti T, Zanella A, Pérez-Torres D, Grasselli G, Ranieri VM. Current knowledge gaps in extracorporeal respiratory support. Intensive Care Med Exp. 2023;11(1):77.
15. Giraud R, Banfi C, Assouline B, De Charrière A, Cecconi M, Bendjelid K. The use of extracorporeal CO_2 removal in acute respiratory failure. Ann Intensive Care. 2021;11(1):43.
16. Morales-Quinteros L, Del Sorbo L, Artigas A. Extracorporeal carbon dioxide removal for acute hypercapnic respiratory failure. Ann Intensive Care. 2019;9(1):79.
17. Combes A, Fanelli V, Pham T, Ranieri VM. European Society of Intensive Care Medicine Trials Group and the "strategy of ultra-protective lung ventilation with extracorporeal CO2 removal for new-onset moderate to severe ARDS" (SUPERNOVA) investigators. Feasibility and safety of extracorporeal CO_2 removal to enhance protective ventilation in acute respiratory distress syndrome: the SUPERNOVA study. Intensive Care Med. 2019;45(5):592–600.
18. Grasselli G, Calfee CS, Camporota L, Poole D, Amato MBP, Antonelli M, Arabi YM, Baroncelli F, Beitler JR, Bellani G, Bellingan G, Blackwood B, Bos LDJ, Brochard L, Brodie D, Burns KEA, Combes A, D'Arrigo S, De Backer D, Demoule A, Einav S, Fan E, Ferguson ND, Frat JP, Gattinoni L, Guérin C, Herridge MS, Hodgson C, Hough CL, Jaber S, Juffermans NP, Karagiannidis C, Kesecioglu J, Kwizera A, Laffey JG, Mancebo J, Matthay MA, McAuley DF, Mercat A, Meyer NJ, Moss M, Munshi L, Myatra SN, Ng Gong M, Papazian L, Patel BK, Pellegrini M, Perner A, Pesenti A, Piquilloud L, Qiu H, Ranieri MV, Riviello E, Slutsky AS, Stapleton RD, Summers C, Thompson TB, Valente Barbas CS, Villar J, Ware LB, Weiss B, Zampieri FG, Azoulay E, Cecconi M; European Society of Intensive Care Medicine Taskforce on ARDS. ESICM guidelines on acute respiratory distress syndrome: definition, phenotyping and respiratory support strategies. Intensive Care Med. 2023;49(7):727–59.
19. Del Sorbo L, Pisani L, Filippini C, Fanelli V, Fasano L, Terragni P, Dell'Amore A, Urbino R, Mascia L, Evangelista A, Antro C, D'Amato R, Sucre MJ, Simonetti U, Persico P, Nava S, Ranieri VM. Extracorporeal Co2 removal in hypercapnic patients at risk of noninvasive ventilation failure: a matched cohort study with historical control. Crit Care Med. 2015;43(1):120–7. Pisani L, Fasano L, Corcione N, Comellini V, Guerrieri A, Ranieri MV, Nava S. Effects of extracorporeal CO2 removal on inspiratory effort and respiratory pattern in patients who fail weaning from mechanical ventilation. Am J Respir Crit Care Med 2015; 192(11):1392–4
20. Braune S, Sieweke A, Brettner F, Staudinger T, Joannidis M, Verbrugge S, Frings D, Nierhaus A, Wegscheider K, Kluge S. The feasibility and safety of extracorporeal carbon dioxide removal to avoid intubation in patients with COPD unresponsive to noninvasive ventilation

for acute hypercapnic respiratory failure (ECLAIR study): multicentre case-control study. Intensive Care Med. 2016;42(9):1437–44.
21. Duggal A, Conrad SA, Barrett NA, Saad M, Cheema T, Pannu S, Romero RS, Brochard L, Nava S, Ranieri VM, May A, Brodie D. Hill NS; VENT-AVOID investigators. Extracorporeal carbon Dioxide removal to avoid invasive ventilation during exacerbations of chronic obstructive pulmonary disease: VENT-AVOID trial – a randomized clinical trial. Am J Respir Crit Care Med. 2024;209(5):529–42.
22. Pisani L, Fasano L, Corcione N, Comellini V, Guerrieri A, Ranieri MV, Nava S. Effects of extracorporeal CO2 removal on inspiratory effort and respiratory pattern in patients who fail weaning from mechanical ventilation. Am J Respir Crit Care Med. 2015;192(11):1392–4.
23. Schellongowski P, Riss K, Staudinger T, Ullrich R, Krenn CG, Sitzwohl C, Bojic A, Wohlfarth P, Sperr WR, Rabitsch W, Aigner C, Taghavi S, Jaksch P, Klepetko W, Lang G. Extracorporeal CO2 removal as bridge to lung transplantation in life-threatening hypercapnia. Transpl Int. 2015;28(3):297–304.
24. Ruberto F, Alessandri F, Piazzolla M, Zullino V, Bruno K, Celli P, Diso D, Venuta F, Bilotta F, Pugliese F. Intraoperative use of extracorporeal CO_2 removal ($ECCO_2R$) and emergency ECMO requirement in patients undergoing lung transplant: a case-matched cohort retrospective study. J Anesth Analg Crit Care. 2022;2(1):22.
25. Ekechukwu N, Batra S, Orsi D, Rahmanian M, Bangar M, Mohamed A. Outcomes of extracorporeal life support (ECLS) in acute severe asthma: a narrative review. Lung. 2024;202(2):91–6.
26. Redant S, De Bels D, Barbance O, Loulidi G, Honoré PM. Extracorporeal CO2 removal integrated within a continuous renal replacement circuit offers multiple advantages. Blood Purif. 2021;50(1):9–16.

Wearable and Portable Blood Purification Devices

12

Silvia De Rosa, Giuseppe Marini, and Anna Lorenzin

12.1 Introduction

End-stage renal disease (ESRD) is becoming an increasingly common health problem around the world [1]. The number of people who depend on dialysis or a kidney transplant continues to grow, mainly because life expectancy is increasing and chronic conditions like diabetes and high blood pressure are more widespread [2]. Today, more than two million patients rely on renal replacement therapies to survive [3]. Although current treatment options have saved countless lives, they still come with important limitations. Traditional hemodialysis is usually performed in a clinic several times per week and requires large machines, specialized staff, and significant infrastructure. Because it is intermittent, this type of dialysis causes repeated swings in fluid balance, toxins, and electrolytes in the body, changes that can lead to fatigue, cardiovascular stress, and reduced overall well-being [4]. Kidney transplantation remains the most effective treatment, but donor organs are limited and not all patients are eligible [5]. Even home-based dialysis, designed to offer more

S. De Rosa
Centre for Medical Sciences, University of Trento, Trento, Italy

Anesthesia and Intensive Care, Santa Chiara Hospital, Azienda Provinciale per i Servizi Sanitari di Trento, Trento, Italy
e-mail: silvia.derosa@unitn.it

G. Marini
Anesthesia and Intensive Care, Santa Chiara Hospital, Azienda Provinciale per i Servizi Sanitari di Trento, Trento, Italy
e-mail: giuseppe.marini@apss.tn.it

A. Lorenzin (✉)
Department of Nephrology Dialysis and Transplantation, San Bortolo Hospital, Vicenza, Italy

International Renal Research Institute of Vicenza (IRRIV), San Bortolo Hospital, Vicenza, Italy

S. De Rosa, S. Lassola (eds.), *Next-Gen Blood Purification*, https://doi.org/10.1007/978-3-032-27033-7_12

independence, can still feel restrictive due to equipment size, supply needs, and caregiver involvement. In response to these challenges, there has been growing interest in alternative solutions that allow treatment to be more flexible, continuous, and integrated into daily life. Wearable and portable blood purification devices are among the most promising innovations in this area [6]. Instead of requiring patients to be physically connected to large machines, these technologies aim to make dialysis lighter, mobile, and more frequent, more closely mimicking the natural behavior of a healthy kidney [7]. The purpose of this chapter is to provide a clear and updated overview of these emerging technologies. We will explore how wearable and portable devices work, the scientific advances that make them possible, where current development stands, and what barriers still need to be overcome before they become widely available. Understanding these innovations is important, because devices that are now prototypes and early clinical trials may soon reshape how we deliver kidney care, offering patients more freedom, better treatment stability, and a more normal life.

12.2 Rationale for Next-Generation Renal Replacement Therapy

Traditional dialysis only cleans the blood a few times per week, which means that toxins and excess fluid gradually build up between treatments and are then removed in a short period of time. This "stop-and-start" pattern can be hard on the body. Many patients experience fatigue, drops in blood pressure, cramps, and other uncomfortable symptoms because their system is constantly adjusting to these fluctuations. Home hemodialysis gives patients more flexibility, but the machines are still large and complicated, so not everyone feels comfortable or able to manage the process independently. Peritoneal dialysis (PD) offers a gentler and more continuous form of treatment, but it brings other challenges, including a risk of infection and the possibility that the peritoneal membrane may stop working over time [8]. For many patients, a kidney transplant would be the best solution because it can restore natural kidney function, including hormonal and metabolic regulation [2]. Unfortunately, donor organs are limited, waiting lists are long, and not all patients can undergo transplantation due to their health condition [5]. These limitations make it clear that new solutions are needed. Wearable and implantable dialysis systems offer a different approach, one that aims to provide treatment continuously or more frequently, without tying the patient to a hospital or large machine [9]. The goal is to make therapy gentler on the body, more compatible with everyday life, and less disruptive to physical and emotional well-being [10]. If successful, these next-generation devices could allow people living with kidney failure to have more independence, greater stability, and a better overall quality of life. A summary comparison of current renal replacement options and emerging technologies is shown in Table 12.1.

Table 12.1 Comparison of renal replacement modalities

Feature	In-center HD	Home HD	PD	Wearable/portable	Implantable
Treatment frequency	3/week	Variable	Variable	Continuous/ frequent	Continuous
Mobility	None	Limited	Moderate	High	Full
Infrastructure required	High	Moderate	Low	Low	Minimal
Dialysate needs	High	High	Moderate	Very low	None
Mimics native kidney	No	Partial	Partial	Partial	Yes

Summary of key clinical and functional characteristics of conventional and emerging renal replacement options

12.3 How Wearable Kidney Devices Work

Wearable artificial kidney systems combine several medical and engineering technologies to make dialysis smaller, lighter, and more adaptable to daily life. Although different prototypes use slightly different designs, they share the same goal: to clean the blood continuously or more frequently, without requiring patients to stay connected to a large dialysis machine [6]. To achieve this, wearable systems include a few essential components [6, 9]:

1. A filter (membrane) that removes toxins and extra fluid from the blood.
2. A pump to move blood and/or dialysate through the system.
3. A fluid management system, often using sorbents, to clean and reuse dialysate instead of relying on large volumes of new fluid.
4. Sensors and alarms to monitor pressure, flow, and safety.
5. A battery powerful enough to operate for many hours without needing a power outlet.

One of the biggest breakthroughs has been the development of advanced membranes and sorbent-based regeneration systems. These technologies allow the dialysate, the fluid used to clean the blood, to be continuously purified and reused, instead of being discarded [11]. This dramatically reduces the amount of fluid needed, which is one of the main barriers preventing portability. Another important area of progress is miniaturization [11]. Advances in microfluidics, nanomaterials, and battery technology have helped shrink components that once filled an entire clinic into compact, wearable units. Some experimental systems now weigh only a few kilograms and can be worn around the waist like a medical belt.

Modern prototypes are also being designed to interact with digital health systems. Built-in sensors can monitor blood flow, pressure, and treatment performance in real time. In the future, these devices may connect to smartphones or remote medical platforms, allowing healthcare teams to adjust treatment settings or safety parameters without the patient being physically present in a clinic [12].

Although these systems are still under development and testing, the technology is rapidly advancing. Each improvement brings wearable dialysis closer to becoming a safe, practical alternative to conventional treatment.

12.4 Current Wearable and Portable Devices in Development

In recent years, several prototype devices have been created and tested to explore whether dialysis can be delivered in a more mobile and patient-friendly way. While each design follows a slightly different approach, they all share a common goal: to make kidney therapy continuous, portable, and easier to integrate into everyday life. A summary of the main device categories and their current development status is shown in Table 12.2.

12.4.1 Wearable Artificial Kidney (WAK)

The Wearable Artificial Kidney (WAK) is one of the most recognized early prototypes. It is designed to be worn around the waist like a belt and to provide continuous dialysis using a sorbent-based system to regenerate dialysate. Early pilot studies have shown encouraging results. Patients using the WAK during testing were able to walk, sit, and carry out normal activities while the device performed dialysis in the background. The prototypes successfully removed toxins and helped regulate fluid balance, demonstrating that continuous ambulatory dialysis is technically possible outside a clinical setting. However, early trials also revealed areas that need further refinement. Some challenges included variability in flow control, device reliability over extended use, and patient comfort while wearing the system. In addition, long-term safety and stability still require more research before the device can move beyond experimental use. These findings are not unusual for early-stage medical technology, and they have guided ongoing engineering improvements and next-generation designs [6, 9]. Despite these challenges, the WAK remains a key milestone in the evolution of portable dialysis. Its development has proven that continuous, movement-compatible dialysis is feasible, and it has paved the way for newer wearable and implantable solutions that continue to build on its foundation.

12.4.2 Portable Hemodialysis Systems

Another area of innovation involves portable hemodialysis machines that are designed for use at home or while traveling. These systems are not wearable, but they are significantly smaller and more user-friendly than conventional dialysis equipment [6]. Their main advantage is flexibility: patients can dialyze more often or for longer sessions, which can lead to better toxin control, fewer symptoms after treatment, and overall improved well-being. Portable systems aim to reduce the logistical barriers of home dialysis. Many are built to use less water, fewer supplies,

Table 12.2 Overview of wearable and portable blood purification technologies

Device type	Technology Used	Dialysis mode	Development stage	Key advantages	Main challenges
Wearable artificial kidney (WAK)	Sorbent-based dialysate regeneration	Hemodialysis	Early human trials	Continuous therapy, patient mobility	Flow variability, comfort, long-term safety
Portable hemodialysis systems	Miniaturized hemodialysis components, reduced water requirement	Hemodialysis	Early clinical use	Travel/home use, increased frequency flexibility	Not wearable, still requires supplies
Automated wearable artificial kidney (AWAK)	Sorbent regeneration in closed-loop system	Peritoneal dialysis	Pilot human study	Low dialysate use, wearable PD	Abdominal discomfort, ultrafiltration control
Portable peritoneal dialysis systems	Automated fluid control, reduced dialysate volume	Peritoneal dialysis	Prototype	Simpler workflow, remote monitoring potential	Infection risk, durability testing ongoing
Vicenza wearable artificial kidney for peritoneal dialysis (ViWAK PD)	Sorbent regeneration in closed-loop system	Peritoneal dialysis	Prototype	Low dialysate use, wearable PD	Infection risk, sorbent saturation, and chemical stability of regenerated dialysate
Artificial diuresis (AD1)	Miniaturized elements, spontaneous ultrafiltration	Ultrafiltration	Prototype	Easy-to-use device	Infection risk, safety, and efficacy testing are ongoing in a clinical trial
Implantable renal assist device (iRAD)	Silicon nanopore membrane + renal cell bioreactor	Continuous hemofiltration	Preclinical	Physiologic replacement potential, no dialysate	Biocompatibility, regulatory pathway

Comparison of key characteristics of current prototype devices and emerging systems

and shorter setup times, making them easier to manage without professional assistance. Some devices are designed to fit on a bedside table or inside a small suitcase, which means patients can maintain treatment even when away from home. A key benefit of increasing treatment frequency is that it more closely mimics how healthy kidneys work, steadily and continuously, rather than in large intermittent shifts. This can help stabilize blood pressure, reduce cardiovascular stress, and prevent the uncomfortable physical fluctuations that many patients experience after traditional dialysis sessions. Although portable machines are already in use in some regions, ongoing work is focused on making them even more automated, intuitive, and compatible with digital monitoring platforms. In the future, these systems may be paired with telemedicine support and remote clinical supervision, giving patients more independence while still maintaining safety. Portable hemodialysis devices occupy an important middle step in the evolution of renal replacement therapy: they do not yet offer complete mobility like wearable systems, nor the biological integration of implantable devices, but they represent meaningful progress toward more patient-centered and flexible care [6].

12.4.3 Automated Wearable Artificial Kidney (AWAK)

The Automated Wearable Artificial Kidney (AWAK) takes a different approach from the WAK because it uses *PD rather than hemodialysis* [6]. Like the WAK, the AWAK relies on sorbent-based regeneration technology, which allows the dialysate to be cleaned and reused rather than discarded. This reduces the need for large volumes of fluid and makes the device much more portable than conventional PD systems [6]. Early feasibility work suggested that AWAK could provide a gentler and more physiologic treatment cycle, potentially making dialysis more compatible with everyday activities. To better understand its safety and performance, a preliminary clinical study was conducted in Singapore involving patients already receiving PD [13]. Fifteen participants completed up to nine AWAK treatments over a 72-hour period and were followed for one month. The study reported *no serious adverse events*, which is an encouraging safety indicator. Some users did experience side effects—mainly abdominal discomfort and bloating, which affected around half of the participants [13]. Despite this, the treatment showed *meaningful reductions in urea, creatinine, phosphate, and β2-microglobulin levels*, demonstrating that the device was effective at clearing toxins [13]. The median peritoneal weekly Kt/V of urea achieved during the study was 3.0, a range consistent with adequate dialysis. Device adjustments were needed during early testing to address flow occlusions, reflecting the iterative nature of early-stage engineering and clinical refinement. Overall, the trial showed that AWAK is safe in short-term use, but further improvements are still required to enhance comfort, ultrafiltration performance, and usability [13]. With continued development, the AWAK has the potential to offer a lightweight and practical alternative to conventional PD, especially for patients seeking more independence and mobility.

12.4.4 Vicenza Wearable Artificial Kidney for Peritoneal Dialysis (ViWAK PD)

The Vicenza Wearable Artificial Kidney for Peritoneal Dialysis (ViWAK PD) is a wearable system designed to enable continuous ambulatory peritoneal dialysis (CAPD) for patients with chronic kidney disease [14]. Unlike previous wearable peritoneal dialysis systems such as AWAK, this prototype is designed to operate as a fully continuous closed-loop platform, more closely approximating natural renal physiology while enhancing patient mobility and autonomy. The device includes: (1) a double-lumen peritoneal catheter, (2) an outflow line for dialysate removal, (3) a compact rotary pump, (4) a regeneration circuit containing a waterproof module with four parallel sorbent cartridges filled with activated carbon and polystyrene resins, (5) a safety filter for air removal and microbiological protection, (6) an inflow line to return the regenerated dialysate to the peritoneal cavity, and (7) a handheld computer used as a remote controller [14]. Recent efforts to improve the performance of standard CAPD and automated peritoneal dialysis (APD) have encouraged the development of continuous-flow peritoneal dialysis systems. However, one of the main challenges of continuous-flow approaches is the need for large volumes of dialysate to significantly improve solute clearance. An alternative solution is the regeneration of small dialysate volumes that are continuously recirculated within the peritoneal cavity [14]. Using sorbents in combination with advanced catheter designs offers the possibility to regenerate dialysate directly within the system, reducing the overall consumption of dialysis fluid and improving toxin removal. This strategy may significantly enhance the efficiency of peritoneal dialysis.

With further refinement, this technology has the potential to become a practical alternative to current CAPD or APD therapies, offering higher weekly solute clearance (up to 1100 liters) and increased patient independence. Although several technical and clinical challenges remain, preliminary results demonstrate feasibility. We anticipate that this approach will stimulate further development and miniaturization of dialysis systems, ultimately improving treatment options and quality of life for patients.

12.4.5 Portable Peritoneal Dialysis Systems

Alongside wearable and portable hemodialysis innovations, several research teams and companies are also developing solutions to make PD more mobile and easier to manage. The goal of these systems is to reduce the amount of equipment patients need, simplify setup, and automate key steps in the treatment process, such as fluid exchanges and monitoring [6]. Portable PD systems are designed to give patients more freedom compared with standard home equipment, which can be bulky and require multiple bags of sterile dialysate. By integrating *compact fluid regeneration technology, reusable components, and automated controls***,** these devices aim to make PD more practical for daily life and travel [6].

Another important focus is user experience. Many patients report that current PD routines can feel repetitive, time-consuming, or intimidating, especially for those who live alone or have mobility challenges. Portable systems may help overcome these barriers by offering:

- Fewer manual connections.
- Simpler workflows.
- Automated alarms and safety checks.
- Digital tools that track treatment progress.

Some prototypes already include wireless connectivity features that allow clinicians to review treatment data remotely. This could improve confidence for both patients and healthcare providers, especially during the transition to more independent dialysis care. While these devices are still in development and testing, they represent an important step between conventional home dialysis and fully wearable solutions. As the technology matures, portable PD systems may help expand access to home-based treatment and give patients more flexibility and control over their therapy.

12.4.6 Artificial Diuresis AD1

There is a growing clinical need for new extracorporeal ultrafiltration technologies capable of providing safe and effective fluid removal through a simpler and more accessible approach. Current ultrafiltration systems are typically adapted from hemodialysis machines and remain complex, bulky, and outdated in design. Their use requires specialized staff, controlled environments, and large-bore vascular access, limiting their applicability in routine or decentralized care [15]. In response to these limitations, the concept of a smaller, user-friendly ultrafiltration device has become increasingly relevant. Advances in miniaturized components now make it possible to integrate compact and ergonomic elements into ultrafiltration circuits [15]. The AD1 system represents this evolution. It performs continuous ultrafiltration at low blood flow rates (approximately 60 mL/min) using a single peristaltic pump. The disposable component is a closed, sterile, saline-primed circuit that includes a hollow-fiber polysulfone filter, tubing, pressure and flow sensors, and detectors for air and blood leaks, all fully integrated [15].

Ultrafiltration occurs passively, with transmembrane pressure generated by the height difference between the filter outlet and the collection bag. This simple mechanism, combined with compact design and ease of use, highlights the potential of AD1 as a practical alternative to conventional ultrafiltration systems.

12.5 Implantable Artificial Kidney Technologies

While wearable and portable dialysis devices are important steps toward more flexible treatment, the long-term goal of innovation in this field is to move beyond external equipment altogether. Implantable artificial kidneys represent the next major stage of development and aim to function continuously inside the body, much more like a natural organ [6]. One of the most notable projects in this area is the Implantable Renal Assist Device (iRAD), which combines a synthetic hemofilter with a bioreactor containing living renal epithelial cells. The hemofilter uses silicon nanopore membranes engineered to mimic the filtration properties of the natural glomerulus. Blood passes through these microchannels using the patient's own blood pressure, without requiring external pumps. The filtrate then flows into the bioreactor, where the living cells perform some of the metabolic and regulatory functions of kidney tubules, including solute transport and electrolyte balance [6].

Early preclinical testing has shown promising results, including stable filtration, biocompatibility, and reliable cell function over time. Importantly, because the iRAD is designed to work without systemic immunosuppression, it may be suitable for patients who are not eligible for traditional organ transplantation. Research teams are now working to optimize membrane durability, energy independence, and long-term integration with the host circulatory system before moving into larger-scale human trials [6]. Although implantable systems are still in early development and remain years away from routine clinical use, they represent a major shift in how kidney failure may be treated in the future. If successful, these devices could one day eliminate the need for external dialysis therapy entirely. The usability, efficacy, and safety of the device were first evaluated in a prolonged in vivo study in animals [16]. A subsequent first-in-human, single-center, randomized, open-label crossover pilot trial is currently underway to further assess safety and clinical efficacy [17].

12.6 Challenges and Barriers

Although recent developments in wearable and implantable blood purification technologies are promising, several important challenges still need to be addressed before these devices can be widely adopted in clinical practice. Many of these limitations relate to safety, usability, regulation, and long-term performance. A major technical challenge is *vascular access*. Wearable hemodialysis requires repeated or continuous blood flow through small catheters or ports. Maintaining reliable access without infection, clot formation, or damage to blood vessels remains difficult. Similar challenges exist in peritoneal dialysis devices, where long-term use increases the risk of peritonitis and membrane failure. Another key issue is *device durability and biocompatibility*. Wearable systems must operate safely for many hours or days at a time, often subjected to movement, temperature changes, and varying pressure. Components such as membranes, pumps, and sorbents must function reliably without degrading, leaking, or generating harmful byproducts. Energy supply is also a barrier. Continuous dialysis requires a stable power source, yet batteries must remain lightweight, safe, and long-lasting. While energy-efficient pumps and microfluidic systems have reduced power demands, further optimization is needed before fully autonomous systems become practical. There are also *human-factor considerations*. Devices must be easy to use, comfortable to wear, and intuitive enough for patients with limited technical skills or physical limitations. Anxiety related to alarms, malfunctions, or accidental disconnection remains a concern in early user feedback. Finally, regulatory pathways are complex. These devices combine elements of dialysis machines, implantable medical devices, and biologic systems, creating new requirements for safety testing and approval. Cost will also play an important role, as large-scale adoption will depend on affordability and integration into existing healthcare systems.

12.7 Conclusion

Wearable, portable, and implantable blood purification technologies represent a major step forward in the evolution of renal replacement therapy. They aim to provide continuous or more frequent treatment, greater independence, and better alignment with the rhythms of daily life. While significant technical, logistical, and regulatory challenges remain, early clinical results demonstrate that these systems are feasible and increasingly effective. As research advances, these technologies may reshape care models, expanding home-based treatment and reducing reliance on large dialysis centers. In time, fully implantable, autonomous artificial kidneys could offer a transformative alternative to conventional dialysis and possibly reduce the need for organ transplantation. For patients living with kidney failure, these innovations offer not just a new treatment approach but the possibility of restored mobility, dignity, and quality of life.

References

1. Francis A, Harhay MN, Ong ACM, Tummalapalli SL, Ortiz A, Fogo AB, et al. Chronic kidney disease and the global public health agenda: an international consensus. Nat Rev Nephrol [Internet]. 3 aprile 2024 [citato 24 maggio 2024]; Disponibile su: https://www.nature.com/articles/s41581-024-00820-6
2. Shi B, Ying T, Chadban SJ. Survival after kidney transplantation compared with ongoing dialysis for people over 70 years of age: a matched-pair analysis. Am J Transpl. 2023;23(10):1551–60.
3. Robinson BM, Akizawa T, Jager KJ, Kerr PG, Saran R, Pisoni RL. Factors affecting outcomes in patients reaching end-stage kidney disease worldwide: differences in access to renal replacement therapy, modality use, and haemodialysis practices. Lancet. 2016;388(10041):294–306.
4. Canaud B. Recent advances in dialysis membranes. Curr Opin Nephrol Hypertens. 2021;30(6):613–22.
5. Anderson DJ, Locke JE. Progress towards solving the donor organ shortage. Nat Rev Nephrol. 2023;19(2):83–4.
6. Ramada DL, De Vries J, Vollenbroek J, Noor N, Ter Beek O, Mihăilă SM, et al. Portable, wearable and implantable artificial kidney systems: needs, opportunities and challenges. Nat Rev Nephrol. 2023;19(8):481–90.
7. Haleem A, Javaid M, Singh RP, Suman R. Telemedicine for healthcare: capabilities, features, barriers, and applications. Sensors Int. 2021;2:100117.
8. Davies S. The future of peritoneal dialysis. Clin Kidney J. 2024;17(Supplement_2):ii9–18.
9. Armignacco P, Lorenzin A, Neri M, Nalesso F, Garzotto F, Ronco C. Wearable devices for blood purification: principles, miniaturization, and technical challenges. Sem Dial. 2015;28(2):125–30.

10. Davenport A, Ronco C, Gura V. Portable and wearable dialysis: where are we now? Hemodialysis International [Internet]. ottobre 2010 [citato 24 novembre 2025];14(s1). Disponibile su: https://onlinelibrary.wiley.com/doi/10.1111/j.1542-4758.2010.00486.x
11. Fabiani T, Zarghamidehaghani M, Boi C, Dimartino S, Kentish S, De Angelis MG. Sorbent-based dialysate regeneration for the wearable artificial kidney: advancing material innovation via experimental and computational studies. Separat Purificat Technol. 2025;360:130776.
12. Shajari S, Kuruvinashetti K, Komeili A, Sundararaj U. The emergence of AI-based wearable sensors for digital health technology: a review. Sensors. 2023;23(23):9498.
13. Htay H, Gow SK, Jayaballa M, Oei EL, Chan CM, Wu SY, et al. Preliminary safety study of the automated wearable artificial kidney (AWAK) in peritoneal dialysis patients. Perit Dial Int luglio. 2022;42(4):394–402.
14. Ronco C, Fecondini L. The Vicenza wearable artificial kidney for peritoneal dialysis (ViWAK PD). Blood Purif. 2007;25(4):383–8.
15. Ramírez-Guerrero G, Ronco C, Lorenzin A, Brendolan A, Sgarabotto L, Zanella M, et al. Development of a new miniaturized system for ultrafiltration. Heart Fail Rev. 2024;29(3):615–30.
16. Lorenzin A, Sgarabotto L, Bacci ML, Elmi A, Ventrella D, Aniballi C, et al. Artificial diuresis: animal studies on efficacy and safety of a new miniaturized device for extracorporeal ultrafiltration. Cardiorenal Med. 2023:167–75.
17. Reis T, Sgarabotto L, Brendolan A, Lorenzin A, Corradi V, Marchionna N, et al. New miniaturized system for ultrafiltration: rationale and Design of a Single-Center, crossover, randomized, open-label, pilot study protocol. Cardiorenal Med. 2023:176–83.

Nanotechnology for Blood Purification 13

Flavia Carton, Paola Feraco, and Silvia De Rosa

Abbreviations

AO	Alcohol oxidase
BP	Blood purification
BPTs	Blood purification therapies
CAT	Catalase
CDCs	Carbon-derived carbons
CNTs	Carbon nanotubes
CU^{2+}	Copper ions
DIC	Disseminated intravascular coagulation
E. coli	*Escherichia coli*
EDTA	Ethylenediaminetetraacetic acid
EDTA-Fe_3O_4	Ethylenediaminetetraacetic acid magnetic particles
E-liposomes	Enzyme-loaded liposomes
FNs	Ferromagnetic NPs
GO	Graphene oxide
Hcy	Homocysteine
HD	Hemodialysis
HPAM	Hyperbranched poly(amidoamine)s
IAA	Indole-3-acetate

F. Carton (✉)
Centre for Medical Sciences (CISMed), University of Trento, Trento, Italy

Department of Cellular, Computational and Integrative Biology (CIBIO), University of Trento, Trento, Italy
e-mail: flavia.carton@unitn.it

P. Feraco · S. De Rosa
Centre for Medical Sciences (CISMed), University of Trento, Trento, Italy
e-mail: paola.feraco@unitn.it; silvia.derosa@unitn.it

S. De Rosa, S. Lassola (eds.), *Next-Gen Blood Purification*,
https://doi.org/10.1007/978-3-032-27033-7_13

IL-1β	Interleukin-1β
IL-6	Interleukin-6
IS	Indole sulfate
LA-liposomes	Linoleic acid-modified liposomes
LCMs	Lysine-modified cellulose/carbon nanotube microspheres
LMCMs	Lysine-modified macroporous cellulose/carbon nanotube microspheres
LPS	Lipopolysaccharides
MAHD	Magnetically assisted hemodialysis
MD	Magnetic dialyzer
MOF	Multiple organ failure
NATMs	Nanoporous atomically thin membranes
NMs	Nanomaterials
NO	Nitric oxide
NPs	Nanoparticles
PBUTs	Protein-bound uremic toxins
PCA-g-MWCNTs	Poly (citric acid)-grafted-multiwalled carbon nanotubes
PCS	p-Cresol sulfate
PDCs	Preceramic polymers
PEG	Polyethylene glycol
PEI	Polyethyleneimine
PES	Polyethersulfone
PFTs	Pore-forming toxins
RGO	Reduced graphene oxide
S. aureus	*Staphylococcus aureus*
S-HA	Sulfonated-hyaluronic acid
Si-C-N	Silicon carbonitride
TEM	Transmission electron microscopy
TEOS	Tetraethyl orthosilicate
TNF-α	Tumor necrosis factor alpha
UO_2^{2+}	Uranyl ions

13.1 Nanotechnology in Blood Purification

Blood purification (BP) is a medical therapy designed to "remove" dangerous compounds like waste products, toxins, drugs, or excess substances from the bloodstream. Blood purification therapies (BPTs) are commonly used when the body's own organs are dysfunctional, or in specific conditions such as hepatic dysfunction, autoimmune diseases, renal failure, sepsis, or acute intoxications. The main goal of BP is to treat metabolic organ dysfunction by stabilizing the patient's condition. In the case of sepsis, this involves restoring homeostasis of circulating mediators, rather than selectively inhibiting proinflammatory or anti-inflammatory mediators. Nowadays, different extracorporeal and intracorporeal BPTs have been developed, such as hemofiltration, hemoadsorption, hemodialysis, and peritoneal dialysis. Their efficacy varies according to the principle of function [1, 2]. Crucially, while promising and increasingly studied, these treatments are generally considered adjunctive to antibiotic therapy and organ support. Moreover, despite their widespread use, BPTs come with a number of significant weaknesses, including: (I) vascular complications (e.g., infection, vessel damage, stenosis), (II) bleeding (e.g., anticoagulation), (III) hemodynamic instability, (IV) nonselective removal, (V) loss of plasma components, (VI) modality-related complications (e.g., allergic reaction, air embolism), (VII) complexity, and (VIII) high costs [3–5].

In this regard, nanotechnology offers a promising field for overcoming the current limitations of BPTs. Nanotechnology employs engineered nanoparticles (NPs), which are 1–100 nm in size, to target and remove undesirable compounds from the blood more effectively than conventional methods.

For instance, nanotechnology can improve the specificity and selectivity of BP. This is accomplished by functionalizing the surface of nanomaterials (NMs) with ligands (e.g., antibodies, peptides, aptamers) to specifically interact with target substances (e.g., bacterial endotoxin, inflammatory cytokines, drug molecules, etc.) [6, 7]. This approach addresses the poor specificity of BPTs, which often risk removing both harmful and beneficial substances from the blood. To reduce bleeding risk, NMs can also be coated with molecules that slow the blood's clotting process or loaded with anticoagulant agents. Moreover, the high surface area-to-volume ratio of NMs makes them excellent adsorbents, thus enhancing removal efficiency. For instance, nanoporous materials like carbon nanotubes, silica- and graphene-based NMs offer a vast internal surface area that increases the adsorption capacity [8, 9]. To further improve hemocompatibility and reduce unwanted interactions, NMs are often engineered with a surface layer derived from a patient's own blood cells or leukocyte membrane fragments [10, 11]. Finally, NMs can be used as "theranostic systems", which combine the therapeutic function of BP with real-time diagnostic monitoring of toxins, pathogens, or biomarkers. The ability to combine therapeutic and diagnostic capabilities in a single nanodevice allows for more personalized and dynamic treatment adjustments [11]. In BPTs, NMs can be used in both extracorporeal and intracorporeal settings. The extracorporeal settings require specific phases: (I) blood sampling, (II) passage of blood through an extracorporeal loop, (III) introduction of NMs into the circuit, (IV) removal of NMs loaded with toxic agents from the device, and finally (V) return of purified blood to the patient [12–14]. The intracorporeal setting, conversely, involves direct injection of NMs into the patient's bloodstream to neutralize or clear undesirable compounds without an external circuit. Of these two approaches, the extracorporeal strategy is considered the safest and most practical pathway. It avoids major unresolved in vivo challenges, such as controlling biodistribution, preventing accumulation in organs like liver or spleen, long-term toxicity, immunological response, and embolism risk [15].

Nanotechnology is also being used to create new types of nanostructured membranes with enhanced stability, strength, selectivity, and permeability. These properties can be controlled by tailoring pore size and porosity, often using NMs like carbon nanotubes or graphene. Additionally, nanoadditives like titanium dioxide

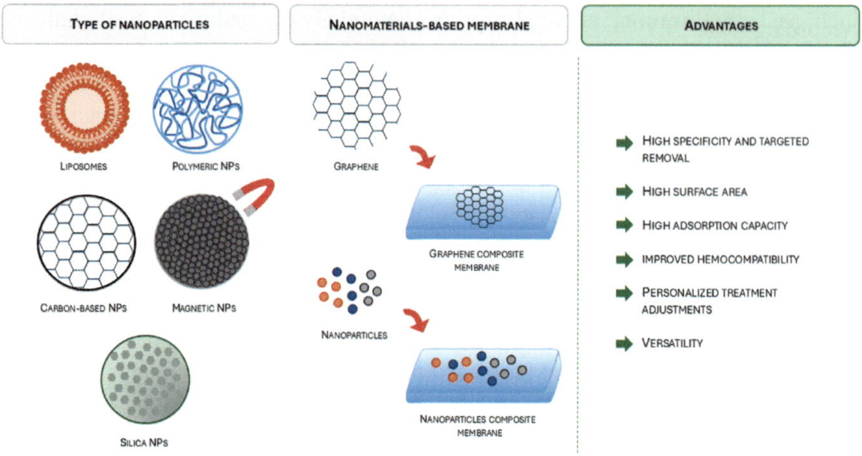

Fig. 13.1 NMs commonly utilized in BPTs with their associated advantages

can be integrated into membranes or applied as a coating to prevent biofilm formation, which compromises filtering efficiency [16–18]. All these approaches improve filtration efficiency, enhancing BPTs outcomes (Fig. 13.1).

This chapter endeavors to provide a comprehensive examination of nanotechnology's role in BPTs. The investigation covers the design principles, application strategies, outcomes, and challenges associated with nanotechnology-driven BP systems. Specifically, attention has been focused on the most used types of NMs and nanostructured membranes for BP in a variety of clinical conditions: acute intoxications, sepsis, bloodstream infections, chronic kidney disease, viral clearance, and other persistent conditions.

13.2 Magnetic Manomaterials

One of the most studied approaches for BP is magnetic bioseparation, which uses magnetic materials, typically alloys, oxides, or composites of iron, cobalt, and nickel. To be effective, these materials must be biocompatible, highly magnetic, and exhibit high target affinity. These properties can be achieved by functionalizing their surfaces with specific molecules to target and clear dangerous substances from the blood. Their magnetic nature enables the manipulation of these materials via an external magnetic field, facilitating the real-time removal of harmful compounds without disrupting blood flow dynamics [11, 13, 19] (Fig. 13.2).

As early as 2005, Kaminski et al. proposed a conceptual technology based on the development of polymeric nanospheres encapsulating nanocrystals of magnetic iron oxides. The nanospheres, coated with polyethylene glycol (PEG) to prolong circulation, were functionalized with receptors (e.g., antibodies or chelators) for selective toxin targeting. The system was designed to be directly injected into the bloodstream. Subsequently, an extracorporeal magnetic filter separated the toxin-loaded

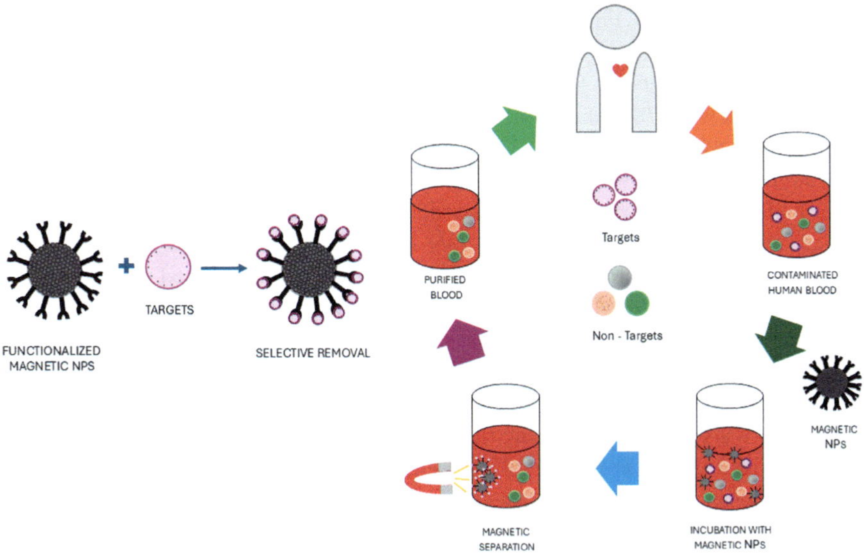

Fig. 13.2 Principle of BP using magnetic nanocomposites

nanospheres from the clean blood before returning it to the patient [20]. In the following years, various authors implemented this idea, testing different magnetic nanocomposites in vitro and in vivo. For instance, Hermann and co-workers developed carbon-coated iron carbide nanomagnets functionalized with ethylenediaminetetraacetic acid (EDTA)-like chelators, antidigoxin antibody fragments (digoxin immune FAB antigen-binding), and anti-human interleukin-6 antibodies. This system removed various agents from contaminated blood, including heavy metal ions Pb^{2+}, the steroid drug digoxin, and the protein interleukin-6 (IL-6) [7]. Similarly, Wang et al. successfully developed bisphosphonate-modified magnetite (Fe_3O_4) NPs for removing radionuclides from a biological fluid. In detail, a conjugate of dopamine and bisphosphonate was used to modify Fe_3O_4 NPs for binding uranyl ions (UO_2^{2+}). The designed NPs removed 69% of UO_2^{2+} from blood using a small bar magnet [21]. Using an extracorporeal BP circuit, Hermann et al. developed carbon-encapsulated iron carbide nanomagnets functionalized to capture lead ions and digoxin. This method achieved approximately 40% removal of lead and digoxin within 10 minutes, and over 75% within 40 minutes [22]. In a similar way, the same group developed an extracorporeal BP system that uses high-gradient magnetic separation to quickly and efficiently remove toxins directly from whole blood. Carbon-coated iron nanomagnets with core/shell geometry were functionalized with anti-digoxin and anti-interleukin-1β (IL-1β) antibodies as capturing moieties. The magnetic separation demonstrated a high removal efficiency, promising for clinical applications [12]. An article by Wan et al. described the synthesis of a new blood lead remover using Fe_3O_4 NPs as the core and amine-enriched hyperbranched poly(amidoamine)s (HPAM) as a template/co-adsorbent. The proposed magnetic remover first entered red blood cells to bind the lead, fixing it within the NPs' mesoporous channels. Finally, the remover was separated from the blood using a simple magnetic separation technology. In simulated blood, Pb^{2+} removal reached 80.1% in just 0.5 hours. When tested on rabbit and human blood samples, the removal rates were 78% and 76%, respectively. In a live pig, subjected to an extracorporeal circulation, the removal efficiency reached 75% after a single 50-minute operation [23]. Beyond heavy metals and drugs, magnetic NMs can also be used to clear endotoxins, which can cause uncontrolled inflammatory response, including sepsis, shock, disseminated intravascular coagulation (DIC), and multiple organ failure (MOF). For example, Hermann et al. successfully developed ultra-magnetic cobalt/iron alloy NPs and a polymyxin B-functionalized nanomagnet approach to eliminate endotoxin from human blood in vitro [24]. In another approach, lipopolysaccharides (LPS) sequestration was achieved using iron oxide NPs and macrophage membranes acting as a bait to specifically adsorb LPS. In an endotoxic mouse model, NPs significantly weakened the immune response, reduced inflammation, and improved the survival rate [25]. Kang et al. developed magnetic nanobeads coated with an engineered human opsonin, mannose-binding lectin, designed to sequestrate pathogens and toxins without activating complement or coagulation factors. In vitro studies proved that the fluidic device effectively eliminated over 90% of gram-negative and gram-positive bacteria, fungi, and endotoxins from whole human blood. In rat models of endotoxic shock, the extracorporeal BP device cleared over 90% of bacteria (e.g., *Staphylococcus aureus* (*S. aureus*) and *Escherichia coli* (*E. coli*)) from the blood. This led to reduced pathogen and immune cell infiltration, decreased inflammatory cytokine levels, and improved survival rates and physiological responses [26]. Xu and co-workers developed an integrated platform for the diagnosis and treatment of *S. aureus* bloodstream infection. The platform used magnetic mesoporous silica NPs modified with sulfonated-hyaluronic acid (S-HA) and an *S. aureus* antibody, loaded with the antibiotic vancomycin. In this system, *S. aureus* was specifically recognized by NPs. Once bound, the bacteria secreted an enzyme that degrades the S-HA coating of NPs, triggering the release of the encapsulated vancomycin, which showed a bacteriostatic efficiency of up to 98% against *S. aureus* [27].

Another area of interest in BP involves using an external magnetic field for blood cell identification and/or removal, which allows for the rapid and efficient detection and treatment of diseases. For instance, Ding et al. synthesized ethylenediaminetetraacetic acid-modified magnetic NPs (EDTA-Fe_3O_4) charged with copper ions (Cu^{2+}-EDTA-Fe_3O_4) for specific sequestration of hemoglobin from blood samples for biomedical diagnostic purposes. The removal process combined the selectivity of immobilized copper ions on NPs—targeting histidine-rich proteins such as hemoglobin—with the magnetic properties that allowed for easy separation. The particles demonstrated high efficiency and excellent selectivity for removing hemoglobin from both bovine and human blood samples. The maximum adsorption capacity for bovine hemoglobin was measured to be 1250 mg/g [28]. Similarly, Shi et al. developed Fe_3O_4 NPs coated with silica shell (SiO_2) using tetraethyl orthosilicate (TEOS) with copper ions (Cu^{2+}) grafted on the surface. The system showed

Table 13.1 Summary of the main compounds removed from whole blood by using different types of NMs including magnetic NPs, carbon-based NPs, polymeric NPs, and liposomes

Main target	Type of NPs	Model	References
Heavy metal ions (e.g., Pb^{2+}, $UO_2{}^{2+}$)	Magnetic NPs	In vitro In vivo	[7, 21–23]
Drugs (e.g., digoxin)	Magnetic NPs	In vitro (ex vivo) In vivo	[7, 12, 22]
Cytokine (e.g., tumor necrosis factor alpha (TNF-α), Interleukin-6 (IL-6), interleukin-1b (IL-1b)	Magnetic NPs Carbon-based NPs Polymeric NPs	In vitro (ex vivo) In vivo	[7, 12, 31–33, 42]
Endotoxin, gram-positive, and gram-negative bacteria	Magnetic NPs Polymeric NPs	In vitro In vivo	[24–27, 43]
Potentially toxic compounds (e.g., homocysteine, alpha toxin, uremic toxin, pore-forming toxins, protein-bound uremic toxins, p-cresol sulfate, indole sulfate, indole-3-acetate)	Magnetic NPs Polymeric NPs Liposomes	In vitro In vivo	[30, 39–41, 45, 46]
Blood cells (e.g., hemoglobin)	Magnetic NPs	In vitro	[28, 29]
Nitric oxide	Polymeric NPs	In vivo	[42]
Bilirubin	Carbon-based NPs Liposomes	In vitro	[34, 45]
Alcohol poisoning	Liposomes	In vitro In vivo	[44]

high affinity and selectivity for bovine hemoglobin, reaching a maximum adsorption capacity of 116.3 mg/g within 30 minutes [29]. Table 13.1 summarizes the main compounds removed using magnetic nanomaterials.

Magnetic NMs have also been studied to enhance the performance of conventional membrane filtration. Stamopoulos et al. introduced magnetically assisted hemodialysis (MAHD) as a new method for the selective and more efficient removal of toxins that conventional hemodialysis (HD) cannot adequately filter. The authors developed biocompatible ferromagnetic NPs (FNs) combined with a targeted binding substance (bovine serum albumin) for homocysteine (Hcy), a toxin not efficiently removed by conventional dialyzers. These NPs were administered to the patient before the MAHD session and then removed by a "magnetic dialyzer" (MD). The findings showed that the removal rate and efficiency of MAHD were significantly greater than those of conventional HD, suggesting that MAHD can be a promising method for specific toxin extraction [30].

In summary, magnetic NMs show great promise for BP, primarily because their efficient and targeted removal capabilities are coupled with the significant advantage of external manipulation via magnetic fields, which minimizes the disruption of blood flow dynamics. However, achieving the necessary biocompatibility and high magnetism remains a costly and complex synthesis challenge. Moreover, the potential for organ accumulation and long-term toxicity represents a critical safety concern if the NMs escape the extracorporeal circuit. These limitations could restrict the clinical translation of magnetic NMs, motivating further research into the discovery of carbon-based NMs.

13.3 Carbon-Based Nanomaterials

Another technology developed to optimize BP concerns the use of carbon-based NMs as nanoadsorbent materials. Their high surface-area-to-volume ratio, porous structure, tunable surface properties, and customizable functionality make them ideal for removing a wide range of toxins, pathogens, or unwanted molecules from the bloodstream. Several works outlined the importance of pore size and surface area accessibility for controlling the rate and effectiveness of the adsorption process. For instance, Yachamaneni et al. developed porous carbon-derived carbons (CDCs) as an effective material for cytokine adsorption, such as tumor necrosis factor alpha (TNF-α), IL-6, and IL-1β from plasma samples. This research underscores that the removal efficiency of cytokines was directly influenced by the relationship between the size of the cytokine molecule and the pore size of the CDCs. This relationship can be optimized by tuning the synthesis temperature, carbon particle size, and annealing conditions [31]. Presser et al. explored the potential of a specific type of CDCs, derived from silicon carbonitride (Si-C-N) preceramic polymers (PDCs), to separate inflammatory cytokines from human blood plasma. They found that cytokine removal was directly linked to the specific surface area of pores. In particular, the CDCs with a surface area of pores wider than 9.4 nm removed a maximum of 60% of TNF-α and up to 80% of IL-6 [32]. Similarly, Yushin and coworkers produced CDCs from ternary MAX-phase carbides, with an optimized pore structure with a large volume of slit-shaped mesopores. This porosity allowed large biological molecules to diffuse into the bulk of the adsorbent particles. This contrasts with conventional, primarily microporous activated carbons, where adsorption typically occurs only on the external surface. This study also confirmed that pore size control is a crucial factor for the effective removal of large cytokines from blood plasma [33]. These carbon-based NMs have also been developed to clear other potentially toxic agents from the blood. For instance, lysine-modified cellulose/carbon nanotube microspheres have been developed to treat conditions like liver disease, where excess bilirubin accumulates in the blood. Experimental results revealed that lysine-modified macroporous cellulose/carbon nanotube microspheres (LMCMs) had higher permeability, faster adsorption kinetics, and a higher adsorption capacity for bilirubin. This performance was superior to that of lysine-modified cellulose/carbon nanotube microspheres (LCMs) without macropores. The results show that LMCMs removed approximately 79% of the bilirubin in rabbit serum, whereas the LCMs (without macropores) removed only 67% of the bilirubin in rabbit serum [34]. Table 13.1 summarizes the main compounds removed using carbon-based nanomaterials.

Carbon-based NMs such as graphene oxide (GO), reduced graphene oxide (RGO), and carbon nanotubes (CNTs) have also been extensively investigated to develop novel membranes with high filtration efficiency. In several studies, graphene nanocoating, graphene oxide-based membranes, and CNTs have shown a range of beneficial properties. These include antibacterial effects, good hemocompatibility, improved solute transport, and heavy metal ion removal ability [35, 36]. For instance, Kidambi et al. describe a method for fabricating large-area nanoporous atomically thin membranes (NATMs) from graphene for dialysis applications. The graphene NATMs showed 1–2 orders of magnitude increase in permeance and a selective size separation over the commercial polymeric membrane, offering new opportunities in BP [37]. Abidin et al. developed a biocompatible and safe hemodialysis membrane using polyethersulfone (PES) embedded with poly(citric acid)-grafted multiwalled carbon nanotubes (PCA-g-MWCNTs). The study concluded that the developed PES/PCA-g-MWCNT nanocomposite membrane had the potential to be a safe and high-performance hemodialysis membrane [38].

In summary, carbon-based NMs offer the main advantage of highly efficient adsorption capacity and targeted toxin removal, enabled by their high surface area and tunable pore structure. However, a key limitation is represented by the critical dependence of removal effectiveness on the target molecule/carbon-based NMs pore size ratio, which requires precise synthesis tuning for optimal performance. Considering the potential issues with pore architecture, polymeric NMs are being investigated as an effective alternative for highly specific drug release and toxin sequestration.

13.4 Polymeric Nanomaterials

Polymeric NMs are being investigated for their potential in BP, particularly in the context of extracorporeal BPTs. These materials are solid, colloidal particles, made of natural or synthetic polymers that remove harmful substances through several key mechanisms. The first mechanism involves the use of NMs with a sponge-like structure to directly bind toxins from the blood. For instance, Ben-Akiva and coworkers developed biomimetic anisotropic polymeric NPs coated with red blood cell membranes as potential nanosystems for BP. The pharmacokinetic properties of the anisotropic coated particle contributed to a stronger capability to mediate detoxification of systemically administered bacterial toxin (alpha toxin). This capability was further supported by the increased surface area resulting from the anisotropic shape [39]. Similarly, engineers at the University of California designed a biomimetic "nanosponge" capable of safely removing pore-forming toxins (PFTs) from the bloodstream. These nanosponges consisted of a polymeric core enveloped by red blood cell bilayer membranes. In this system, the red blood cell membrane acted as a targeted "absorber," capturing and neutralizing toxins before they could cause cellular damage. In vitro studies demonstrated that nanosponges successfully prevented the destruction of red blood cells caused by PFTs. Meanwhile, in vivo experiments on mice showed that nanosponges could prevent skin and muscle tissue damage and increase survival rates in mice given a lethal dose of PFTs. Unlike anti-toxin platforms that require custom synthesis for individual toxin types, this innovative approach absorbs different pore-forming toxins regardless of their molecular structures [40]. Another method uses NMs functionalized with ligands to target specific compounds, like pathogens or malignant cells, which are then physically removed. Patel et al. developed polymeric NPs functionalized with heparin mimicking moieties capable of binding uremic toxins such as indoxyl sulfate and p-cresyl sulfate. The in vitro experiments showed a significant reduction in toxin levels without altering key blood parameters [41]. Lastly, polymeric NMs can deliver therapeutic agents that neutralize or break down toxins, offering an indirect BP method. Mishra developed polymer-encapsulated NPs loaded with ciprofloxacin, designed to target LPS in vivo. These NPs significantly reduced the production of TNF-α and nitric oxide (NO) in a LPS-induced sepsis model [42]. Similarly, Mas-Moruno et al. developed acylated peptide nanostructures with longer acyl chains to enhance LPS neutralization. Transmission electron microscopy (TEM) analysis showed that long-chain N-acylation promoted micellar and fibrous nanostructure formation, correlated with increased anti-LPS activity [43]. Table 13.1 summarizes the main compounds removed using polymeric nanomaterials.

In summary, the major advantage of polymeric NMs in BP stems from their broad mechanisms of action, ranging from direct adsorption (using sponge-like structures) and selective removal (via surface functionalization) to indirect benefit through therapeutic agent delivery. However, the clinical translation of these NMs is hampered by critical challenges such as safety concerns, the need to ensure long-term stability and shelf life, as well as the risk of secondary release of captured toxins or therapeutic agents. To overcome these limitations, other types of NMs have been explored as alternatives.

13.5 Other Nanomaterials for Blood Purification

In addition to the nanocarriers previously detailed, other NMs have been developed for BP purposes, including inorganic NMs such as silica NPs and organic nanovesicles such as liposomes.

Silica NPs are tiny particles of silicon dioxide (SiO_2), characterized by chemical and physical stability, high biocompatibility, and large surface area. Similarly to CNTs, silica NPs can be synthesized with different shapes, sizes, diameters, and porosities, making them versatile for different types of applications. In membrane technology, silica NPs have been widely applied as antimicrobial coatings. For instance, Wu et al. developed a polyamide thin-film composite membrane covalently bonded with silica NPs. The results proved that adding an optimal concentration of silica NPs significantly improved membrane performance and anti-fouling surface properties [17].

Another type of nanocarrier that has recently shown promising results in BPT strategies is the liposomes. Liposomes are made of phospholipids that form uni- or multilamellar spherical vesicles composed of a hydrophobic lipid bilayer and an aqueous inner core. Due to their unique structure, liposomes can enhance dialysis efficacy through two main mechanisms. First, the inner core can be modified or loaded with enzymes able to trap and extract specific toxins. Second, the lipid bilayers act as natural binders for lipophilic toxins and can be further modified and functionalized (e.g., by adjusting surface charge, liposolubility, and functional groups) to enhance binding capacity [8]. Pratsinis et al. developed enzyme-loaded liposomes (E-liposomes), containing alcohol oxidase (AO) and catalase (CAT), as direct nanoadsorbents to support peritoneal dialysis in a model of acute alcohol poisoning. The results revealed that E-Liposomes were able to enhance ethanol elimination in vitro and in rats [44]. In another study, Shen et al. developed linoleic acid-modified liposomes (LA-liposomes) as indirect adsorbents in the dialysate for protein-bound uremic toxins (PBUTs) and cholestatic solutes (e.g., bilirubin and bile acids). LA-liposome dialysate showed higher solute reduction rates of PBUTs and cholestatic solutes than traditional dialysate or dialysate supported by the unmodified plain liposomes [45]. In another study, the same authors developed polyethyleneimine (PEI)-anchored, linoleic acid-decorated liposomes to improve the clearance of PBUTs like p-cresol sulfate (PCS), indole sulfate (IS), and indole-3-acetate (IAA). This anchoring also improved biocompatibility and reduced the risk of hemolysis [46]. Table 13.1 summarizes the main compounds removed using liposomes.

In summary, silica NMs are advantageous due to their high stability, biocompatibility, and large surface area, making them versatile for improving membrane performance and anti-fouling properties. On the other hand, liposomes offer unique benefits via a dual-action structure, facilitating both the loading of enzymes in their core to trap toxins as well as the use of modified lipid bilayers to bind lipophilic toxins. However, advancing both nanosystems faces critical obstacles in clinical translation. These are primarily related to ensuring safety and stability in the bloodstream, and mitigating nonspecific adsorption, a process that risks complications like hemolysis.

13.6 Conclusion

This chapter focuses on the potential of nanotechnology for BPTs. Nanotechnology represents a transformative leap forward in BP, offering solutions to the significant limitations of traditional methods. By leveraging the unique physicochemical properties of NMs, such as their small size, high surface area, and tunable surface chemistry, it is possible to overcome key challenges. These challenges include nontargeted removal, low efficiency, poor hemocompatibility, and the risk of bleeding complications. The development of precisely engineered NMs to target and remove specific compounds, alongside the creation of advanced nanostructured membranes, promises to make BPTs more effective, safer, and tailored to the individual patient. Despite their great potential, the clinical translation of these systems remains constrained by unresolved challenges. The primary hurdles include safety concerns (toxicity, immunogenicity, blood clotting) and the practical use of these technologies in a clinical setting. While extracorporeal strategies, which use an external circuit, are considered the safest and most practical approach, the long-term effects of using these materials still require extensive research. Specifically, issues such as biodistribution, immunological responses, and potential organ accumulation need further investigation. In addition, the lack of standardized regulatory pathways, scalable good manufacturing practices, and cost-effective implementation must be addressed before these therapies reach clinical use. For these reasons, a greater focus on overcoming these challenges will be crucial for realizing the full potential of nanotechnology to revolutionize BP and improve patients' outcomes.

References

1. Mehta Y, Paul R, Ansari AS, et al. Extracorporeal blood purification strategies in sepsis and septic shock: an insight into recent advancements. World J Crit Care Med. 2023;12:71–88.
2. Bellomo R, Honoré P, Matson J, Ronco C, Winchester J. Extracorporeal blood treatment (EBT) methods in SIRS/sepsis. Int J Artif Organs. 2005;28:450–8.
3. Dianaty S, Khodadadi S, Alimoghaddam R, Mirzaei A. Comparison of outcomes and costs of extracorporeal blood purification therapies in critically ill COVID-19 patients. Ther Apher Dial. 2022;27:505–16.
4. Yessayan L, Pino CJ, Humes HD. Extracorporeal therapies in sepsis: a comprehensive review of the selective Cytopheretic device, Polymyxin B and seraph cartridges. Ren Fail. 2025;47:2459349.
5. Saha M, Allon M. Diagnosis, treatment, and prevention of hemodialysis emergencies. Clin J Am Soc Nephrol. 2017;12:357–69.
6. Phuong-Dung Ly K, Ly H-LP, Nguyen HHT, Duong V-A, Nguyen HV. Recent advances in surface decoration of nanoparticles in drug delivery. Front Nanotechnol. 2024;6
7. Herrmann IK, Urner M, Koehler FM, Hasler M, Roth-Z'Graggen B, Grass RN, Ziegler U, Beck-Schimmer B, Stark WJ. Blood purification using functionalized core/shell nanomagnets. Small. 2010;6:1388–92.
8. Shen Y, Shen Y, Bi X, Shen A, Wang Y, Ding F. Application of nanoparticles as novel adsorbents in blood purification strategies. Blood Purif. 2024;53:743–54.
9. Li Q, Ma L, Ma T, Cao S, Zhu B, Chen F, Qiu L, He C, Cheng C. Development trends of blood purification-related adsorbents: from novel adsorbents to functional porous materials. Blood Purif Mat. 2025;19:267–94.
10. Shen H, Ouyang Y, Zhang L, Li J, Wang S. Blood cell membrane-coated nanomaterials as a versatile biomimetic Nanoplatform for antitumor applications. Nano. 2024;14:1757.
11. Fahmawi S, Abu-Dalu AE-R. Application of nanoparticles in blood detoxification and viral clearance: development of Nanodevices for blood filtration in chronic kidney disease and other persistent conditions. Int J Innov Sci Res Technol. 2025:2500–5.
12. Herrmann IK, Bernabei RE, Urner M, Grass RN, Beck-Schimmer B, Stark WJ. Device for continuous extracorporeal blood purification using target-specific metal nanomagnets. Nephrol Dial Transplant. 2011;26:2948–54.
13. Herrmann IK, Schlegel AA, Graf R, Stark WJ, Beck-Schimmer B. Magnetic separation-based blood purification: a promising new approach for the removal of disease-causing compounds? J Nanobiotechnol. 2015;13:49.
14. Doswald S, Stark WJ, Beck-Schimmer B. Biochemical functionality of magnetic particles as nanosensors: how far away are we to implement them into clinical practice? J Nanobiotechnol. 2019;17:73.
15. Yuk SA, Kim H, Abutaleb NS, Dieterly AM, Taha MS, Tsifansky MD, Lyle LT, Seleem MN, Yeo Y. Nanocapsules modify membrane interaction of polymyxin B to enable safe systemic therapy of Gram-negative sepsis. Sci Adv. 2021;7:eabj1577.
16. Wójtowicz D, Stodolak-Zych E. Strategies to mitigate biofouling of nanocomposite polymer-based membranes in contact with blood. Membranes (Basel). 2023;13:762.

17. Wu H, Tang B, Wu P. Optimizing polyamide thin film composite membrane covalently bonded with modified mesoporous silica nanoparticles. J Membr Sci. 2013;428:341–8.
18. Adiga SP, Jin C, Curtiss LA, Monteiro-Riviere NA, Narayan RJ. Nanoporous membranes for medical and biological applications. Wiley Interdiscip Rev Nanomed Nanobiotechnol. 2009;1:568–81.
19. Yang Q, Dong Y, Qiu Y, Yang X, Cao H, Wu Y. Design of Functional Magnetic Nanocomposites for bioseparation. Colloids Surf B Biointerfaces. 2020;191:111014.
20. Kaminski MD, Rosengart AJ. Detoxification of blood using injectable magnetic nanospheres: a conceptual technology description. J Magn Magn Mater. 2005;293:398–403.
21. Wang L, Yang Z, Gao J, Xu K, Gu H, Zhang B, Zhang X, Xu B. A biocompatible method of Decorporation: bisphosphonate-modified magnetite nanoparticles to remove uranyl ions from blood. J Am Chem Soc. 2006;128:13358–9.
22. Herrmann IK, Schlegel A, Graf R, et al. Nanomagnet-based removal of lead and digoxin from living rats. Nanoscale. 2013;5:8718–23.
23. Wan MM, Xu TT, Chi B, et al. A safe and efficient strategy for the rapid elimination of blood Lead in vivo based on a capture–fix–separate mechanism. Angew Chem Int Ed. 2019;58:10582–6.
24. Herrmann IK, Urner M, Graf S, Schumacher CM, Roth-Z'graggen B, Hasler M, Stark WJ, Beck-Schimmer B. Endotoxin removal by magnetic separation-based blood purification. Adv Healthc Mater. 2013;2:829–35.
25. Shen S, Han F, Yuan A, Wu L, Cao J, Qian J, Qi X, Yan Y, Ge Y. Engineered nanoparticles disguised as macrophages for trapping lipopolysaccharide and preventing endotoxemia. Biomaterials. 2019;189:60–8.
26. Kang JH, Super M, Yung CW, et al. An extracorporeal blood-cleansing device for sepsis therapy. Nat Med. 2014;20:1211–6.
27. Xu T, Li J, Zhang S, Jin Y, Wang R. Integration of diagnosis and treatment in the detection and kill of *S. aureus* in the whole blood. Biosens Bioelectron. 2019;142:111507.
28. Ding C, Ma X, Yao X, Jia L. Facile synthesis of copper(II)-decorated magnetic particles for selective removal of hemoglobin from blood samples. J Chromatogr A. 2015;1424:18–26.
29. Shi L, Tang Y, Hao Y, He G, Gao R, Tang X. Selective adsorption of protein by a high-efficiency Cu2+-cooperated magnetic imprinted nanomaterial. J Sep Sci. 2016;39:2876–83.
30. Stamopoulos D, Bouziotis P, Benaki D, Kotsovassilis C, Zirogiannis PN. Utilization of nanobiotechnology in haemodialysis: mock-dialysis experiments on homocysteine. Nephrol Dial Transplant. 2008;23:3234–9.
31. Yachamaneni S, Yushin G, Yeon S-H, Gogotsi Y, Howell C, Sandeman S, Phillips G, Mikhalovsky S. Mesoporous carbide-derived carbon for cytokine removal from blood plasma. Biomaterials. 2010;31:4789–94.
32. Presser V, Yeon S-H, Vakifahmetoglu C, Howell CA, Sandeman SR, Colombo P, Mikhalovsky S, Gogotsi Y. Hierarchical porous carbide-derived carbons for the removal of cytokines from blood plasma. Adv Healthc Mater. 2012;1:796–800.
33. Yushin G, Hoffman EN, Barsoum MW, Gogotsi Y, Howell CA, Sandeman SR, Phillips GJ, Lloyd AW, Mikhalovsky SV. Mesoporous carbide-derived carbon with porosity tuned for efficient adsorption of cytokines. Biomaterials. 2006;27:5755–62.
34. Liangzhi Q, Shanshan W, Kaifeng D. Macroporous cellulose/carbon nanotube microspheres prepared by surfactant micelle swelling strategy for rapid and high-capacity adsorption of bilirubin. Cellulose. 2021;28:8419–28.
35. Agarwalla SV, Ellepola K, Sorokin V, Ihsan M, Silikas N, Neto AC, Seneviratne CJ, Rosa V. Antimicrobial-free graphene nanocoating decreases fungal yeast-to-hyphal switching and maturation of cross-kingdom biofilms containing clinical and antibiotic-resistant bacteria. Biomater Biosyst. 2022;8:100069.
36. Basile C, Davenport A, Mitra S, Pal A, Stamatialis D, Chrysochou C, Kirmizis D. Frontiers in hemodialysis: innovations and technological advances. Artif Organs. 2021;45:175–82.

37. Kidambi PR, Jang D, Idrobo J-C, Boutilier MSH, Wang L, Kong J, Karnik R. Nanoporous atomically thin graphene membranes for desalting and dialysis applications. Adv Mater. 2017; https://doi.org/10.1002/adma.201700277.
38. Abidin MNZ, Goh PS, Ismail AF, Othman MHD, Hasbullah H, Said N, Kadir SHSA, Kamal F, Abdullah MS, Ng BC. Development of biocompatible and safe polyethersulfone hemodialysis membrane incorporated with functionalized multi-walled carbon nanotubes. Mater Sci Eng C Mater Biol Appl. 2017;77:572–82.
39. Ben-Akiva E, Meyer RA, Yu H, Smith JT, Pardoll DM, Green JJ. Biomimetic anisotropic polymeric nanoparticles coated with red blood cell membranes for enhanced circulation and toxin removal. Sci Adv. 2020;6:eaay9035.
40. Hu C-MJ, Fang RH, Copp J, Luk BT, Zhang L. A biomimetic nanosponge that absorbs pore-forming toxins. Nature Nanotech. 2013;8:336–40.
41. Patel AK, Singhania RR, Chen C-W, Tseng Y-S, Kuo C-H, Wu C-H, Dong CD. Advances in micro- and nano bubbles technology for application in biochemical processes. Environ Technol Innovation. 2021;23:101729.
42. Mishra PR. An investigation on the approach to target lipopolysaccharide through polymeric capped nano-structured formulation for the management of sepsis. J Biomed Nanotechnol. 2011;7:47–9.
43. Mas-Moruno C, Cascales L, Cruz LJ, Mora P, Pérez-Payá E, Albericio F. Nanostructure formation enhances the activity of LPS-neutralizing peptides. ChemMedChem. 2008;3:1748–55.
44. Pratsinis A, Zuercher S, Forster V, Fischer EJ, Luciani P, Leroux J-C. Liposome-supported enzymatic peritoneal dialysis. Biomaterials. 2017;145:128–37.
45. Shen Y, Shen Y, Bi X, Li J, Chen Y, Zhu Q, Wang Y, Ding F. Linoleic acid-modified liposomes for the removal of protein-bound toxins: an in vitro study. Int J Artif Organs. 2021;44:393–403.
46. Shen Y, Shen Y, Li J, Ding F, Wang Y. Polyethyleneimine-anchored liposomes as scavengers for improving the efficiency of protein-bound uremic toxin clearance during dialysis. J Biomed Mater Res A. 2022;110:976–83.

14 Extracorporeal Blood Purification and Cancer Therapy

Novella Conti, Stefania Bianzina, and Pasquale Esposito

14.1 Introduction

The term "extracorporeal blood purification" (EBP) refers to various techniques that utilize an extracorporeal circuit to remove chemical or biological molecules from the circulation, thereby supporting specific organ functions or modulating immune and inflammatory responses.

The most used EBP is kidney replacement therapy (KRT), which itself can be delivered intermittently (intermittent kidney replacement therapy, IKRT) or continuously (continuous kidney replacement therapy, CKRT), through various methodologies, such as continuous veno-venous hemofiltration (CVVH), continuous veno-venous hemodialysis (CVVHD), and continuous veno-venous hemodiafiltration (CVVHDF) [71]. Further techniques include the use of sorbent cartridges and plasmapheresis-based therapies. According to the clinical scenario, these methods can be applied individually or in combination.

N. Conti
IRCCS Azienda Ospedaliera Metropolitana Policlinico San Martino, Nephrology, Dialysis and Transplantation, Genoa, Italy
e-mail: novella.conti@aomliguria.it

S. Bianzina
IRCCS Istituto Giannina Gaslini, Neonatal and Pediatric Intensive Care Unit, Emergency Department, Genoa, Italy
e-mail: stefaniabianzina@gaslini.org

P. Esposito (✉)
IRCCS Azienda Ospedaliera Metropolitana Policlinico San Martino, Nephrology, Dialysis and Transplantation, Genoa, Italy

Department of Internal Medicine and Medical Specialties (DIMI), University of Genova, Genoa, Italy
e-mail: pasquale.esposito@unige.it

S. De Rosa, S. Lassola (eds.), *Next-Gen Blood Purification*,
https://doi.org/10.1007/978-3-032-27033-7_14

The main underlying physiological mechanisms are diffusion, convection, ultrafiltration, and hemoadsorption, which are technical discussions far beyond the scope of this chapter (for more details, see other chapters of this book and Claure-Del Granado and Clark [18].

EBP has been mostly employed in specific clinical settings for conditions such as acute kidney injury (AKI), sepsis, and autoimmune diseases [103]. However, growing evidence suggests a role for these techniques in a broader range of conditions, such as necrotizing meningococcal sepsis, hyperbilirubinemia, rhabdomyolysis, poisoning, and, more recently, cytokine release syndrome (CRS) [12, 28].

This evidence has highlighted the potential utility of EBP in the management of cancer patients, who often present with distinctive cancer and treatment-related features.

Cancer therapy is a rapidly evolving field, and recent years have seen the development of new approaches, such as targeted therapies, immunotherapies, and cell-based treatments [5, 101]. While these strategies offer more personalized and effective therapeutic opportunities, they also introduce new challenges in managing treatment-related side effects [52, 102].

In this complex landscape, EBP may be useful not only as a supportive intervention to face treatment-related complications but also to counteract systemic inflammation and toxicity, and in specific settings, acting as a direct intervention in specific settings.

In this chapter, we discuss the current and potential applications of EBP in cancer therapy and consider interesting future perspectives.

14.2 Extracorporeal Blood Purification as a Supportive Strategy in the Management of Cancer Therapy Complications

Cancer is a global health issue with significant clinical, social, and economic effects. Over the last 20 years, structured screening programs, advances in cancer treatments, and improvements in supportive care have been adopted into clinical practice [56]. Despite these developments, patients receiving cancer treatment still face a high risk of systemic and organ-specific complications, many of which can greatly affect prognosis, reduce quality of life, and limit the success or feasibility of ongoing therapy [52]. The development of these complications results from a complex interaction of patient-specific, disease-specific, and treatment-specific factors, making their management challenging [81]. It often requires stopping the offending medication, the use of targeted drug therapies such as corticosteroids for immune-related adverse events, careful assessment and management of hemodynamics, and the implementation of comprehensive supportive strategies [61]. Among these interventions, EBP techniques, especially KRT, may provide valuable additional support in reducing the severity of complications and maintaining cancer treatment.

AKI is one of the most common and clinically important conditions, with the potential to not only worsen cancer prognosis but also to limit access to potentially life-saving oncologic therapies, extend hospitalization, and increase healthcare resource use [29]. Reported AKI incidence in cancer patients varies widely, from 12% to over 50%, with consistently higher rates in hematologic malignancies compared to solid tumors, and the highest frequencies seen in critically ill patients [17, 67]. Observational data show that, in adult groups, AKI occurs in up to 60% of patients with hematologic cancers, around 45% of those with kidney cancer, and about 30% in liver cancer and multiple myeloma [79]. In pediatric populations, the highest incidences are linked to urinary tract cancers, liver cancer, and retroperitoneal malignancies [100]. Known risk factors include advanced disease stage, female sex, intravascular volume depletion, renal hypoperfusion, preexisting chronic kidney disease, and diabetes mellitus. Severity of illness, age, and baseline functional status also significantly influence prognosis [46].

In addition to all causes encountered in the general population, the etiology of AKI in cancer patients includes cancer-specific mechanisms and treatment-induced nephrotoxicity (Table 14.1).

Chemotherapy-induced injury is a major contributor, with platinum-based compounds such as cisplatin, alkylating agents (including cyclophosphamide and

Table 14.1 Main causes of AKI in cancer patients

Category	Cause	Description
Patient-related factors	Hypovolemia	Mostly due to vomiting, diarrhea, or poor intake.
	Sepsis and systemic inflammation	Can cause renal hypoperfusion and direct injury.
	Preexisting CKD	Baseline renal impairment increases AKI risk.
	Use of nephrotoxic drugs	Includes NSAIDs and aminoglycosides.
Cancer-related factors	Urinary tract obstruction/direct renal infiltration	Postrenal AKI due to tumors or lymphadenopathy; common in lymphomas and leukemias (60–90% renal involvement in autopsy series).
	Multiple myeloma	Cast nephropathy from light chain deposition; causes tubular obstruction and toxicity.
	Membranous nephropathy	Most common malignancy-associated glomerular disease; often linked with lung, breast, renal/prostate, and colon cancers.
	ANCA vasculitis	Autoimmune glomerular inflammation linked to malignancy.
	Amyloidosis	Commonly secondary to multiple myeloma.
	Light chain deposition disease	Deposition of monoclonal light chains in kidneys.
	Hypercalcemia	From bone metastases or paraneoplastic syndromes; common in multiple myeloma, lymphoma, breast, lung, kidney cancers.
Treatment-related factors	Nephrotoxicity from different drugs [41]	Different mechanisms [89].

Abbreviations: *AKI* acute kidney injury, *CKD* chronic kidney disease, *NSAIDs* non-steroidal anti-inflammatory drugs ifosfamide), and antifolates such as methotrexate among the most implicated drugs. These agents may cause acute tubular toxicity, crystal-induced obstruction, or hemorrhagic cystitis, with risk influenced by dose intensity, age, comorbidities, and concomitant therapies [63]. Novel targeted agents and immune checkpoint inhibitors have introduced new nephrotoxic patterns, including immune-related adverse events manifesting as acute interstitial nephritis, glomerulonephritis, or electrolyte disturbances, and cellular immunotherapies have also recently been associated with distinct renal toxicities [72, 74]. In addition to direct renal injury, indirect mechanisms such as rhabdomyolysis and tumor lysis syndrome (TLS) can precipitate severe kidney damage and lead to life-threatening systemic derangements. TLS, an oncologic emergency most frequently associated with hematologic malignancies but also occurring in solid tumors, results from rapid tumor cell breakdown and release of intracellular contents, producing metabolic abnormalities including hyperuricemia, hyperkalemia, hyperphosphatemia, and hypocalcemia, which can lead to AKI, cardiac arrhythmias, and neurological complications [59].

Effective management of AKI in cancer patients requires prompt recognition, rapid initiation of specific therapeutic measures, and optimization of hydration, hemodynamic stability, and urinary output [21].

KRT, delivered as IKRT or CKRT, follows the same general indications of non-oncologic population (i.e., oligoanuria with fluid overload, hyperkalemia, severe metabolic acidosis, or uremic manifestations) while also addressing specific oncologic needs such as managing cancer-related hypercalcemia, TLS, chemotherapy- or immunotherapy-induced nephrotoxicity, and drug- or malignancy-associated thrombotic microangiopathy [60]. Utilization rates of KRT in critically ill patients with cancer range from 8–13% for solid tumors to 10–34% for hematologic malignancies, with reported short-term mortality rates of up to 66% [17, 20].

Facing the issue of AKI treatment in oncological patients, a potential question is whether performing KRT may be considered a suitable intervention.

In this regard, a large retrospective study analyzed 296,424 Intensive Care Unit (ICU) patients, specifically examining 35,356 patients with cancer of different origins [20]. Among them, 1408 (4.0%) developed AKI requiring KRT compared to 13,637 (5.2%) in the noncancer group. While overall mortality was higher in patients with cancer, deaths directly attributable to AKI were lower compared with noncancer patients. The authors concluded that the incidence and outcomes of KRT-requiring AKI in ICU patients with solid cancers are broadly comparable to those in other ICU populations, underscoring that cancer itself should not preclude KRT initiation.

In practice, while current evidence and clinical experience support applying the same indications for EBP in patients with cancer as in the general population of AKI patients, robust data to guide specific choices regarding timing, modality, and prescription are still lacking. As in noncancer patients, hemodynamically stable patients may be managed with intermittent hemodialysis (HD), while CKRT is often preferred in those who are unstable. However, the choice of therapy and dialysis membrane should also be guided by specific clinical indications [60].

So, while standard membranes and conventional HD are effective in replacing kidney function, advanced and specific EBP techniques or devices are increasingly being explored as adjunctive therapies in oncology. These approaches may help in removing proinflammatory mediators or circulating cellular components, modulating dysregulated immune responses, and reducing treatment-related toxicities (more details in the following paragraphs).

In this context, hemoadsorption has recently drawn attention for its potential role in managing cancer-related complications such as rhabdomyolysis-associated AKI, liver failure, and multiorgan dysfunction, particularly when triggered by endotoxemia, sepsis, or hyperinflammatory states [75].

Finally, it should be mentioned that EBP may be useful not only for the treatment of AKI or conditions such as rhabdomyolysis and tumor lysis syndrome, but it can also be employed in cases of drug overdose. Historically, this approach has been described in patients with cisplatin intoxication, which may manifest with nephrotoxicity, gastrointestinal toxicity, neurotoxicity, ototoxicity, and myelotoxicity [77]. In this context, standard HD is ineffective, whereas therapeutic plasma exchange (TPE) has been shown to reduce serum cisplatin concentrations and mitigate related toxicity [35]. More recently, similar strategies have been proposed as a second-line option for neurological complications following immunotherapy [58]. Nevertheless, even for this specific EBP application, no strong recommendations currently exist, and clinical experience remains very limited.

14.3 Extracorporeal Blood Purification as an Adjuvant Component of Cancer Therapy

As discussed above, and as well established by clinical practice and scientific evidence, EBP plays a primary role as a kidney-specific supportive therapy in the management of AKI and other conditions that affect renal function, such as rhabdomyolysis or drug-induced toxicity. However, it is increasingly evident that various EBP modalities can also modulate physiological and pathological processes, extending their application well beyond conventional kidney replacement therapy.

The paradigmatic example of this conceptual shift from supportive to therapeutic use is represented by sepsis, where current guidelines and recommendations acknowledge that EBP may be employed not only for renal support but also to attenuate the dysregulated inflammatory response and modulate immune function [103].

A similar evolution is now emerging in oncology. Indeed, beyond the management of treatment-related complications, modern perspectives suggest that EBP techniques may represent an active component of the therapeutic armamentarium, with potential to influence disease biology and complement existing pharmacological or cellular treatments.

In these contexts, EBP can be seen as an adjuvant strategy that may enhance and accelerate clinical responses. Examples of this application are monoclonal gammopathies and the modulation of the tumor microenvironment, which may facilitate the use of novel immunomodulatory therapeutic approaches.

14.3.1 EBP Application in Monoclonal Gammopathies

Monoclonal gammopathies, particularly multiple myeloma (MM), represent one of the most prevalent and challenging hematologic malignancies, often requiring a multimodal therapeutic approach [24]. In this setting, the removal of serum-free light chains (sFLCs) through EBP has been proposed as an adjunctive intervention to clone-directed therapies, which remain the cornerstone of treatment.

The rationale for sFLC removal lies in their nephrotoxic potential. Excessive production and subsequent glomerular filtration of sFLCs can exceed the proximal tubule's reabsorptive capacity, leading to intratubular accumulation [87]. This may cause AKI triggered by the formation of obstructive casts in the distal nephron (a process mostly known as cast nephropathy). Additional precipitating factors, including hypercalcemia, hypovolemia, and nephrotoxic medications, may contribute to this pathophysiology [65]. In these settings, EBP offers the potential advantage of physically removing the circulating pathogenic stimulus responsible for cast formation [30].

Candidates for extracorporeal sFLC removal are patients with MM who present with AKI and have biopsy-proven or strongly suspected cast nephropathy [26]. The primary therapeutic objective is to reduce the cast burden and limit further renal damage. Since cast nephropathy typically presents acutely, the appropriate timing of therapeutic intervention plays a critical role. Previous studies have shown that a reduction exceeding 50% in serum sFLC levels within the first 21 days after diagnosis significantly increases the likelihood of renal function recovery [39].

Once the indication for sFLC removal is established, the choice of EBP modality remains under debate. Due to their molecular weights, sFLCs (approximately 22.5 kDa for kappa and 45 kDa for lambda chains, often circulating as dimers) are poorly cleared by standard diffusive HD, including high-flux membranes, which typically have a molecular weight cut-off around 20 kDa [88]. Therefore, effective sFLC removal requires dialyzers with substantially higher cut-offs, such as high-cutoff (HCO) or medium-cutoff (MCO) membranes, or techniques based on adsorption, or plasma exchange.

The earliest clinical approach to sFLC removal involved plasmapheresis. However, early randomized controlled trials evaluating TPE produced inconsistent results, limiting its widespread use [42, 107]. The efficacy of TPE is constrained by the fact that sFLCs are predominantly distributed in the extravascular compartment, which is not accessed during plasma exchange. Furthermore, the reduction in sFLC levels is often transient, and the lack of integrated KRT in AKI reduces its clinical utility. For these reasons, TPE is not currently recommended as a routine treatment in MM-related AKI, though it may retain a role in selected cases, such as hyperviscosity syndrome [19].

Technological advances in dialysis membrane design have led to the development of more effective modalities for sFLC clearance. HCO membranes, characterized by larger pore sizes and cut-offs around 50–60 kDa, have shown high efficacy in early in vitro studies, with approximately 90% clearance of sFLCs over 3 weeks [38]. These promising results prompted the design of two randomized controlled trials, MYRE and EuLITE, which assessed the clinical impact of HCO compared to standard high-flux HD, both performed together with clone-directed chemotherapy.

In the MYRE trial, 98 patients with biopsy-confirmed myeloma cast nephropathy requiring dialysis were randomized to treatment with either HCO or high-flux HD. Although HCO dialysis resulted in greater sFLC reduction, the primary outcome, i.e., dialysis independence at 3 months, did not significantly differ between groups (41% vs. 33%) [14]. Similarly, in the EuLITE trial, involving 90 patients, dialysis independence rates were comparable between HCO and high-flux HD groups, with the HCO group experiencing a higher incidence of infections [37]. While these findings tempered the initial enthusiasm surrounding HCO membranes, these two trials were considered underpowered to detect modest but clinically meaningful differences, and currently they are considered not conclusive about the actual therapeutic value of this approach [99]. Furthermore, concerns have been raised regarding the unintended removal of essential plasma proteins, such as albumin and immunoglobulins, which may limit the tolerability of HCO membranes in prolonged use [44].

In response to these limitations, MCO has been developed to balance effective sFLC removal with preservation of albumin and other critical plasma components [48].

These membranes are made of polyarylethersulfone/polyvinylpyrrolidone and have a tighter pore distribution with larger pores compared to high-flux and low-flux membranes.

This porosity allows greater removal of the larger middle molecular uremic toxins (25–58 kDa) with controlled albumin clearance [36].

The potential utility of MCO in the context of the so-called expanded hemodialysis (HDx) has been demonstrated in clinical studies showing that MCO increased the reduction rate of FLC when compared to hemodiafiltration, with no significant difference in albumin loss into the dialysate [45].

Furthermore, the prospective REMOVAL-HD trial further confirmed that MCO dialysis does not significantly lower serum albumin levels and is associated with effective early sFLC clearance [49].

In a retrospective study of 60 patients with MM-associated dialysis-dependent AKI, MCO HD achieved a reduction of 58% in kappa and 39% in lambda light chains, while creatinine levels improved significantly over 12 months. Importantly, no significant alterations were observed in total protein, immunoglobulin, or lactate dehydrogenase levels, supporting the biochemical safety of MCO membranes [82].

Additional extracorporeal techniques, such as adsorption-based HD and hemodiafiltration with endogenous reinfusion (HFR), have also been explored. HFR, which combines convection and resin-based adsorption, has shown removal rates of approximately 54% and 36.7% for kappa and lambda chains, respectively [38]. Similarly, polymethylmethacrylate (PMMA) membranes, which possess intrinsic adsorptive properties, have demonstrated removal efficiencies of up to 88% for kappa and 73% for lambda chains [91]. However, this last treatment may be limited by the rapid saturation of the membrane due to sFLC adhesion. This limitation was the rationale leading to the development of the so-called enhanced adsorption dialysis (EAD), which employs two PMMA membranes in parallel to overcome the early saturation that occurs with single-membrane systems [27]. Although in vitro studies have confirmed the ability of EAD to adsorb significant quantities of sFLCs, clinical data remain limited.

In a multicenter retrospective study of 25 patients with MM-related AKI requiring renal replacement therapy, those treated with intensive dialysis—defined as six sessions per week during the first 2 weeks using PMMA or HFR—had significantly higher rates of kidney function recovery. Among patients who became dialysis-independent, 92.9% had received intensive dialysis compared to 36.4% of those who remained dialysis-dependent. These findings support the hypothesis that early and aggressive sFLC removal, when combined with effective anti-myeloma therapy, may improve renal outcomes [90].

In conclusion, the progression from plasmapheresis to advanced membranes has significantly expanded the range of therapeutic options for sFLC removal in MM. Although various modalities have demonstrated efficacy in sFLC clearance and retrospective data suggest a potential benefit on renal recovery, robust evidence from randomized trials remains limited and inconclusive. The evolving landscape of MM therapy, driven by novel agents such as proteasome inhibitors, immunomodulatory drugs, and anti-CD38 monoclonal antibodies, has led to improved hematological responses and survival, and may reduce the additional benefit of EBP [55]. While the rationale for extracorporeal sFLC removal remains strong, especially in the setting of cast nephropathy, its definitive role in improving clinical outcomes in the era of modern MM treatment is yet to be fully established (Table 14.2).

14.3.2 EBP Strategies to Modulate the Tumor Microenvironment

Modern theories of cancer biology emphasize the role of the tumor microenvironment (TME) in influencing the disease course.

TME is a dynamic and interactive network of cellular elements, vascular structures, and soluble factors that can support cancer cell proliferation, favor local invasion, and facilitate distant metastasis [6, 98].

Given the recognition of these roles, TME components are now being explored as potential new therapeutic targets [78].

Tumor cell-derived exosomes (TDEs) have drawn particular interest in this regard.

These nanometer-sized extracellular vesicles, typically ranging from 30 to 150 nm, originate from the endosomal compartment and carry nucleic acids, proteins, and lipids [64]. Once into the circulation, they exert autocrine and paracrine effects, interacting with adjacent cancer cells, immune populations, and

Table 14.2 Extracorporeal blood purification for sFLC removal in multiple myeloma-associated AKI

Modality	Advantages	Disadvantages	Clinical outcomes/ evidence (References in the text)
Plasma exchange	Rapid intravascular sFLC reduction	Limited to intravascular compartment Short-lived effect No integrated KRT Procedure-intensive	Early RCTs showed conflicting results Not associated with improved renal recovery Not recommended as standard therapy
High-cutoff hemodialysis (HCO-HD)	High sFLC clearance (~90% in vitro) Pore size allows dimeric LC removal	Loss of albumin and immunoglobulins Higher infection risk Requires albumin supplementation	MYRE and EuLITE trials: significant LC reduction, but no significant benefit in dialysis independence Trials underpowered
Medium-cutoff hemodialysis (MCO-HD)	Selective sFLC clearance Preserves albumin Well tolerated	Long-term efficacy not fully established Less studied than HCO	Retrospective studies: effective sFLC removal Improved renal function in dialysis-dependent AKI
HFR (Hemodiafiltration with endogenous reinfusion)	Combines convection and adsorption Effective sFLC removal Biocompatible	Less accessible Not standardized across centers	LC reduction: 54% (kappa), 36.7% (lambda) Associated with improved renal recovery in retrospective studies
PMMA membrane dialysis	High adsorptive capacity for sFLC Preserves albumin	Rapid membrane saturation Adsorption effectiveness variable	Kappa/lambda LC removal: 88%/73% Requires frequent membrane changes or dual-membrane circuits (EAD)
EAD (enhanced adsorption dialysis)	Dual-membrane system increases adsorptive efficiency	Requires complex setup Data still limited	~23% sFLC reduction in early studies with single membrane Promising with dual-membrane system

Abbreviations: *sFLC* serum free light chains, *MM* multiple myeloma, *AKI* acute kidney injury, *EBP* extracorporeal blood purification, *RCT* randomized controlled trial, *KRT* kidney replacement therapy, *HCO-HD* high-cutoff hemodialysis, *MCO-HD* medium-cutoff hemodialysis, *PMMA* polymethylmethacrylate, *HFR* hemodiafiltration with endogenous reinfusion, *EAD* enhanced adsorption dialysis cancer-associated fibroblasts [97]. Experimental and clinical data have associated TDEs with many pathological processes, such as cancer progression, angiogenic remodeling, immune evasion, metastatic colonization, and resistance to pharmacological agents [53].

One particularly relevant concern implicates their involvement in the resistance to immune checkpoint inhibitors. Indeed, while antibodies targeting the PD-1/PD-L1 axis have become a key therapeutic tool in the management of several malignancies, resistance to the treatment remains a significant clinical problem [16]. TDEs have been shown to transport PD-L1 on their surface, providing an alternative route to engage PD-1 on effector lymphocytes and thereby attenuating antitumor immunity [57]. Coherently, manipulating exosomes to reduce or neutralize PD-L1 content has been demonstrated in preclinical systems to restore immune responsiveness [73]. These findings suggest that TDEs themselves may constitute a novel therapeutic target [54].

Several strategies with the aim of interfering with TDE activity are currently under exploration [50]. Molecular approaches, including genetic modification and small-molecule inhibitors, aim to prevent exosome biogenesis or release. At the same time, physical removal of circulating vesicles offers additional therapeutic opportunities (Fig. 14.1).

In a proof-of-concept study, TPE was applied in patients with advanced melanoma receiving immunotherapy, achieving a marked reduction in circulating PD-L1–positive exosomes [70]. Although the clinical meaning of this reduction remains uncertain, the study provided initial evidence that extracorporeal techniques may be used to modulate the systemic exosomal load.

Other EBP modalities have been investigated in preclinical and early translational settings. Adsorptive technologies, for example, have been used to capture tumor-associated cytokines. Polyvinyl alcohol microspheres coupled with heparin have demonstrated the capacity to selectively bind the vascular endothelial growth factor and transforming growth factor-β released by breast cancer cells, with inhibition of proliferation and promotion of apoptosis [96].

A further innovative approach involves the use of the Hemopurifier® (Aethlon Medical, San Diego, CA), a hollow-fiber plasma separator containing a lectin-based affinity resin able to capture glycoprotein-rich vesicles and viral particles. Initially developed for infectious diseases such as HIV and hepatitis C, the device has also been tested in the context of COVID-19 [4]. Building on this rationale, a clinical trial was initiated to evaluate the feasibility of an approach based on the combination of the Hemopurifier with pembrolizumab, a PD-1 checkpoint inhibitor, as first-line therapy for head and neck squamous cell carcinoma. The trial was terminated early due to insufficient patient enrolment, but it provided a clear translational framework for integrating extracorporeal exosome removal with immunotherapy [109].

Most recently, attention has shifted toward adsorption cartridges, such as the Seraph®-100 Microbind® Affinity Blood Filter (ExThera Medical, Martinez, CA). This filter, composed of ultrahigh molecular weight polyethylene beads covalently coated with heparin, has demonstrated activity in clearing bacteria and viruses from

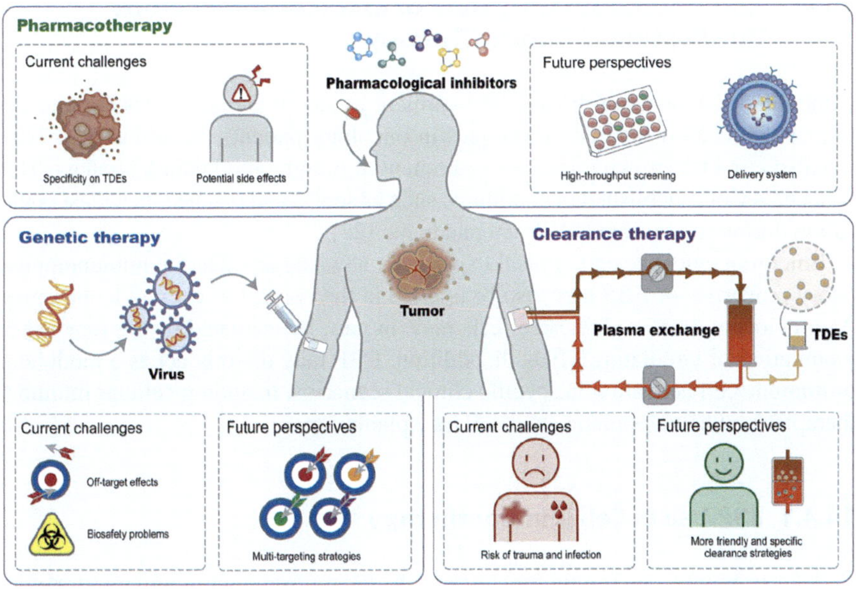

Fig. 14.1 Current strategies and future perspectives for the inhibition and clearance of tumor-derived exosomes (TDEs) to support cancer therapy. Current drug-based approaches focus on gene manipulation or pharmaceutical inhibition, but these can sometimes cause off-target effects and side effects. Extracorporeal blood purification offers a potential means of directly removing TDEs from circulation. Early findings with plasma exchange are promising, but more precise and tailored methods should be developed to pave the way for future clinical applications. (Reprinted under the terms of the Creative Commons Attribution License (https://creativecommons.org/licenses/by/4.0/). Li et al. [54])

the circulation [85]. Preliminary exploratory data suggest that it may also adsorb subsets of extracellular vesicles and tumor-associated proteins, thus potentially affecting the cancer course [94]. While the relevance of these effects for cancer treatment remains speculative, the concept broadens the potential application of EBP as an adjunctive modality in oncology.

Taken together, the emerging evidence indicates that TME manipulation or removal of TDEs may represent promising frontiers in the management of cancer. By targeting extracellular communication pathways, EBP-based interventions could complement pharmacological therapies and contribute to more durable clinical responses. However, systematic clinical evaluation is still ongoing, and rigorous trials are required to establish safety, efficacy, and appropriate patient selection.

14.4 Immunomodulatory Role of Extracorporeal Blood Purification in Cancer Therapy

Although the removal of disease- or treatment-related toxic molecules remains the primary indication for EBP techniques in oncology patients, in recent years EBP has also attracted growing interest as a potential immunomodulatory strategy. This concept is well established in conditions such as sepsis and reached its widest application during the recent COVID-19 pandemic [22].

Emerging evidence and clinical experience now suggest that the immunomodulatory properties of EBP may also be applied in the context of oncologic therapies. As previously discussed, these effects may, in part, be mediated by the removal or modulation of circulating TEDs. In addition, EBP may directly act as a modulator of immune cell activation in specific clinical scenarios, including cellular immunotherapies and hematopoietic stem cell transplantation.

14.4.1 EBP Use in Cell Immunotherapy

Cellular immunotherapy represents one of the most recent and promising strategies in the evolving landscape of cancer treatment. This approach utilizes living cells—most commonly T lymphocytes—that are engineered, expanded, or selected ex vivo and subsequently reinfused into the patient to recognize and eradicate malignant cells [108]. While the therapeutic potential of these modalities is considerable, they are also associated with a broad spectrum of severe inflammatory and immune-related toxicities.

Among cellular therapies, chimeric antigen receptor T-cell (CAR-T) therapy is currently the most widely adopted and extensively studied [3]. Approved indications include relapsed or refractory B-cell malignancies such as acute lymphoblastic leukemia, diffuse large B-cell lymphoma, mantle cell lymphoma, and MM [95]. CAR-T therapy has demonstrated remarkable efficacy in inducing remission and improving survival outcomes. However, it is frequently complicated by significant toxicities [10]. These include immune effector cell-associated neurotoxicity syndrome (ICANS), hematologic cytopenias, cardiac dysfunction, and AKI. The most common and clinically impactful adverse event is cytokine release syndrome (CRS), a systemic hyperinflammatory state that occurs in up to 90% of treated patients [33].

CRS results from excessive release of proinflammatory cytokines, most notably interleukin-6 (IL-6), tumor necrosis factor-alpha (TNF-α), and interferon-gamma. Its clinical manifestations range from mild symptoms to life-threatening multiorgan dysfunction. AKI is also frequently observed and may arise from direct cytokine-mediated injury, hemodynamic instability, or nephrotoxic pharmacotherapy [51, 80]. A recent systematic review involving more than 3300 CAR-T recipients reported an overall AKI incidence of approximately 18.6%, affecting both pediatric and adult cohorts [43].

The current standard of care for moderate to severe CRS includes supportive measures, corticosteroids, and cytokine-targeted therapies such as tocilizumab, an

IL-6 receptor antagonist [68]. However, in refractory or fulminant cases, pharmacologic interventions alone may be insufficient. In this setting, EBP techniques, primarily TPE and hemoadsorption, have gained interest.

There is a strong rationale for using these EBP modalities in severe CRS, based on evidence demonstrating their capacity to remove circulating cytokines and attenuate systemic inflammation. Interestingly, also in these cases, the majority of the supporting data originates from studies in sepsis and, more recently, from clinical experience during the COVID-19 pandemic. In both in vitro and in vivo models of sepsis, high cut-off membranes and hemoadsorption cartridges have been shown to significantly reduce circulating levels of key inflammatory cytokines, including IL-6 and IL-8 [34, 106]. These reductions are often accompanied by improvements in hemodynamic stability and decreased requirements for vasopressor support [15]. Similar findings have been reported in severe COVID-19, where hemoadsorption has been associated with diminishing of the cytokine storm and improved clinical trajectories [62, 104].

Despite this strong biological rationale and supportive evidence from other hyperinflammatory conditions, experience with EBP techniques for refractory CRS after CAR T-cell therapy remains limited. To date, reports consist mainly of anecdotal cases and small case series, although clinical trials are currently underway to define their efficacy, optimal timing, and patient selection [25].

In a multicenter study of 17 patients undergoing TPE for refractory CRS, with or without concomitant ICANS, rapid clinical improvement was observed, including defervescence, reduction of inflammatory markers, and improved hemodynamic status [76].

About hemoadsorption, beyond a few isolated case reports [13, 84], we recently described a series of four hematologic patients who experienced rapid clinical deterioration—within 1–2 days after CAR-T infusion—characterized by marked elevations in IL-6 and ferritin levels [23]. These patients, unresponsive to standard therapies including corticosteroids, tocilizumab, and anakinra (an interleukin-1 receptor antagonist), were treated with CVVHD combined with CytoSorb® (CytoSorbents Corporation) hemoadsorption cartridges. This intervention was well tolerated and led to substantial reductions in IL-6 levels (from 18% to 95%), resolution of CRS, and discontinuation of vasopressor support in three of the four cases (Fig. 14.2).

Although these preliminary findings are constrained by the retrospective nature and the small sample sizes, they suggest that hemoadsorption may represent a safe and potentially effective adjunctive strategy for managing severe CAR-T-related toxicities.

Notably, similar principles apply to T-cell receptor-engineered T-cell (TCR-T) therapies, which are currently under clinical development, particularly for solid tumors such as melanoma, sarcoma, and mesothelioma [92]. The toxicity profile of TCR-T therapy resembles that of CAR-T therapy, including the risk of severe CRS. However, evidence regarding EBP use in this context is even more limited, with only a single case report describing a patient with hepatocellular carcinoma

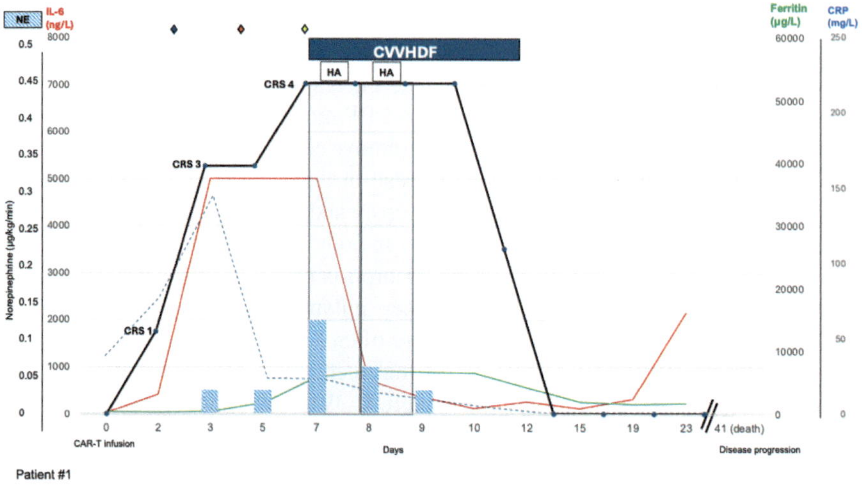

Fig. 14.2 Exemplificative individual clinical course and management of CAR-T patients treated with hemoadsorption. Black line = CRS grading, Red line = IL-6 levels, Green line = Ferritin levels, Blue line = CRP levels. Light blue columns denote the NE dose. Light blue columns depict the NE dose. Treatment initiation dates are marked by colored rhombuses: black for tocilizumab, red for corticosteroids, and yellow for anakinra. Each hemoadsorption cycle is indicated by an "HA" box. Abbreviations: Chimeric Antigen Receptor T-cell (CAR-T), Hemoadsorption (HA), Continuous Veno-Venous Hemodiafiltration (CVVHDF), Norepinephrine (NE), Interleukin-6 (IL-6), C-Reactive Protein (CRP), Cytokine Release Syndrome (CRS). For IL-6, the level of 5000 ng/L represents the upper limit of the laboratory reference range. (Reproduced under the terms of the Creative Commons Attribution License Esposito et al. [23])

treated with TPE, in whom inflammatory markers and hemodynamics improved significantly [105].

In conclusion, EBP techniques hold promise as adjunctive strategies for managing severe complications associated with cellular immunotherapies. However, at present, reliable data are insufficient to guide clinical decision-making or to establish standardized treatment algorithms, and management therefore continues to be based largely on clinical judgment. This lack of robust evidence is likely related to the limited availability of CAR-T therapy worldwide and to the fact that current pharmacologic treatments are generally effective in controlling CRS. As a result, strictly refractory cases requiring EBP are relatively uncommon. Nevertheless, as the use of CAR-T therapy expands and indications broaden, beyond oncology, defining the role of EBP in CRS management becomes increasingly clinically relevant [83].

Accordingly, larger prospective studies are needed to validate the indications for EBP in this setting, refine patient selection, and determine optimal timing and treatment protocols. Such efforts will be essential to maximize therapeutic benefit while ensuring that extracorporeal interventions do not compromise the antitumor efficacy of these innovative therapies.

14.4.2 Extracorporeal Photopheresis

Although restricted to specific clinical indications, extracorporeal photopheresis (ECP) represents one of the most established immunomodulatory EBP techniques. In this procedure, mononuclear cells are separated from whole blood by centrifugation, exposed to the photosensitizing agent 8-methoxypsoralen (8-MOP), and subsequently irradiated with ultraviolet A light before being reinfused into the patient [7].

This process results in photoactivation of lymphomonocytes, which exerts profound immunomodulatory effects, primarily targeting T lymphocytes [69].

ECP induces significant alterations in the cytokine milieu, including reductions in proinflammatory mediators such as interleukin-12, TNF-α, and interleukin-1, alongside increases in anti-inflammatory cytokines such as interleukin-10 and interleukin-4 [31]. This shift promotes a transition from a Th1-dominant to a Th2-dominant immune response and enhances the expansion and functional activity of regulatory T cells [1].

Clinically, ECP has demonstrated efficacy across a range of T cell–mediated autoimmune disorders, including pemphigus vulgaris, systemic sclerosis, Crohn's disease, multiple sclerosis, and transplanted organ rejection [9, 11, 47]. In oncology, ECP holds an important role in the treatment of cutaneous T-cell lymphoma and in the management of complications following hematopoietic stem cell transplantation [2]. Specifically, it is recommended for patients with acute and chronic graft-versus-host disease (GVHD) after allogeneic transplantation, particularly in cases refractory to corticosteroids and conventional immunosuppressive therapy [8, 32].

In this context, by providing a controlled form of immune modulation, ECP constitutes a well-established adjunctive treatment to modify disease trajectory and improve long-term outcomes [66] (Table 14.3).

Table 14.3 Immunomodulatory extracorporeal blood purification in cancer patients according to the current evidence and experience

Clinical scenario	Modality selection	Mechanistic rationale	Clinical benefits	Current limitations
General immunomodulatory use of EBP in oncology	TPE; Hemoadsorption	TED removal/ modulation; hyperinflammation control	Conceptually promising; experience extrapolated from sepsis/ COVID-19	Heterogeneous applications; no cancer-specific clinical trials
Severe CRS after CAR-T therapy (refractory)	TPE; Hemoadsorption + CVVHD	Cytokine removal (IL-6, TNF-α), inflammatory mediator reduction	Rapid IL-6 reduction, hemodynamic stabilization, CRS resolution	Small cohorts, no RCTs, heterogeneous protocols

(continued)

Table 14.3 continued

Clinical scenario	Modality selection	Mechanistic rationale	Clinical benefits	Current limitations
ICANS associated with CAR-T therapy	TPE; Hemoadsorption	Immune activation modulation	Neurologic improvement in select cases	Sparse evidence; limited mechanistic clarity
CRS in TCR-T therapy	TPE	Reduction of circulating cytokines	Clinical improvement reported	Insufficient data (one single case report)
Graft-versus-host disease (GVHD)	Extracorporeal Photopheresis (ECP)	Treg expansion; IL-12↓ TNF-α↓ IL-10↑; Th1 → Th2 shift	Steroid-sparing; improved survival; established therapy	Multiple sessions required
Cutaneous T-cell lymphoma	ECP	Immune reprogramming; apoptosis of malignant T-cells	Disease control; symptom improvement	Slow responsiveness; variable efficacy

Abbreviations: *AKI* acute kidney injury, *CAR-T* chimeric antigen receptor T-cell therapy, *CRS* cytokine release syndrome, *CVVHD* continuous veno-venous hemodiafiltration, *ECP* extracorporeal photopheresis, *EBP* extracorporeal blood purification, *GVHD* graft-versus-host disease, *ICANS* immune effector cell–associated neurotoxicity syndrome, *IL-6* interleukin-6, *TCR-T* T-cell receptor–engineered T-cell therapy, *TPE* therapeutic plasma exchange, *TEDs* tumor- or treatment-related extracellular determinants

14.5 Extracorporeal Blood Purification as a Cancer Therapy

Up to this point, we have described the use of EBP as an adjunctive approach in oncology, primarily aimed at managing cancer- and treatment-related complications, or as a permissive and supportive strategy to enhance the effectiveness of pharmacological and cellular therapies.

Beyond these applications, the potential role of EBP as a direct therapeutic modality in oncology is emerging as a new frontier.

In this context, recent attention has been focused on the potential role of hemoadsorption techniques for the removal of circulating tumor cells (CTCs). Ex vivo studies have shown that a membrane composed of polyethylene beads covalently coated with heparin (e.g., Seraph®-100, ExThera Medical) can effectively clear CTCs from the blood of patients with pancreatic ductal adenocarcinoma [86].

So far, clinical experience remains limited to case reports and small case series [93]. Ilic and colleagues recently reported their results in 10 patients with metastatic solid tumors whose liquid biopsy was positive for the epithelial cell adhesion molecule. All patients also had positive bacterial or fungal isolates. The Seraph100® filter was placed in series with a standard dialyzer, with an average treatment duration of 120 min. Following this treatment, all blood cultures turned negative, while the median reduction in CTCs was 71% (IQR 67–100%) [40]. Based on these early findings, prospective clinical trials are now underway aiming to explore the safety and clinical impact of this approach. These include evaluations of ONCObind, a platform based on the Seraph®-100 Filter technology, for CTC removal in patients with metastatic pancreatic ductal adenocarcinoma (mPDAC).

The first trial, OSCAR I (ONCObind CTC Removal Study; [110]), has recently completed enrollment of 30 patients, with awaited results. A larger feasibility study, OSCAR II [111], is planned and will expand inclusion to patients with metastatic colorectal carcinoma.

14.6 Final Remarks

Extracorporeal blood purification is emerging as a multifaceted adjunctive therapy in oncology, bridging supportive care, immune modulation, and direct anticancer interventions (Fig. 14.3). While its clinical utility is well recognized in managing treatment-related complications, ongoing research highlights its potential to actively

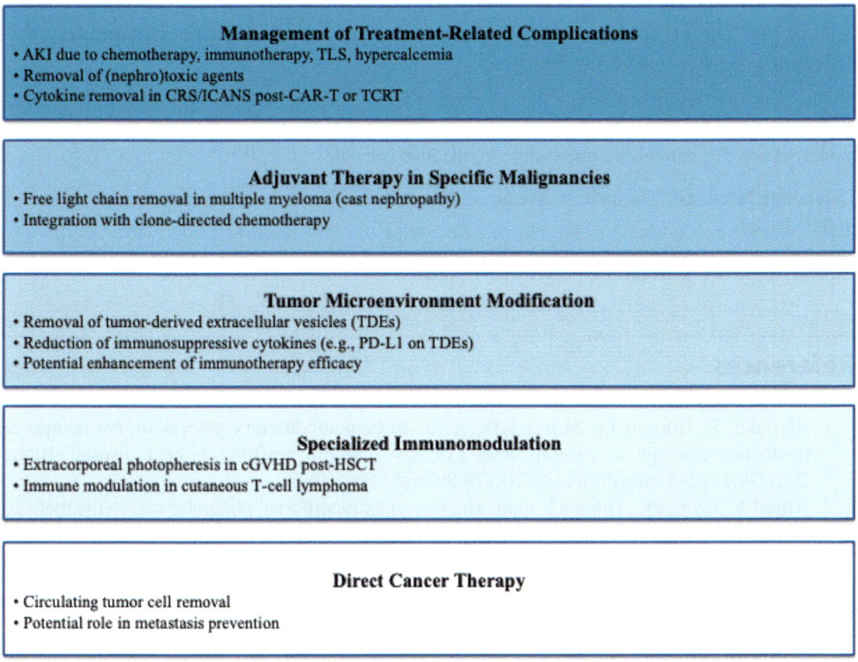

Fig. 14.3 Applications of extracorporeal blood purification in cancer therapy. Abbreviations: AKI acute kidney injury, CRS cytokine release syndrome, ICANS immune effector cell–associated neurotoxicity syndrome, CAR-T chimeric antigen receptor T-cell therapy, TCRT T cell receptor–T cell therapy, cGVHD chronic graft-versus-host disease, HSCT hematopoietic stem cell transplantation

influence tumor biology through modulation of circulating mediators, extracellular vesicles, and tumor cells. The development of adsorption-based technologies and high- or medium-cut-off membranes has extended the therapeutic armamentarium.

Looking ahead, future research directions may include integrating EBP with immunotherapies to overcome therapeutic resistance, refining extracorporeal strategies targeting tumor-derived exosomes, and exploring the removal of circulating tumor cells as a potential approach to limit metastatic spread.

However, although the expanded indications of EBP in cancer patients are promising, several knowledge gaps and barriers currently obstruct broader clinical implementation. These include the marked heterogeneity of cancer populations and oncologic treatments, the absence of uniform approaches to guide modality selection, timing, and treatment intensity, and the scarcity of data on how EBP can be optimally integrated with pharmacologic or cellular therapies. The development of device- and disease-specific registries, improved patient phenotyping enabling phenotype-based trials, and the establishment of standardized protocols could all represent key strategies to facilitate implementation of EBP in routine oncologic care. Likewise, innovative study designs, such as platform trials, trial emulation frameworks, and the use of multidimensional endpoints beyond mortality, may help strengthen the evidence base.

Ultimately, EBP may evolve from a supportive measure into an integral component of precision oncology, offering new opportunities to enhance therapeutic tolerance and improve patient outcomes.

Acknowledgments English editing support was provided with the assistance of a large language model (LLM). The authors are responsible for the final content.

Competing Interests The authors have no conflicts of interest to declare that are relevant to the content of this chapter.

Ethical Approval No ethics approval was required.

References

1. Alcindor T, Gorgun G, Miller KB, et al. Immunomodulatory effects of extracorporeal photochemotherapy in patients with extensive chronic graft-versus-host disease. Blood. 2001;98:1622–5. https://doi.org/10.1182/blood.V98.5.1622.
2. Alfred A, Taylor PC, Dignan F, et al. The role of extracorporeal photopheresis in the management of cutaneous T-cell lymphoma, graft-versus-host disease and organ transplant rejection: a consensus statement update from the UK Photopheresis Society. Br J Haematol. 2017;177:287–310. https://doi.org/10.1111/bjh.14537.
3. Alnefaie A, Albogami S, Asiri Y, et al. Chimeric antigen receptor T-cells: an overview of concepts, applications, limitations, and proposed solutions. Front Bioeng Biotechnol. 2022;10:797440.
4. Amundson DE, Shah US, de Necochea-Campion R, et al. Removal of COVID-19 spike protein, whole virus, exosomes, and exosomal micrornas by the hemopurifier® lectin-affinity cartridge in critically ill patients with COVID-19 infection. Front Med (Lausanne). 2021;8:744141. https://doi.org/10.3389/fmed.2021.744141.

5. Anand U, Dey A, Chandel AKS, Sanyal R, Mishra A, Pandey DK, De Falco V, Upadhyay A, Kandimalla R, Chaudhary A, Dhanjal JK, Dewanjee S, Vallamkondu J, Pérez de la Lastra JM. Cancer chemotherapy and beyond: Current status, drug candidates, associated risks and progress in targeted therapeutics. Genes Dis. 2023;10(4):1367–401. https://doi.org/10.1016/j.gendis.2022.02.007.
6. Anderson NM, Simon MC. The tumor microenvironment. Curr Biol. 2020;30(16):R921–R25. https://doi.org/10.1016/j.cub.2020.06.081.
7. Arora S, Setia R. Extracorporeal photopheresis: review of technical aspects. Asian J Transfus Sci. 2017;11:81–6. https://doi.org/10.4103/ajts.AJTS_87_16.
8. Asensi Cantó P, Sanz Caballer J, Solves Alcaína P, et al. Extracorporeal photopheresis in graft-versus-host disease. Transplant Cell Ther. 2023;29:556–66. https://doi.org/10.1016/j.jtct.2023.07.001.
9. Barten MJ, Fisher AJ, Hertig A. The use of extracorporeal photopheresis in solid organ transplantation—current status and future directions. Am J Transplant. 2024;24:1731–41. https://doi.org/10.1016/j.ajt.2024.03.012.
10. Bellal M, Malherbe J, Damaj G, Du Cheyron D. Toxicities, intensive care management, and outcome of chimeric antigen receptor T cells in adults: an update. Crit Care. 2024;28:69.
11. Bisaccia E, Palangio M, Gonzalez J. Extracorporeal photochemotherapy for the treatment of refractory Crohn's disease. Transfus Apher Sci. 2007;37:171–4. https://doi.org/10.1016/j.transci.2007.08.001.
12. Bouchard J, Shepherd G, Hoffman RS, Gosselin S, Roberts DM, Li Y, Nolin TD, Lavergne V, Ghannoum M; EXTRIP workgroup. Extracorporeal treatment for poisoning to beta-adrenergic antagonists: systematic review and recommendations from the EXTRIP workgroup. Crit Care. 2021;25(1):201. doi: 10.1186/s13054-021-03585-7. PMID: 34112223; PMCID: PMC8194226.
13. Bottari G, Merli P, Guzzo I, et al. Multimodal therapeutic approach of cytokine release syndrome developing in a child given chimeric antigen receptor-modified T cell infusion. Crit Care Explor. 2020;2:e0071. https://doi.org/10.1097/CCE.0000000000000071.
14. Bridoux F, Carron PL, Pegourie B, et al. Effect of high-cutoff hemodialysis vs conventional hemodialysis on hemodialysis Independence among patients with myeloma cast nephropathy: a randomized clinical trial. JAMA. 2017;318:2099–110. https://doi.org/10.1001/jama.2017.17924.
15. Broman ME, Hansson F, Vincent J-L, Bodelsson M. Endotoxin and cytokine reducing properties of the oXiris membrane in patients with septic shock: a randomized crossover double-blind study. PLoS One. 2019;14:e0220444. https://doi.org/10.1371/journal.pone.0220444.
16. Chocarro de Erauso L, Zuazo M, Arasanz H, et al. Resistance to PD-L1/PD-1 blockade immunotherapy. A tumor-intrinsic or tumor-extrinsic phenomenon? Front Pharmacol. 2020;11:441. https://doi.org/10.3389/fphar.2020.00441.
17. Christiansen CF, Johansen MB, Langeberg WJ, et al. Incidence of acute kidney injury in cancer patients: a Danish population-based cohort study. Eur J Intern Med. 2011;22:399–406. https://doi.org/10.1016/j.ejim.2011.05.005.
18. Claure-Del Granado R, Clark WR. Continuous renal replacement therapy principles. Semin Dial. 2021;34(6):398–405. https://doi.org/10.1111/sdi.12967. Epub 2021 Apr 5.
19. Dima D, Khouri J. The role of therapeutic plasma exchange in plasma cell disorders. Ann Hematol. 2024;103:3941–6. https://doi.org/10.1007/s00277-024-05712-0.
20. Druml W, Zajic P, Schellongowski P, et al. Association of acute kidney injury receiving kidney replacement therapy with prognosis of critically ill patients with and without cancer: a retrospective study. Crit Care Med. 2021;49:1932–42. https://doi.org/10.1097/CCM.0000000000005102.
21. Esposito P, Cappadona F, Prenna S, et al. Acute kidney injury in hospitalized patients with real-life analysis of incidence and clinical impact in Italian hospitals (the SIN-AKI study). Sci Rep. 2025;15:14261. https://doi.org/10.1038/s41598-025-96236-8.

22. Esposito P, Cipriani L, Verzola D, et al. Effects of different dialysis strategies on inflammatory cytokine profile in maintenance hemodialysis patients with covid-19: a randomized trial. J Clin Med. 2021;10:1383. https://doi.org/10.3390/jcm10071383.
23. Esposito P, Gambella M, Russo E, et al. Hemoadsorption as a supportive strategy for severe toxicity associated with chimeric antigen receptor T-cell therapy: a case series. Kidney Med. 2025;7:101001. https://doi.org/10.1016/j.xkme.2025.101001.
24. Esposito P, Macciò L, Cagnetta A, et al. Monoclonal gammopathy of renal significance (MGRS): retrospective monocentric analysis of clinical outcomes and treatment strategies. Clin Exp Med. 2025;25:118. https://doi.org/10.1007/s10238-025-01646-7.
25. Extracorporeal Cytokine Adsorption as Additive Treatment of CAR-T Associated Cytokine Release Syndrome (CRS) (CYTORELEASE) https://www.clinicaltrials.gov/study/NCT04048434. In: Extracorporeal cytokine adsorption as additive treatment of CAR-T associated Cytokine Release Syndrome (CRS) (CYTORELEASE).
26. Fabbrini P, Finkel K, Gallieni M, et al. Light chains removal by extracorporeal techniques in acute kidney injury due to multiple myeloma: a position statement of the Onconephrology Work Group of the Italian Society of Nephrology. J Nephrol. 2016;29:735–46. https://doi.org/10.1007/s40620-016-0347-9.
27. Fabbrini P, Sirtori S, Casiraghi E, et al. Polymethylmethacrylate membrane and serum free light chain removal: enhancing adsorption properties. Blood Purif. 2013;35:52–8. https://doi.org/10.1159/000350849.
28. Ferrari F, Carletti A, Peroni N, Mongodi S, Esposito P, Orlando A, Mojoli F, Ronco C, Belliato M, Iotti GA. Brief Report: A Case of Tramadol Overdose: Extracorporeal Life Support and Hemoperfusion as Life-Saving Treatment. Blood Purif. 2020;49(4):509–12. https://doi.org/10.1159/000505845.
29. Floris M, Trevisani F, Angioi A, et al. Acute kidney disease in oncology: a new concept to enhance the understanding of the impact of kidney injury in patients with cancer. Kidney Blood Press Res. 2024;49:745–52. https://doi.org/10.1159/000540908.
30. Geraldes C, Roque A, Sarmento-Ribeiro AB, et al. Practical management of disease-related manifestations and drug toxicities in patients with multiple myeloma. Front Oncol. 2024;14. https://doi.org/10.3389/fonc.2024.1282300.
31. Gorgun G, Miller KB, Foss FM. Immunologic mechanisms of extracorporeal photochemotherapy in chronic graft-versus-host disease. Blood. 2002;100:941–7. https://doi.org/10.1182/blood-2002-01-0068.
32. Greinix HT, Worel N, Just U, Knobler R. Extracorporeal photopheresis in acute and chronic graft-versus-host disease. Transfus Apher Sci. 2014;50:349–57. https://doi.org/10.1016/j.transci.2014.04.005.
33. Grigor EJM, Fergusson D, Kekre N, et al. Risks and benefits of chimeric antigen receptor T-cell (CAR-T) therapy in cancer: a systematic review and meta-analysis. Transfus Med Rev. 2019;33:98–110. https://doi.org/10.1016/j.tmrv.2019.01.005.
34. Harm S, Schildböck C, Hartmann J. Cytokine removal in extracorporeal blood purification: an in vitro study. Blood Purif. 2020;49:33–43. https://doi.org/10.1159/000502680.
35. Hofmann G, Bauernhofer T, Krippl P, et al. Plasmapheresis reverses all side-effects of a cisplatin overdose–a case report and treatment recommendation. BMC Cancer. 2006;6:1. https://doi.org/10.1186/1471-2407-6-1.
36. Hulko M, Dietrich V, Koch I, et al. Pyrogen retention: comparison of the novel medium cut-off (MCO) membrane with other dialyser membranes. Sci Rep. 2019;9:6791. https://doi.org/10.1038/s41598-019-43161-2.
37. Hutchison CA, Cockwell P, Moroz V, et al. High cutoff versus high-flux haemodialysis for myeloma cast nephropathy in patients receiving bortezomib-based chemotherapy (EuLITE): a phase 2 randomised controlled trial. Lancet Haematol. 2019;6:e217–28. https://doi.org/10.1016/S2352-3026(19)30014-6.
38. Hutchison CA, Cockwell P, Reid S, et al. Efficient removal of immunoglobulin free light chains by hemodialysis for multiple myeloma. J Am Soc Nephrol. 2007;18:886–95. https://doi.org/10.1681/ASN.2006080821.

39. Hutchison CA, Cockwell P, Stringer S, et al. Early reduction of serum-free light chains associates with renal recovery in myeloma kidney. J Am Soc Nephrol. 2011;22:1129–36. https://doi.org/10.1681/ASN.2010080857.
40. Ilic S, Premuzic V. First-in-human rapid removal of circulating tumor cells in solid metastatic neoplasia by microbind affinity blood filter. Blood Purif. 2024;1–3. https://doi.org/10.1159/000542325.
41. Izzedine H, Perazella MA. Anticancer drug-induced acute kidney injury. Kidney Int Rep. 2017;2:504–14. https://doi.org/10.1016/j.ekir.2017.02.008.
42. Johnson WJ, Kyle RA, Pineda AA, et al. Treatment of renal failure associated with multiple myeloma. Plasmapheresis, hemodialysis, and chemotherapy. Arch Intern Med. 1990;150:863–9.
43. Kanduri SR, Cheungpasitporn W, Thongprayoon C, et al. Systematic review of risk factors and incidence of acute kidney injury among patients treated with CAR-T cell therapies. Kidney Int Rep. 2021;6:1416–22. https://doi.org/10.1016/j.ekir.2021.02.013.
44. Karakala N, Juncos LA. High-cutoff hemodialysis therapy for patients with light chain cast nephropathy and AKI requiring dialysis: CON. Kidney360. 2023;4:1024–6.
45. Kirsch AH, Lyko R, Nilsson L-G, et al. Performance of hemodialysis with novel medium cut-off dialyzers. Nephrol Dial Transplant. 2016;gfw310. https://doi.org/10.1093/ndt/gfw310.
46. Kitchlu A, McArthur E, Amir E, et al. Acute kidney injury in patients receiving systemic treatment for cancer: a population-based cohort study. J Natl Cancer Inst. 2019;111:727–36. https://doi.org/10.1093/jnci/djy167.
47. Knobler RM, French LE, Kim Y, et al. A randomized, double-blind, placebo-controlled trial of photopheresis in systemic sclerosis. J Am Acad Dermatol. 2006;54:793–9. https://doi.org/10.1016/j.jaad.2005.11.1091.
48. Koniman R, Teo SH, Kaushik M, et al. The use of medium cutoff dialyzers in patients with multiple myeloma and acute kidney injury requiring hemodialysis: a systematic review. Semin Dial. 2023;36:12–7. https://doi.org/10.1111/sdi.13115.
49. Krishnasamy R, Hawley CM, Jardine MJ, et al. A tRial evaluating mid cut-off value membrane clearance of albumin and light chains in HemoDialysis patients: a safety device study. Blood Purif. 2020;49:468–78. https://doi.org/10.1159/000505567.
50. Kuang L, Wu L, Li Y. Extracellular vesicles in tumor immunity: mechanisms and novel insights. Mol Cancer. 2025;24:45. https://doi.org/10.1186/s12943-025-02233-w.
51. Lee MD, Strohbehn IA, Seethapathy HS, et al. Acute kidney injury after the CAR-T therapy tisagenlecleucel. Am J Kidney Dis. 2021;77:990–2.
52. Leng G, Duan B, Liu J, et al. The advancements and prospective developments in anti-tumor targeted therapy. Neoplasia. 2024;56:101024. https://doi.org/10.1016/j.neo.2024.101024.
53. Li I, Nabet BY. Exosomes in the tumor microenvironment as mediators of cancer therapy resistance. Mol Cancer. 2019;18:32. https://doi.org/10.1186/s12943-019-0975-5.
54. Li Y, Chen Z-K, Duan X, et al. Targeted inhibition of tumor-derived exosomes as a novel therapeutic option for cancer. Exp Mol Med. 2022;54:1379–89. https://doi.org/10.1038/s12276-022-00856-3.
55. Lin CH-T, Tariq MJ, Ullah F, et al. Current novel targeted therapeutic strategies in multiple myeloma. Int J Mol Sci. 2024;25. https://doi.org/10.3390/ijms25116192.
56. Liu B, Zhou H, Tan L, et al. Exploring treatment options in cancer: tumor treatment strategies. Signal Transduct Target Ther. 2024;9:175. https://doi.org/10.1038/s41392-024-01856-7.
57. Liu J, Peng X, Yang S, et al. Extracellular vesicle PD-L1 in reshaping tumor immune microenvironment: biological function and potential therapy strategies. Cell Commun Signal. 2022;20:14. https://doi.org/10.1186/s12964-021-00816-w.
58. Lopes S, Pabst L, Bahougne T, et al. Central nervous system complications of immune checkpoint inhibitors: a comprehensive review. Crit Rev Oncol Hematol. 2025;206:104595. https://doi.org/10.1016/j.critrevonc.2024.104595.
59. Lupuşoru G, Ailincăi I, Frăţilă G, et al. Tumor lysis syndrome: an endless challenge in onco-nephrology. Biomedicine. 2022;10:1012. https://doi.org/10.3390/biomedicines10051012.

60. Lupuşoru M, Lupuşoru G, Ailincăi I, et al. Renal replacement therapy in cancer patients with acute kidney injury (review). Exp Ther Med. 2021;22:864. https://doi.org/10.3892/etm.2021.10296.
61. Lustberg MB, Kuderer NM, Desai A, et al. Mitigating long-term and delayed adverse events associated with cancer treatment: implications for survivorship. Nat Rev Clin Oncol. 2023;20:527–42. https://doi.org/10.1038/s41571-023-00776-9.
62. Ma J, Xia P, Zhou Y, et al. Potential effect of blood purification therapy in reducing cytokine storm as a late complication of critically ill COVID-19. Clin Immunol. 2020;214:108408. https://doi.org/10.1016/j.clim.2020.108408.
63. Mao X, Wu S, Huang D, Li C. Complications and comorbidities associated with antineoplastic chemotherapy: rethinking drug design and delivery for anticancer therapy. Acta Pharm Sin B. 2024;14:2901–26. https://doi.org/10.1016/j.apsb.2024.03.006.
64. Mathew M, Zade M, Mezghani N, et al. Extracellular vesicles as biomarkers in cancer immunotherapy. Cancers (Basel). 2020;12:2825. https://doi.org/10.3390/cancers12102825.
65. Menè P, Stoppacciaro A, Lai S, Festuccia F. Light chain cast nephropathy in multiple myeloma: prevalence, impact and management challenges. Int J Nephrol Renovasc Dis. 2022;15:173–83. https://doi.org/10.2147/IJNRD.S280179.
66. Michallet M, Sobh M, Deloire A, et al. Second line extracorporeal photopheresis for corticoresistant acute and chronic GVHD after allogeneic hematopoietic cell transplantation for hematological malignancies: long-term results from a real-life study. Transfus Apher Sci. 2024;63:103899. https://doi.org/10.1016/j.transci.2024.103899.
67. Miyamoto Y, Andes LJ, Koyama AK, et al. Association between cancer and incident acute kidney injury among medicare fee-for-service population. Kidney Med. 2025;7:101069. https://doi.org/10.1016/j.xkme.2025.101069.
68. Murthy H, Iqbal M, Chavez JC, Kharfan-Dabaja MA. Cytokine release syndrome: current perspectives. Immunotargets Ther. 2019;8:43–52. https://doi.org/10.2147/ITT.S202015.
69. Ni M, Wang L, Ding Y, et al. Response to extracorporeal photopheresis therapy of patients with steroid-refractory/-resistant GvHD is associated with up-regulation of Th22 cells and Tfh cells. Cytotherapy. 2022;24:311–9. https://doi.org/10.1016/j.jcyt.2021.09.008.
70. Orme JJ, Enninga EAL, Lucien-Matteoni F, et al. Therapeutic plasma exchange clears circulating soluble PD-L1 and PD-L1-positive extracellular vesicles. J Immunother Cancer. 2020;8:e001113. https://doi.org/10.1136/jitc-2020-001113.
71. Ostermann M, Ankawi G, Cantaluppi V, Madarasu R, Dolan K, Husain-Syed F, Kashani K, Mehta R, Prowle J, Reis T, Rimmelé T, Zarbock A, Kellum JA, Ronco C; Nomenclature Standardization Faculty. Nomenclature of Extracorporeal Blood Purification Therapies for Acute Indications: The Nomenclature Standardization Conference. Blood Purif. 2024;53(5):358–72. https://doi.org/10.1159/000533468. Epub 2023 Nov 3.
72. Picciotto D, Genova C, Costigliolo F, et al. An updated focus on immune checkpoint inhibitors and tubulointerstitial nephritis. In: Cancer treatment: an interdisciplinary approach. Cham: Springer Nature Switzerland; 2022. p. 157–84.
73. Poggio M, Hu T, Pai C-C, et al. Suppression of exosomal PD-L1 induces systemic anti-tumor immunity and memory. Cell. 2019;177:414–427.e13. https://doi.org/10.1016/j.cell.2019.02.016.
74. Porta C, Cosmai L, Gallieni M, et al. Renal effects of targeted anticancer therapies. Nat Rev Nephrol. 2015;11:354–70. https://doi.org/10.1038/nrneph.2015.15.
75. Premuzic V, Forni LG. The use of hemoadsorption in cancer-related complications. Blood Purif. 2025;1–9. https://doi.org/10.1159/000547348.
76. Pu Y, Zhao Y, Qi Y, et al. Multi-centers experience using therapeutic plasma exchange for corticosteroid/tocilizumab-refractory cytokine release syndrome following CAR-T therapy. Int Immunopharmacol. 2024;130:111761. https://doi.org/10.1016/j.intimp.2024.111761.
77. Qi L, Luo Q, Zhang Y, et al. Advances in toxicological research of the anticancer drug cisplatin. Chem Res Toxicol. 2019;32:1469–86. https://doi.org/10.1021/acs.chemrestox.9b00204.
78. Quail DF, Joyce JA. Microenvironmental regulation of tumor progression and metastasis. Nat Med. 2013;19:1423–37. https://doi.org/10.1038/nm.3394.

79. Rosner MH, Perazella MA. Acute kidney injury in patients with cancer. N Engl J Med. 2017;376:1770–81. https://doi.org/10.1056/NEJMra1613984.
80. Russo E, Gambella M, Raiola AM, et al. Acute kidney injury in hematological patients treated with CAR-T cells: risk factors, clinical presentation and impact on outcomes. Sci Rep. 2024;14:26886. https://doi.org/10.1038/s41598-024-77720-z.
81. Sarfati D, Koczwara B, Jackson C. The impact of comorbidity on cancer and its treatment. CA Cancer J Clin. 2016;66:337–50. https://doi.org/10.3322/caac.21342.
82. Schaaf CW, Braunisch MC, Holzmann-Littig C, et al. Extracorporeal light-chain elimination in myeloma with simple medium cutoff membrane hemodialysis: a retrospective cohort study. Front Oncol. 2023;13. https://doi.org/10.3389/fonc.2023.1193504.
83. Schett G, Mackensen A, Mougiakakos D. CAR T-cell therapy in autoimmune diseases. Lancet. 2023;402:2034–44. https://doi.org/10.1016/S0140-6736(23)01126-1.
84. Schultz P, Schwier E, Eickmeyer C, et al. High-dose CytoSorb hemoadsorption is associated with improved survival in patients with septic shock: a retrospective cohort study. J Crit Care. 2021;64:184–92. https://doi.org/10.1016/j.jcrc.2021.04.011.
85. Seffer M-T, Cottam D, Forni LG, Kielstein JT. Heparin 2.0: a new approach to the infection crisis. Blood Purif. 2021;50:28–34. https://doi.org/10.1159/000508647.
86. Shishido SN, Suresh D, Courcoubetis G, et al. Determining the efficacy of ExThera Seraph100 blood filtration in patients diagnosed with pancreatic cancer through the liquid biopsy. BJC Rep. 2024;2:47. https://doi.org/10.1038/s44276-024-00069-3.
87. Sirac C, Batuman V, Sanders PW. The proximal tubule toxicity of immunoglobulin light chains. Kidney Int Rep. 2021;6:1225–31. https://doi.org/10.1016/j.ekir.2021.02.026.
88. Solomon A. Light chains of human immunoglobulins. Methods Enzymol. 1985;116:101–21. https://doi.org/10.1016/s0076-6879(85)16008-8.
89. Tang J, Yang N, Pan S, et al. The renal damage and mechanisms relevant to antitumoral drugs. Front Oncol. 2023;13:1331671. https://doi.org/10.3389/fonc.2023.1331671.
90. Terrades NR, Senin A, Azancot MA, et al. Role of light chain clearance in the recovery of renal function in multiple myeloma: another point of view. Clin Kidney J. 2023;16:1014–21. https://doi.org/10.1093/ckj/sfad022.
91. Testa A, Dejoie T, Lecarrer D, et al. Reduction of free immunoglobulin light chains using adsorption properties of hemodiafiltration with endogenous reinfusion. Blood Purif. 2010;30:34–6. https://doi.org/10.1159/000316684.
92. Tsimberidou A-M, Van Morris K, Vo HH, et al. T-cell receptor-based therapy: an innovative therapeutic approach for solid tumors. J Hematol Oncol. 2021;14:102. https://doi.org/10.1186/s13045-021-01115-0.
93. Ulahannan S, Smith P, Rios J, Chawla L. Extracorporeal blood filtration leading to tumor growth arrest and reduced analgesic requirements in stage IV poorly differentiated pancreatic adenocarcinoma: a case report. Oncotarget. 2025;16:582–6. https://doi.org/10.18632/oncotarget.28756.
94. Waldron RT, Wang R, Shishido SN, et al. Selective removal of proteins and microvesicles ex vivo from blood of pancreatic cancer patients using bioengineered adsorption filters. Cancer Lett. 2025;614:217546. https://doi.org/10.1016/j.canlet.2025.217546.
95. Wang J-Y, Wang L. CAR-T cell therapy: where are we now, and where are we heading? Blood Sci. 2023;5:237–48. https://doi.org/10.1097/BS9.0000000000000173.
96. Wang L, Chen J, Chai Y, et al. Targeting regulation of the tumour microenvironment induces apoptosis of breast cancer cells by an affinity hemoperfusion adsorbent. Artif Cells Nanomed Biotechnol. 2021;49:325–34. https://doi.org/10.1080/21691401.2021.1902337.
97. Wang X, Zhou Y, Wang Y, et al. Overcoming cancer treatment resistance: unraveling the role of cancer-associated fibroblasts. J Natl Cancer Cent. 2025;5:237–51. https://doi.org/10.1016/j.jncc.2025.03.002.
98. Whiteside TL. Tumor-derived exosomes and their role in cancer progression. Adv Clin Chem. 2016;74:103–41.
99. Xing Y, Yan J, Yu Z, et al. High-cutoff hemodialysis in multiple myeloma patients with acute kidney injury. Front Oncol. 2022;12:1024133.

100. Xiong M, Wang L, Su L, et al. Acute kidney injury among hospitalized children with cancer. Pediatr Nephrol. 2021;36:171–9. https://doi.org/10.1007/s00467-020-04678-1.
101. Yuzhalin AE. Redefining cancer research for therapeutic breakthroughs. Br J Cancer. 2024;130(7):1078–82. https://doi.org/10.1038/s41416-024-02634-6.
102. Zafar A, Khan MJ, Abu J, Naeem A. Revolutionizing cancer care strategies: immunotherapy, gene therapy, and molecular targeted therapy. Mol Biol Rep. 2024;51(1):219. https://doi.org/10.1007/s11033-023-09096-8.
103. Zarbock A, Nadim MK, Pickkers P, et al. Sepsis-associated acute kidney injury: consensus report of the 28th Acute Disease Quality Initiative workgroup. Nat Rev Nephrol. 2023;19:401–17. https://doi.org/10.1038/s41581-023-00683-3.
104. Zhang H, Zhu G, Yan L, et al. The absorbing filter Oxiris in severe coronavirus disease 2019 patients: a case series. Artif Organs. 2020;44:1296–302. https://doi.org/10.1111/aor.13786.
105. Zheng X, Zhang S, Wu H, et al. Plasma exchange as an effective treatment for cytokine release syndrome following T cell receptor-engineered T cell immunotherapy: a case report. Oncol Lett. 2024;28:607. https://doi.org/10.3892/ol.2024.14740.
106. Zuccari S, Damiani E, Domizi R, et al. Changes in cytokines, haemodynamics and microcirculation in patients with sepsis/septic shock undergoing continuous renal replacement therapy and blood purification with CytoSorb. Blood Purif. 2020;49:107–13. https://doi.org/10.1159/000502540.
107. Zucchelli P, Pasquali S, Cagnoli L, Ferrari G. Controlled plasma exchange trial in acute renal failure due to multiple myeloma. Kidney Int. 1988;33:1175–80. https://doi.org/10.1038/ki.1988.127.
108. Zugasti I, Espinosa-Aroca L, Fidyt K, et al. CAR-T cell therapy for cancer: current challenges and future directions. Signal Transduct Target Ther. 2025;10:210. https://doi.org/10.1038/s41392-025-02269-w.
109. https://clinicaltrials.gov/study/NCT04453046.
110. https://clinicaltrials.gov/study/NCT06481397.
111. https://clinicaltrials.gov/study/NCT06655142.

Gene Therapy and Blood Purification: A Future Perspective

15

Valentina Corradi, Nenzi Marzano, Carlotta Caprara, and Fiorenza Ferrari

15.1 The Intersecting Frontiers of Genetic Medicine and Extracorporeal Support

The confluence of gene therapy and extracorporeal blood purification (EBP) represents a pivotal shift in modern medicine, transforming the treatment of complex diseases from a palliative approach to a potentially curative one.

Gene therapy involves the transfer of genetic material to treat or prevent diseases. This can be achieved by gene replacement with an artificial one through homologous recombination, by modulating the expression of a specific gene, or by targeted

V. Corradi
UOC Nefrologia, Dialisi e Trapianto Renale AULSS 8 BERICA Ospedale San Bortolo Vicenza, Vicenza, Italy

Fondazione IRRIV AULSS 8 BERICA Ospedale San Bortolo, Vicenza, Italy
e-mail: valentina.corradi@aulss8.veneto.it

N. Marzano
Fondazione IRRIV AULSS 8 BERICA Ospedale San Bortolo, Vicenza, Italy

UOC Genetica Medica e Genomica AULSS 8 BERICA Ospedale San Bortolo Vicenza, Vicenza, Italy
e-mail: nenzi.marzano@aulss8.veneto.it

C. Caprara
UOC Nefrologia, Dialisi e Trapianto Renale AULSS 8 BERICA Ospedale San Bortolo Vicenza, Vicenza, Italy

Fondazione IRRIV AULSS 8 BERICA Ospedale San Bortolo, Vicenza, Italy

UOC Genetica Medica e Genomica AULSS 8 BERICA Ospedale San Bortolo Vicenza, Vicenza, Italy
e-mail: carlotta.caprara@aulss8.veneto.it

F. Ferrari (✉)
Fondazione IRRIV AULSS 8 BERICA Ospedale San Bortolo, Vicenza, Italy

Dipartimento Area Emergenza-Urgenza, SC Anestesia e Terapia Intensiva Adulti Fondazione IRCCS Cà Granda Ospedale Maggiore Policlinico, Milan, Italy
e-mail: fiorenza.ferrari@policlinico.mi.it

S. De Rosa, S. Lassola (eds.), *Next-Gen Blood Purification*,
https://doi.org/10.1007/978-3-032-27033-7_15

reverse mutation to restore the normal function of a defective gene. Gene therapy strategies are facilitated by diverse gene delivery modalities, ranging from physical and chemical vectors to biological carriers targeted to specific cellular platforms. These genetic modifications are often delivered using *viral vectors* such as adeno-associated viruses (AAV) or lentiviruses, either in vivo (directly into the patient) or ex vivo (modifying patient cells outside the body before reinfusion). CRISPR-Cas technology has been pivotal, enabling more precise genetic modifications and enhancing its utility in applications such as xenotransplantation. Gene therapy has been successful in various monogenic and acquired diseases, including hemophilia (e.g., Hemgenix and Roctavian, AAV5-based) and spinal muscular atrophy (SMA) (Zolgensma, AAV9-based). Gene therapy applications extend to neurological disorders, ocular diseases, muscular diseases, and notably, cancer immunotherapy using chimeric antigen receptor T cells (CAR-T) [1]. Key challenges include the targeted delivery of AAV vectors to specific tissues, packaging limitations, immune responses against viral vectors, and safety concerns such as the risk of insertional mutagenesis and potential oncogenicity. The kidney is a promising target for gene therapy, as up to 30% of chronic kidney disease (CKD) cases are estimated to be caused by inherited monogenic disorders. However, no gene therapies have been approved that specifically target the kidney [2]. The primary challenge in renal gene therapy is the effective delivery of genetic material to specific nephron cell types. Advances in vector engineering, including pseudo-typed AAV and lentiviruses, aim to enhance renal targeting [1].

Recent advances in bioartificial organ and bioreactor technologies are reshaping the landscape of blood purification by extending beyond conventional dialysis and adding biological functionality. Dialysis, despite being lifesaving in end-stage kidney disease (ESKD), addresses only a limited portion of kidney physiology—primarily the removal of small solutes and fluid balance. It fails to replicate the metabolic, endocrine, and secretory functions of renal tissue. Bioreactors attempt to fill this gap by combining mechanical clearance with living cellular components able to mediate selective reabsorption, toxin metabolism, hormone production, and immunomodulation [3].

A leading example is the "implantable bioartificial kidney" under development within the Kidney Project at the University of California, San Francisco (UCSF) and Vanderbilt University. This device couples a hemofilter with a bioreactor seeded with renal cells, thereby performing both mechanical and cellular functions. Recent large-animal studies have shown that bioreactors implanted in pigs maintained viability and exhibited renal-like activity without provoking immune rejection [4]. In immunocompetent pigs, the device remained patent and thrombus-free for 7 days without systemic immunosuppression, supporting the feasibility of an implantable bioreactor for renal cell therapy using silicon nanopore membranes.

In parallel, bioengineered kidney tubules tested under experimental dialysis conditions have been able to clear protein-bound uremic toxins more efficiently than conventional filtration, highlighting the potential clinical value of adding cellular components to extracorporeal therapies [3].

Concurrently, extracorporeal blood purification, traditionally a life-support modality for acute conditions like sepsis or organ failure, is emerging as an indispensable partner, both for mitigating the toxicities of gene therapy and as a platform for engineering next-generation bioartificial systems [5]. This report will explore this evolving relationship, structured in three main sections: first, the supportive and enabling role of blood purification in the context of gene therapy adverse events; second, the innovative application of gene therapy as a direct engineering tool for bioartificial organs; and third, a critical analysis of the future prospects and hurdles at this nexus.

15.2 Extracorporeal Blood Purification as a Critical Enabler for Gene Therapy

The reinterpretation of genetics, traditionally viewed as a specialist discipline primarily confined to the management of rare and potentially life-threatening disorders, has undergone a complete reconfiguration as a fundamental component across the entire continuum of healthcare, profoundly transforming contemporary medical practice. This paradigm shift has enhanced our understanding of the molecular and cellular mechanisms underlying tissue and organ repair and has unveiled new therapeutic opportunities at both genetic and cellular levels. Gene therapies are progressively establishing themselves as strategies capable of correcting or counteracting dysfunctional genes in conditions that compromise patients' quality of life, thereby reducing reliance on conventional pharmacological treatments, radiotherapy, or surgical interventions. At the same time, it has become necessary to mitigate the adverse events associated with gene therapy. In this context, blood purification serves a dual role: it can actively attenuate gene therapy–related toxicity and contribute to the design of organ-support solutions. Thus, the application of gene therapy as an engineering tool for novel blood purification systems represents a profound and bidirectional relationship.

15.2.1 Blood Purification Modalities as Therapy for Adverse Events

Blood purification serves an important supportive function in addressing adverse events related to gene therapy, with particular emphasis on managing systemic complications such as toxicity, organ failure, and inflammatory cascade that may result when genetically modified cells are used in therapeutic support systems.

The era of precision medicine has been profoundly shaped by CAR T-cell therapy, a groundbreaking, personalized cancer immunotherapy. This treatment involves extracting a patient's T-cells, genetically modifying them in a laboratory to express a CAR that specifically recognizes and binds to antigens on cancer cells, and then reinfusing these enhanced cells back into the patient.[4] The modified T-cells proliferate within the patient, identifying and destroying malignant cells with high efficacy, particularly in cases of refractory leukemias and lymphomas [6]. However, this impressive therapeutic power is accompanied by a severe, systemic risk profile.

The primary and most life-threatening adverse effect of CAR-T cell therapy is Cytokine Release Syndrome (CRS) [6]. Upon engaging with cancer antigens, the infused CAR-T cells undergo rapid activation and proliferation, unleashing a massive cascade of pro-inflammatory cytokines, often referred to as a "cytokine storm" [5]. This uncontrolled inflammatory response manifests initially as fever and chills but can quickly escalate to multiple-organ dysfunction syndrome (MODS), capillary leakage, and a state resembling septic shock.

The systemic nature of CRS leads to a wide range of complications across multiple organ systems. Neurological toxicities, collectively known as immune effector cell-associated neurotoxicity syndrome (ICANS), can occur simultaneously with or as a consequence of CRS, leading to confusion, aphasia, seizures, and even cerebral edema [7]. Other common toxicities include cardiovascular complications such as hypotension and cardiogenic shock, respiratory failure, and renal and liver injury [8]. The broad spectrum of these toxicities highlights the need for comprehensive and rapid interventions.

The clinical viability and widespread adoption of transformative gene therapies like CAR-T are fundamentally dependent on the existence of effective extracorporeal interventions to manage their potentially fatal side effects. The ability to "rescue" patients from a cytokine storm is what transforms a highly toxic but effective treatment into a clinically feasible option. The following extracorporeal blood purification modalities are employed to manage these adverse events.

Therapeutic Plasma Exchange (PE) has emerged as a promising adjunctive therapy for severe CRS, particularly when standard treatments like tocilizumab and corticosteroids are insufficient [9]. The mechanism of action involves the rapid removal of the patient's plasma and its replacement with a substitute fluid, which effectively clears a wide range of circulating inflammatory mediators, including high-molecular-weight cytokines, chemokines, and immune complexes that drive CRS progression [9]. This technique holds a distinct advantage over other blood purification methods, such as hemofiltration (HF) and hemodiafiltration (HDF), because of its superior ability to remove larger molecules [9]. PE's ability to alleviate symptoms such as fever, hypotension, and neurotoxicity has been demonstrated in clinical cases, positioning it as a critical safety net for CAR-T therapy [9].

Hemoperfusion, which circulates blood over a sorbent material, and devices like CytoSorb®, which adsorbs cytokines, aim to directly attenuate the inflammatory response [10, 11]. However, the clinical evidence for these therapies is not uniform, with a notable lack of positive multicenter randomized controlled trials confirming their clinical relevance in certain contexts. These modalities, while part of the therapeutic toolkit, remain a subject of ongoing controversy and research.

Extracorporeal membrane oxygenation (ECMO) is a specialized form of extracorporeal life support (ECLS) that functions as a temporary bypass for the heart and lungs [12]. ECMO is critically important for managing the downstream consequences of severe CRS, such as acute respiratory distress syndrome, refractory cardiogenic shock, and other forms of heart or lung failure. By taking over the work of these organs, ECMO allows them to rest and heal, thereby providing the necessary time for other treatments to resolve the underlying inflammatory cascade [12]. The risk of insertional genotoxicity and T-cell leukemia in early gene therapy trials [13] demonstrated the critical need for safer vectors. Similarly, the known risk of severe CRS in CAR-T therapy [6] would make it a nonviable treatment option without a reliable safety net (Table 15.1).

15.2.2 Gene Therapy as an Engineering Tool for New Blood Purification Systems

Gene therapy acts as an engineering catalyst for the development of advanced hybrid blood purification systems (e.g., bioartificial liver, BAL; bioartificial kidney), overcoming the limitations of conventional therapies through genetic modification of organs or cells. Simultaneously, the clinical success of in vivo gene therapy (for example, in monogenic kidney diseases) is measured by its ability to render traditional blood purification methods, such as dialysis or transplantation, unnecessary for end-stage organ failure.

Organ failure remains a leading cause of mortality worldwide, with current treatment options severely limited [14]. While orthotopic organ transplantation is the only effective long-term solution, it is hampered by a critical shortage of donor organs, the lifelong necessity for immunosuppressive medication, and the length of the organ waiting list, which often leads to the necessity of extracorporeal therapy as a bridge to transplantation [14]. Furthermore, nonbiological extracorporeal devices, such as dialysis and plasmapheresis, are limited in their capacity, unable to replicate the complex metabolic and regulatory functions of native organs, such as protein synthesis, hormonal secretion, and waste removal. This pressing need has spurred the development of a new paradigm: bioartificial systems.

Bioartificial organs are sophisticated devices that integrate living cells with a synthetic or mechanical scaffold to replicate the functions of native organs. The ultimate goal is to create a device that can permanently restore a defective organ's functionality [14]. However, the development of these systems is fraught with significant technical challenges, including the need for a mechanically stable architecture, a robust nutrient transport system (vascularization), and the use of biocompatible materials that do not provoke an immune response [15].

Table 15.1 Clinical toxicities of gene therapy and corresponding extracorporeal therapies

Adverse reaction	Main symptoms	Pathophysiological mechanism	Corresponding extracorporeal therapy
Cytokine release syndrome (CRS)	Fever, hypotension, hypoxia, multiorgan dysfunction	Systemic inflammatory reaction due to a "cytokine storm"	Therapeutic plasma exchange (PE), hemoadsorption
Immune effector cell-associated neurotoxicity syndrome (ICANS)	Aphasia, encephalopathy, seizures, brain edema	Pro-inflammatory cytokines and CAR-T cells entering the central nervous system after blood-brain barrier breakdown	Therapeutic plasma exchange (PE)
Cardiovascular toxicity	Cardiogenic shock, arrhythmia, heart failure	Elevation of inflammatory cytokines (e.g., IL-6, TNF-α)	Extracorporeal membrane oxygenation (ECMO)
Pulmonary toxicity	Respiratory failure, pleural effusion[10]	Systemic inflammation and organ dysfunction induced by cytokine release syndrome (CRS)	Extracorporeal membrane oxygenation (ECMO)
Renal and liver toxicity	Kidney failure, liver injury, electrolyte disorders	Inflammation and multiorgan dysfunction induced by cytokine release syndrome (CRS)	Continuous kidney replacement therapy, therapeutic plasma exchange (PE)

A fundamental shift is occurring in the application of gene therapy. Its role is moving beyond simply correcting a genetic defect in a patient's own cells to actively engineering biological components to perform complex, life-sustaining functions outside the body. This represents a paradigm shift from a "corrective" to a "constructive" application of genetic medicine, blurring the lines between therapeutic intervention and bioengineering.

The UCSF Kidney Project exemplifies this constructive approach. The project's goal is to create a small, surgically implantable, and self-regulating bioartificial kidney that serves as a permanent solution to kidney failure. This device has two main components: a silicon hemofilter that uses nanotechnology to filter blood using the body's natural blood pressure, and a cell bioreactor that employs tissue engineering and potentially gene-engineered human renal tubule cells. The cell bioreactor is designed not only to reabsorb vital nutrients but also to perform complex biological functions such as the autoregulation of blood pressure and the production of vitamin D, functions that cannot be replicated by traditional dialysis.

Bioartificial kidney development represents the next generation of renal replacement therapy, specifically designed to overcome the functional and logistical deficiencies of conventional dialysis and limited transplant availability. These engineered systems aim to replace the kidney's critical metabolic, endocrine, and homeostatic regulatory functions, which are lost in standard filtration therapies (Fig. 15.1) [16].

One significant approach is the Renal Assist Device (RAD), an extracorporeal bioartificial kidney. The RAD combines a conventional synthetic hemofilter with a bioreactor containing primary renal cells, specifically tubule cells, grown on immunoisolating hollow fibers. This cell component provides essential activities, such as active vectorial transport, ammoniagenesis, and the synthesis of endocrinologic metabolites like 1,25-dihydroxyvitamin D3. In critically ill human patients, RAD has been successfully tested on acute kidney injury (AKI), demonstrating a statistically significant survival advantage in a Phase II trial (67% survival vs. 39% in controls over 180 days) [17].

Building on this success, further innovations address commercialization hurdles, particularly cell sourcing and storage. The Bioartificial Renal Epithelial Cell System (BRECS) was developed as a compact, cryopreservable extracorporeal device. The BRECS cultures renal epithelial cells on porous carbon disks to enable mass fabrication, storage, and distribution for on-demand clinical use [16]. As a core component of the proposed Wearable Bioartificial Kidney (WEBAK), this system aims to provide continuous therapy for ESKD patients, often integrated with sorbent-based technologies for dialysate regeneration [16].

The long-term goal is the fully implantable device. The Implantable Renal Assist Device (iRAD) utilizes Microelectromechanical Systems (MEMS) technology to miniaturize the components. Its filtration component relies on Silicon Nanopore Membranes (SNM), which offer high hydraulic permeability and precise selectivity, mimicking the native glomerulus. Crucially, the SNM design allows adequate filtration rates (30 mL/min) using only the natural arteriovenous pressure differential, eliminating the need for an internal pump. Furthermore, the SNM acts as an

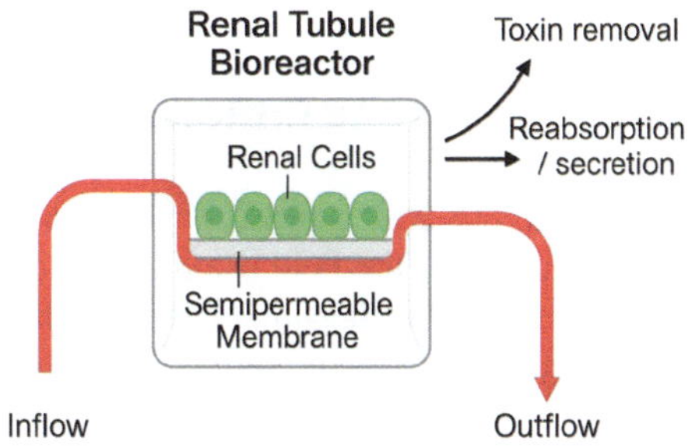

Fig. 15.1 Conceptual illustration of a renal tubule bioreactor in which blood is circulated across a semipermeable membrane seeded with engineered renal tubular cells, mimicking native kidney functions

immunoisolation barrier to protect the seeded renal epithelial cells from the host immune response after implantation [16].

Another groundbreaking application involves the use of genetically modified xenogeneic organs for extracorporeal systems [18]. Researchers have successfully used gene-edited porcine livers in novel BAL systems. Gene editing is used to modify the pig cells to minimize immune rejection and to produce humanized proteins like albumin and coagulation factors, thereby overcoming the metabolic and protein synthesis limitations of traditional nonbiological systems. The use of these genetically modified organs in an extracorporeal circuit, as demonstrated in a 72-h blood filtration study, provides a life-bridge for patients until their own liver can recover or a human donor becomes available.

BAL devices integrate human, porcine, or stem cell-derived hepatocytes into bioreactors designed to provide metabolic and synthetic support in acute liver failure [19]. Unlike dialysis-based detoxification, BAL units can metabolize ammonia, bilirubin, and drugs, while also secreting albumin and coagulation factors. The use of mixed porcine–human repopulated bioengineered livers has shown promise in preclinical models of models of post-resection liver failure, suggesting that hybrid constructs could partially overcome limitations in cell sourcing [20].

From the perspective of blood purification, these devices offer a dual advantage: mechanical clearance of toxins and biologically active processing of complex metabolites. Beyond detoxification of protein-bound molecules, the approach also allows for restoration of endocrine and paracrine functions, as well as the potential modulation of systemic inflammation [4, 18].

Although clinical bioreactors currently rely on unmodified primary or stem cell-derived renal and hepatic cells, the integration of genetic engineering is increasingly recognized as a future development that could significantly enhance their therapeutic capacity. Gene editing technologies such as CRISPR-Cas offer the possibility of tailoring cell populations used within bioreactors to correct specific metabolic defects, enhance resilience to oxidative and inflammatory stress, or optimize secretion of therapeutic proteins [21].

Another promising avenue is the use of patient-derived induced pluripotent stem cells (iPSCs). These cells can be differentiated into renal or hepatic lineages and potentially used in personalized bioreactor cartridges. When combined with gene correction, iPSC-derived cells could not only restore missing functions but also overcome the immunological challenges posed by allogeneic sources. Such strategies open the possibility of autologous, genetically optimized bioartificial organs.

15.3 Trends and Critical Hurdles

By converging with genetic engineering, bioartificial organ technology marks a paradigm shift in the field. Rather than being conceived solely as mechanical substitutes for renal or hepatic clearance, these devices are now seen as dynamic and customizable biological platforms capable of replacing organ functions, modeling disease, and eventually delivering gene- or cell-based therapies in a controlled extracorporeal setting [22]. While major challenges remain—including cell sourcing, long-term viability, immunoprotection, and scalability—the trajectory from mechanical detoxification to genetically optimized bioartificial organs suggests that these systems may become transformative adjuncts, and perhaps even alternatives, to transplantation in the future.

The integration of medicine and engineering is the driving force behind the development of Bioartificial organ systems. This involves ongoing development of appropriate cell sources, better techniques for cell preservation and expansion, the creation of smart bioreactor systems, and standardized production processes to enable large- scale application.

Looking ahead, extracorporeal technology is expected to evolve toward increased portability, improved biocompatibility, and smarter systems. Miniaturized and portable ECMO systems, along with other blood purification devices, are being developed to expand their use beyond the ICU and into broader clinical settings. At the same time, innovations in biocompatible materials aim to reduce the risk of clotting and bleeding complications. Integrating advanced monitoring and data analytics into these systems will give clinicians real-time data to improve decision-making. Together, these technological advancements and growing awareness of their efficacy will drive wider adoption of these lifesaving therapies.

Translating a successful lab prototype into a clinically viable product poses significant logistical challenges. The current fabrication methods, such as bioprinting, often fall short of meeting the large-scale, rapid, and automated production demands of clinical settings. Manual processes not only incur high costs and consume valuable time, but they also introduce unacceptable variability between individual products. For clinical-grade translation, adherence to Good Manufacturing Practice is essential; this includes establishing specialized containment systems and utilizing rigorously tested, standardized bioink materials, which are often scarce or entirely lacking in the current landscape. Unlike traditional small molecules, bioartificial organs are living entities. Therefore, developing effective strategies for long-term preservation and transportation is critical to ensure cell viability and functionality, which are key to achieving a commercially viable and globally accessible technology.

Complex hybrid technologies do not fit neatly into existing regulatory frameworks for either traditional drugs or medical devices. For instance, bioartificial organs are not injectable substances but complex products combining devices with living cells, emphasizing the need for comprehensive regulatory guidance to ensure safe and responsible early-phase clinical trials [23].

Many regulatory agencies don't have a clear and unified classification system in place, which can lead to a lot of uncertainty and increased risk for both developers and investors.

Then there is the question of ethical oversight. When it comes to innovative, irreversible cell-based therapies, the potential for serious risks—like toxicity, infections, or tumor formation—during early-phase clinical trials is real. This situation calls for new ethical guidance and oversight. It is crucial to address issues related to cell sourcing, patient selection, and ensuring that patients give truly informed consent.

On top of that, the financial aspect cannot be ignored. The costs associated with research, development, and the specialized manufacturing processes can make initial investments quite high-risk. Plus, we need to tackle the significant challenge of ensuring that these potentially lifesaving therapies are accessible to all patients, especially given their high costs. This is a moral and societal issue we must address from the outset.

15.4 Conclusion

The relationship between gene therapy and blood purification is evolving from a passive, reactive dynamic to a synergistic, initiative-taking partnership. Gene therapy, once a risky endeavor, is now a proven therapeutic modality whose clinical success is fundamentally enabled by the existence of robust extracorporeal support systems. In this context, blood purification acts not merely as a safety net but as an indispensable pillar enabling revolutionary treatments such as CAR-T cell therapy.

Gene therapies offer strategies to correct dysfunctional genes and reduce dependence on conventional treatments. At the same time, blood purification plays a dual role in mitigating therapy-related toxicity and enabling organ-support designs, highlighting a bidirectional relationship between gene therapy and advanced blood purification systems. Although gene therapy provides the engineering tools (e.g., CRISPR-Cas) to enable next-generation blood purification platforms, including xenogeneic livers and advanced BALs, critical challenges remain in vector capacity, precise renal targeting, and in the long-term validation of efficacy and biosafety for highly engineered cellular and organ products.

Targeted gene delivery to specific cells and tissues remains the primary challenge for gene therapies in complex blood purification organs such as the kidney. Renal gene therapy is hindered by the nephron's structural complexity and the low transduction efficiency of current viral vectors. Overcoming the glomerular barrier—which actively excludes particles larger than 10 nm or 50 kDa—is critical, highlighting the need for novel capsids or nanoparticles. Optimizing administration routes is also essential to maximize therapeutic efficacy while minimizing toxicity and off-target effects [1].

Looking ahead, this relationship is set to deepen further. Gene therapy is moving from a corrective to a constructive tool, actively engineering biological components for extracorporeal devices capable of performing the complex, life-sustaining functions of native organs. From kidneys to livers, these bioartificial systems represent a radical new frontier in treating organ failure, overcoming the critical limitations of transplantation and mechanical support.

Navigating these hurdles will require continued interdisciplinary collaboration among scientists, clinicians, ethicists, and policymakers to ensure that the future of genetic medicine and extracorporeal support delivers broad-based progress and equitable access.

References

1. Peek JL, Wilson MH. Cell and gene therapy for kidney disease. Nat Rev Nephrol. 2023;19:451–62.
2. Gene therapies should be for all. Nat Med. 2021;27:1311. https://doi.org/10.1038/s41591-021-01481-9.
3. Faria J, Ahmed S, Stamatialis D, Verhaar MC, Masereeuw R, Gerritsen KGF, Mihăilă SM. Bioengineered kidney tubules efficiently clear uremic toxins in experimental dialysis conditions. Int J Mol Sci. 2023. https://doi.org/10.3390/ijms241512435.
4. Kim EJ, Chen C, Gologorsky R, et al. Feasibility of an implantable bioreactor for renal cell therapy using silicon nanopore membranes. Nat Commun. 2023;14:4890.
5. Mehta Y, Paul R, Ansari AS, et al. Extracorporeal blood purification strategies in sepsis and septic shock: an insight into recent advancements. World J Crit Care Med. 2023;12:71–88.
6. Garcia Borrega J, Gödel P, Rüger MA, Onur ÖA, Shimabukuro-Vornhagen A, Kochanek M, Böll B. In the eye of the storm: immune-mediated toxicities associated with CAR-T cell therapy. Hemasphere. 2019. https://doi.org/10.1097/HS9.0000000000000191.
7. Müller A. Rare adverse events of CAR T-cell therapy. healthbook TIMES, Oncol hematol. 2024. https://doi.org/10.36000/HBT.OH.2024.19.138.
8. Li Y, Ming Y, Fu R, et al. The pathogenesis, diagnosis, prevention, and treatment of CAR-T cell therapy-related adverse reactions. Front Pharmacol. 2022. https://doi.org/10.3389/fphar.2022.950923.
9. Zhang J, Xie D, Tang M, Gong Q, Huang X, Li J, Xu S, Luo N, Sun H, Tan F. Utilizing plasma exchange for severe cytokine release syndrome after CAR-T cell therapy: clinical experience and literature insights. Front Immunol. 2025. https://doi.org/10.3389/fimmu.2025.1597512.
10. Singbartl K, Rosenthal A, Leis J, Patel B, Sen A. Novel use of extracorporeal blood purification for treatment of severe, refractory neurotoxicity after chimeric antigen receptor T-cell therapy—a case report. Crit Care Explor. 2021;3:e0472.
11. Esposito P, Gambella M, Russo E, et al. Hemoadsorption as a supportive strategy for severe toxicity associated with chimeric antigen receptor T-cell therapy: a case series. Kidney Med. 2025;7:101001.
12. Wang X. Bioartificial organ manufacturing technologies. Cell Transplant. 2019;28:5–17.
13. Nienhuis AW. Development of gene therapy for blood disorders: an update. Blood. 2013;122:1556–64.
14. Corridon PR, Ko IK, Yoo JJ, Atala A. Bioartificial kidneys. Curr Stem Cell Rep. 2017;3:68–76.
15. Geiler C, Andrade I, Clayton A, Greenwald D. Genetically engineered in vitro erythropoiesis. Int J Stem Cells. 2016;9:53–9.
16. Kim S, Fissell WH, Humes DH, Roy S. Current strategies and challenges in engineering a bioartificial kidney. Front Biosci (Elite Ed). 2015;7:215–28.
17. Humes HD, Buffington D, Westover AJ, Roy S, Fissell WH. The bioartificial kidney: current status and future promise. Pediatr Nephrol. 2014;29:343–51.
18. Jiang Q, Su Y, Cao X, Zhang H, Zhang J, Li L. Bioartificial liver: where lies the path ahead—a review. Hepatol Commun. 2025. https://doi.org/10.1097/HC9.0000000000000788.
19. Jasirwan COM, Muradi A, Antarianto RD. Bio-artificial liver support system: a prospective future therapy. Liver. 2023;3:65–75.
20. Felgendreff P, Hosseiniasl SM, Minshew A, et al. First application of a mixed porcine-human repopulated bioengineered liver in a preclinical model of post-resection liver failure. Biomedicine. 2024. https://doi.org/10.3390/biomedicines12061272.
21. Doudna JA, Charpentier E. Genome editing. The new frontier of genome engineering with CRISPR-Cas9. Science. 2014;346:1258096.
22. Bottari G, Ranieri VM, Ince C. et al. Use of extracorporeal blood purification therapies in sepsis: the current paradigm, available evidence, and future perspectives. Crit Care 2024;28:432. https://doi.org/10.1186/s13054-024-05220-7.
23. de Jongh D, Massey EK, Cronin AJ, Schermer MHN, Bunnik EM, VANGUARD Consortium. Early-phase clinical trials of bio-artificial organ technology: a systematic review of ethical issues. Transpl Int. 2022;35:10751.

The Role of Artificial Organs in Blood Purification

16

Réginald Philippe and Silvia Holler

Abbreviations

AO	Artificial organs
BAK	Bio-artificial kidney
BAL	Bio-artificial liver
BP	Blood purification
CKD	Chronic kidney disease
CRRT	Continuous renal replacement therapy
EBP	Extracorporeal Blood Purification
PEG	polyethylene glycol

16.1 Introduction

Blood purification (BP), defined as the removal of waste products, toxins, and other harmful substances from the blood, is a successful example of how artificial organs (AOs), human-made devices designed to substitute for physiological function, can replace vital functions. The field began with the first "artificial kidney" in the mid-twentieth century, enabling survival in end-stage renal failure when no other options existed. Early mechanical filtration devices were rudimentary, but pioneers like Abel, Kolff, and Alwall laid the foundation for modern hemodialysis (HD) and

R. Philippe (✉)
Centre for Medical Sciences, CISMed, University of Trento, Trento, Italy
e-mail: reginald.philippe@unitn.it

S. Holler
Department of Cellular Computational and Integrative Biology, CIBIO, University of Trento, Trento, Italy
e-mail: silvia.holler@unitn.it

S. De Rosa, S. Lassola (eds.), *Next-Gen Blood Purification*,
https://doi.org/10.1007/978-3-032-27033-7_16

hemofiltration, blood purification by diffusion or filtration across a membrane, respectively [1]. These therapies have become life-sustaining for millions, though they cannot fully replicate kidney function. Emerging technologies such as bio-hybrid systems, nanomaterial-functionalized membranes, and synthetic biological constructs seek to address these limitations by integrating bioengineering, materials science, and synthetic biology, thereby moving AO toward more physiologically adaptive and smart designs [2]. This chapter reviews the evolution of AO for BP, comparing conventional extracorporeal systems with emerging technologies such as bio-hybrid devices, functionalized materials, and synthetic biological constructs, and discussing their clinical implications and future perspectives.

16.2 Defining Artificial Organs in Blood Purification

BP technologies span a functional continuum ranging from mechanical extracorporeal support, through partially bioactive hybrid systems integrating living cells, to full organ replacement through transplantation. In this context, an AO replaces or supports kidney function by removing waste, toxins, and excess fluid. Traditional systems use semi-permeable membranes without biological integration, while next-generation devices combine synthetic structures with living components for improved autonomy, biocompatibility, and physiological function. Table 16.1 summarizes key established and emerging technologies along this continuum, highlighting their advantages, limitations, and clinical maturity.

Table 16.1 Artificial organs provide intermediate options between conventional dialysis and organ transplantation, balancing functionality, portability, and clinical challenges

Category	Technologies	Advantages	Limitations	Clinical maturity (TRL)
Mechanical extracorporeal BP support	HD, PD, CRRT	Well-established; lifesaving; suitable for acute and chronic use	Non-curative; limited physiological restoration; risk of clotting, infection, hypotension	Clinical standard (TRL 9)
Miniaturized or implantable mechanical BP systems	Wearable HD, miniaturized dialysis, sorbent PD	Enhanced mobility and independence; home or ambulatory use	Limited toxin removal; partially experimental; requires maintenance	Early clinical trials/ prototype (TRL 6–7)
Hybrid bio-integrated AO	Bio-artificial kidney, bio-artificial liver	Improved toxin/ metabolite removal; partial physiological function; continuous support	Experimental; cell viability and immune challenges; technical complexity; regulatory hurdles	Preclinical stage/early clinical trials (TRL 4–6)
Organ transplantation	Kidney, liver	Complete organ replacement; proven long-term survival	Limited donors; immunosuppression required; risk of rejection	Clinical standard (TRL 9)

TRL Technology Readiness Levels scale

16.3 Membrane Science and Functional Materials

The technological foundations of extracorporeal blood purification (EBP) rely heavily on advances in materials science, membrane engineering, and surface technologies that determine selectivity, efficiency, and biocompatibility.

16.3.1 Evolution of Membrane Technologies

Dialysis membranes have evolved from low-flux designs, with limited permeability, to high-flux and, subsequently, to medium/high-cutoff membranes that can remove larger molecules while posing varying degrees of risk for albumin loss [3]. Current research is moving toward adaptive or responsive membranes, engineered to modulate permeability, charge, or selectivity in real time according to the patient's physiological state [4]. This shift reflects a gradual evolution from purely passive filtration to membranes that support more precise and dynamic BP.

16.3.2 Functionalized Nanomaterials for Selective Toxin Removal

Beyond size-based filtration, nanostructured and functionalized materials expand toxin clearance through targeted adsorption. Polymers with chemical functional groups, affinity ligands, or high-surface-area nanostructures can bind uremic toxins, cytokines, endotoxins, or protein-bound molecules. Representative examples include polymyxin-B–based endotoxin adsorbers and CytoSorb-type broad-spectrum sorbents, which illustrate two main strategies: (1) selective binding of pathogenic molecules and (2) nonspecific adsorption of inflammatory mediators [5]. Hybrid or mixed-matrix membranes incorporating nanomaterials directly into the filtration layer combine diffusion and adsorption in a single device, improving selectivity and reducing pressure drop.

16.3.3 Bio-inspired and Composite Polymers Improving Hemocompatibility

Surface chemistry modifications are crucial for improving hemocompatibility during BP by reducing clot formation, protein fouling, complement activation, and inflammation. Coatings such as heparin, PEG, chitosan, or polydopamine are designed to create more compatible interfaces, yet they still cannot fully prevent long-term coagulation or fouling [6]. The AN69 oXiris® membrane illustrates this approach by combining heparin grafting with adsorptive materials to improve compatibility and cytokine removal [5].

Hydrophilic polymer layers (e.g., PEG or polyphosphoesters) limit platelet adhesion and protein deposition, while chitosan derivatives can reduce complement activation [6]. More advanced nanostructured or zwitterionic surfaces further suppress nonspecific protein adsorption and inflammation, helping extend membrane lifespan in HD and Continuous Renal Replacement Therapy (CRRT) [7].

Future developments focus on adaptive, stimuli-responsive polymers that adjust permeability or adsorption in response to biochemical cues (solute concentration, pH, or oxidative stress), potentially enabling more physiologically responsive and durable extracorporeal devices [8, 9].

16.4 Extracorporeal Circuit Design and Portable Systems

16.4.1 Modular Design of Purification Circuits

The design of BP systems has progressed well beyond traditional HD toward modular EBP circuits that integrate interchangeable components (hemofilters, dialyzers, adsorbers, plasma separators, and pumps) adapted to patient-specific needs. This modularity reflects the new definition of BP, which now encompasses detoxification, fluid management, and immunomodulation in addition to renal replacement. It enables flexible combinations of convective or diffusive CRRT with hemoadsorption or plasma-based therapies, allowing clinicians to rapidly tailor multi-modality treatments for conditions such as acute kidney injury, sepsis, or chronic HD [10].

16.4.2 Sensor Integration and Adaptive Control

Contemporary BP systems increasingly incorporate a range of sensors monitoring pressure, flow, dialysate composition and conductivity, ultrafiltration volume, and circuit integrity (e.g., air/bubble or blood leak detectors) [11]. These sensors provide real-time feedback that supports automatic adjustments of ultrafiltration rates, dialysate flow, and adsorber engagement in response to the patient's physiological status, enhancing safety and treatment precision.

Beyond these established implementations, next-generation BP and CRRT devices are integrating biochemical and metabolic sensing technologies to monitor solute concentrations, electrolyte balance, and acid-base status. When combined with advanced data analytics and artificial intelligence (AI)-based control algorithms, these systems enable adaptive, patient-specific therapies that dynamically respond to changing physiological conditions [12]. AI-driven platforms can optimize device performance, predict circuit dysfunction or component degradation, and guide maintenance or replacement strategies, reducing downtime and treatment interruptions.

The convergence of continuous sensing and intelligent control paves the way toward closed-loop, more autonomous artificial kidney systems. Such approaches aim to improve hemodynamic stability, solute clearance, and overall treatment efficiency.

16.4.3 Portable and Wearable Systems

Wearable and portable BP technologies are rapidly advancing to provide continuous or extended renal support outside traditional dialysis centers, enabled by miniaturized pumps and filters, sorbent-based dialysate regeneration, integrated sensors, and low-power control systems [13, 14]. The Wearable Artificial Kidney (WAK), a HD device, has completed proof-of-concept and small human feasibility trials, demonstrating continuous treatment outside the clinic [15, 16]. In parallel, sorbent-based peritoneal dialysis (PD) platforms illustrate how compact sorbents, microfluidics, and low-energy pumping can support near-continuous therapy for mobile patients [15, 17]. Emerging microfluidic systems, such as the nano-electrokinetic PD dialysate purification device from Seoul National University, further exemplify "artificial kidney on a chip" approaches that may enable ultra-portable or implantable units [18, 19]. These examples illustrate how modern BP systems integrating new technologies could improve patients' quality of life in the future.

16.5 Bio-Hybrid and Artificial Biological Systems

16.5.1 Synthetic Biology and Hemofiltration

The development of AO increasingly relies on engineered compartmentalization to prevent dilution of therapeutic molecules and support complex biochemical networks. Inspired by biological cell organization, modern bioengineering uses membrane-based microcompartments as functional units. These can have two main architectures, lipid-based vesicles [20] and coacervate-based aggregates [21], each offering distinct advantages for creating semi-permeable boundaries and structured microenvironments suitable for integrating synthetic biology components into artificial AO.

Lipid-based vesicles have become central to this approach due to their biocompatibility and functional versatility. Their amphiphilic molecules spontaneously self-assemble into spherical compartments in aqueous environments, forming stable, tunable barriers. Cationic liposomes have been shown to enhance the clearance of anionic protein-bound uremic toxins such as indoxyl sulfate, 3-indoleacetic acid, and p-cresol when used as adsorbents in dialysate [22]. When integrated with engineered proteins, biosensors, or enzymatic modules, lipid compartments could also act as functional modules for detoxification, biosynthesis, or signal processing within AO, while maintaining selective permeability and biochemical organization.

16.5.2 Hybrid Biological Constructs

Hybrid biological constructs, or bio-artificial organs, integrate living cells with synthetic platforms to restore metabolic and regulatory functions beyond the capabilities of conventional dialysis. Typically, these systems pair a filtration or plasma-separation module with a cell-based bioreactor to replicate organ-specific functions. Although both bio-artificial liver (BAL) and bio-artificial kidney (BAK) systems combine living cells with engineered devices, they serve distinct purposes: BAL provides temporary metabolic support for acute liver failure, whereas BAK seeks to continuously restore renal tubular functions and maintain homeostasis.

BAL systems use hepatocytes cultured in hollow-fiber, fluidized-bed, or 3D scaffold platforms to provide detoxification, metabolic activity, and synthetic functions [23]. Early trials in acute and acute-on-chronic liver failure showed temporary improvement and support as a bridge to transplant or recovery. However, despite multiple clinical prototypes, no BAL has demonstrated a consistent survival benefit or obtained regulatory approval; furthermore, its application remains experimental.

BAK devices combine a hemofilter with a renal-cell bioreactor to restore tubular functions, reabsorption, secretion, and metabolic activity [24]. Prototypes confirmed feasibility and suggested potential benefit in acute kidney injury. Current efforts also on replication of cellular 3D proximal tubules to better replicate native kidney architecture [25]. Fully implantable concepts pair a silicon-based nanopore hemofilter with a renal-cell bioreactor to provide pump-free CRRT [26]. Large-animal studies show preserved epithelial viability and function, but long-term patency, immunoprotection, and scalable manufacturing remain major barriers. As a result, implantable BAKs are promising but remain preclinical [27].

16.5.3 Challenges Bridging Synthetic Biology and Hemofiltration

Experimental approaches illustrate this potential: semi-biological modules incorporating renal epithelial cells, enzymatic nanoreactors, or engineered vesicles can actively remove uremic toxins, while multi-compartment microfluidic devices integrate filtration, adsorption, and metabolic processing [28]. Embedded sensors provide continuous monitoring of solutes and feedback control, paving the way for autonomous, closed-loop hemofiltration systems. These strategies demonstrate that bio-hybrid devices could move beyond mere toxin clearance toward active regulation of electrolytes, fluid balance, and metabolic signals. Despite their promise, bio-hybrid artificial kidneys face significant challenges, including long-term stability of living components, hemocompatibility, scalability for clinical use, and regulatory considerations regarding semi-living implants.

16.6 Clinical and Translational Implications

The development of artificial kidneys holds transformative potential across multiple critical clinical scenarios, particularly in chronic kidney disease (CKD), sepsis, and multi-organ failure. In advanced CKD, bio-hybrid devices may act as a bridge to transplantation or offer an alternative for patients not eligible for transplant. In acute settings such as sepsis or cardiorenal syndrome, modular systems combining toxin removal and immunomodulation could influence outcomes by addressing both biochemical and inflammatory pathways.

Compared to conventional HD, artificial kidney offers distinct advantages with enhanced selectivity, improved portability, and bioactivity through the incorporation of living renal cells. A 2023 study demonstrated the feasibility of implantation of a silicon nanopore membrane-based bioreactor in pigs for 7 days without immunosuppression or anticoagulation, with human renal epithelial cells maintaining over 90% viability [26]. Future iterations of these approaches could integrate liposomes and specific adsorbents for enhanced performance. Nowadays, prototypes of implantable kidneys remain largely in preclinical stages; the next critical steps involve building patient-sized prototypes and conducting long-term animal studies. Clinical translation may be achievable in the near future, pending resolution of scalability and long-term biocompatibility challenges.

16.7 Future Perspectives and Ethical Considerations

As illustrated in Fig. 16.1, the development of next-generation artificial kidneys will rely on simultaneous advances in biomaterials, device autonomy, cellular integration, intelligent sensing technologies, and regulatory and ethical governance. Cell-containing systems, including primary renal cells, stem cell-derived progenitors, or genetically modified lines, offer the potential to restore physiological kidney functions beyond what mechanical devices can achieve. These approaches raise important ethical and safety considerations related to cell sourcing, immunogenicity, long-term viability, and the use of genetic modifications, highlighting the need for transparent oversight and standardized reporting.

From a regulatory perspective, hybrid artificial kidneys are likely to be classified as Advanced Therapy Medicinal Products (ATMPs), requiring complex approval

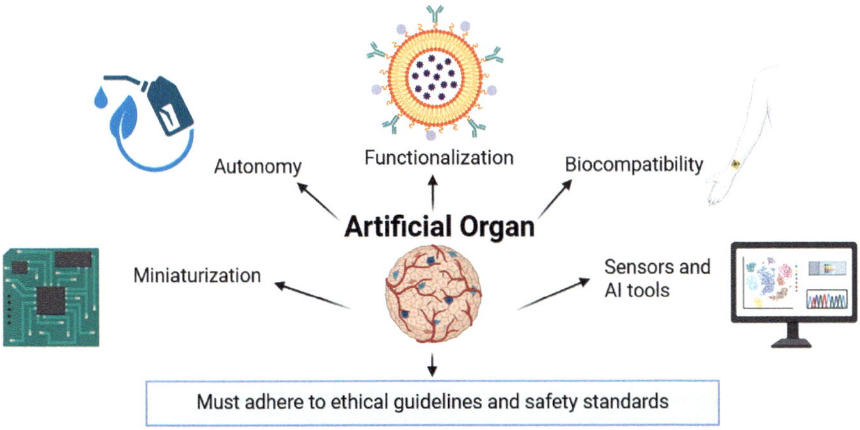

Fig. 16.1 Future challenges in artificial organ development (Created with BioRender.com)

pathways, long-term surveillance, and stringent manufacturing standards [29]. Coordinated engagement with regulatory authorities and harmonization between device and biologic frameworks will be crucial to ensure timely clinical translation while maintaining safety. Equitable access is also essential, as advanced wearable and implantable devices may improve mobility and treatment adherence but risk exacerbating disparities in care without careful planning of pricing, reimbursement, and distribution.

Finally, ethical considerations extend to patient autonomy and data protection, particularly given continuous physiological monitoring in modern devices. Safeguarding sensitive health information, ensuring informed consent, and defining data ownership will be critical for maintaining trust and compliance with evolving regulations. Integrating technological innovation with responsible governance, transparent oversight, and equitable deployment will be essential to realize the full potential of artificial kidneys as safe, effective, and widely accessible therapies.

16.8 Conclusion

AO for BP are rapidly evolving from conventional mechanical filters into adaptive, intelligent systems capable of approximating natural kidney function. Their development requires the integration of advances in materials science, synthetic biology, and clinical nephrology to create devices that are both physiologically effective and safe for patients. Realizing this potential will depend on continued interdisciplinary collaboration to translate innovative technologies into practical, patient-centered therapies that improve outcomes and quality of life.

Acknowledgments ChatGPT (OpenAI) was used to support language editing and to assist with drafting text. All content was reviewed and verified by the authors.

Competing Interests The authors have no conflicts of interest to declare that are relevant to the content of this chapter.

References

1. Fleming GM. Renal replacement therapy review. Organogenesis. 2011;7(1):2–12.
2. Tang YS, Tsai YC, Chen TW, Li SY. Artificial kidney engineering: the development of dialysis membranes for blood purification. Membranes. 2022;12(2):177.
3. Chen YA, Ou SM, Lin CC. Influence of dialysis membranes on clinical outcomes: from history to innovation. Membranes. 2022;12(2):152.
4. Ergun C, Eskizengin H. Recent updates on blood purification: use of smart polymer materials. J Biomed Mater Res. 2025;113(3):e37883.
5. Honore PM, Blackman S, Perriens E, Oueslati I, Haddad C, Al-Sammour C, et al. Adsorptive therapies in sepsis and inflammation: description of the various adsorptive techniques and their failure to improve outcomes. Rev Investig Clin. 2023;75(6):359–76.
6. Ávila E, Sepúlveda RA, Retamal J, Hachim D. Biocompatibility in hemodialysis: artificial membrane and human blood interactions. BMC Nephrol. 2025;26(1):482.
7. Amoako K, Ukita R, Cook KE. Antifouling Zwitterionic polymer coatings for blood-bearing medical devices. Langmuir. 2025;41(5):2994–3006.

8. Uredat S, Gujare A, Runge J, Truzzolillo D, Oberdisse J, Hellweg T. A review of stimuli-responsive polymer-based gating membranes. Phys Chem Chem Phys. 2024;26(4):2732–44.
9. Yoshihara E, Sasaki M, Nabil A, Iijima M, Ebara M. Temperature responsive polymer conjugate prepared by "grafting from" proteins toward the adsorption and removal of uremic toxin. Molecules. 2022;27(3):1051.
10. Ostermann M, Ankawi G, Cantaluppi V, Madarasu R, Dolan K, Husain-Syed F, et al. Nomenclature of extracorporeal blood purification therapies for acute indications: the nomenclature standardization conference. Blood Purif. 2023;53(5):358–72.
11. Randhay A, Eldehni MT, Selby NM. Feedback control in hemodialysis. Semin Dial. 2025;38(1):62–70.
12. Alobaidi S. Emerging biomarkers and advanced diagnostics in chronic kidney disease: early detection through multi-omics and AI. Diagnostics. 2025;15(10):1225.
13. Wieringa FP, Suran S, Søndergaard H, Ash S, Cummins C, Chaudhuri AR, et al. The future of technology-based kidney replacement therapies: an update on portable, wearable, and implantable artificial kidneys. Am J Kidney Dis. 2025;85(6):787–96.
14. Castro AC, Neri M, Nayak Karopadi A, Lorenzin A, Marchionna N, Ronco C. Wearable artificial kidney and wearable ultrafiltration device vascular access—future directions. Clin Kidney J. 2019;12(2):300–7.
15. Stauss M, Htay H, Kooman JP, Lindsay T, Woywodt A. Wearables in nephrology: fanciful gadgetry or Prêt-à-Porter? Sensors. 2023;23(3):1361.
16. Gura V, Rivara MB, Bieber S, Munshi R, Smith NC, Linke L, et al. A wearable artificial kidney for patients with end-stage renal disease. JCI Insight. 2016;1(8):e86397.
17. McGrath SB, Kosalka P, Foo MW, Htay H, Brown EA, Gerritsen KG, Heimbürger O, Jain AK. Advances in sorbent peritoneal dialysis technologies: A narrative review. Perit Dial Int. 2025:8968608251371951. https://doi.org/10.1177/08968608251371951.
18. Kim W, Hong S, Kim K, Lee S, Shin DA, Yang SH, et al. Scalable ion concentration polarization dialyzer for peritoneal dialysate regeneration. J Nanobiotechnol. 2025;23(1):255.
19. Fissell WH, Dubnisheva A, Eldridge AN, Fleischman AJ, Zydney AL, Roy S. High-performance silicon nanopore hemofiltration membranes. J Membr Sci. 2009;326(1):58–63.
20. Elani Y, Law RV, Ces O. Vesicle-based artificial cells as chemical microreactors with spatially segregated reaction pathways. Nat Commun. 2014;5(1):5305.
21. Ghosh B, McCall PM, Le Vay KK, Ghosh A, Hubatsch L, Gonzales DT, et al. RNA-peptide interactions tune the ribozyme activity within coacervate microdroplet dispersions. Nat Commun. 2025;16(1):8765.
22. Shen Y, Wang Y, Shi Y, Bi X, Xu J, Zhu Q, et al. Improving the clearance of protein-bound uremic toxins using cationic liposomes as an adsorbent in dialysate. Colloids Surf B: Biointerfaces. 2020;186:110725.
23. Jiang Q, Su Y, Cao X, Zhang H, Zhang J, Li L. Bioartificial liver: where lies the path ahead-a review. Hepatol Commun. 2025;9(9):e0788.
24. Humes HD, MacKay SM, Funke AJ, Buffington DA. Tissue engineering of a bioartificial renal tubule assist device: in vitro transport and metabolic characteristics. Kidney Int. 1999;55(6):2502–14.
25. Homan KA, Kolesky DB, Skylar-Scott MA, Herrmann J, Obuobi H, Moisan A, et al. Bioprinting of 3D convoluted renal proximal tubules on perfusable chips. Sci Rep. 2016;6(1):34845.
26. Kim EJ, Chen C, Gologorsky R, Santandreu A, Torres A, Wright N, et al. Feasibility of an implantable bioreactor for renal cell therapy using silicon nanopore membranes. Nat Commun. 2023;14(1):4890.
27. Karageorgos FF, Neiros S, Karakasi KE, Vasileiadou S, Katsanos G, Antoniadis N, et al. Artificial kidney: challenges and opportunities. World J Transplant. 2024;14(1):89025.
28. Ramada DL, de Vries J, Vollenbroek J, Noor N, ter Beek O, Mihăilă SM, et al. Portable, wearable and implantable artificial kidney systems: needs, opportunities and challenges. Nat Rev Nephrol. 2023;19:481–90.
29. Frederico C, Conceição A, Nóbrega C, Mendonça LS. Advanced therapy medicinal products development - from guidelines to medicines in the market. Biotechnol Adv. 2025;83:108612.

17 Ethics, Economics, and Global Access to Blood Purification Technologies

Max Bell

17.1 Introduction

Chronic kidney disease (CKD) and acute kidney injury (AKI) represent major global health challenges. CKD prevalence reached 9.1% globally in 2017 (697.5 million cases), increasing 1.2% annually [1]. End-stage kidney disease (ESKD) incidence varies dramatically: 149 per million population (pmp) in high-income countries (HICs) versus 129 pmp in low-income countries (LICs), yet renal replacement therapy (RRT) rates show stark disparities—969 pmp in HICs versus only 4.4 pmp in LICs [2].

AKI affects one-third to half of intensive care unit (ICU) patients, with 20% requiring RRT [3]. Continuous renal replacement therapy (CRRT) is utilized in 75.2% of ICU RRT sessions globally [4]. Despite technological advances, mortality for dialysis-dependent AKI exceeds 50%, and between 2 and 7 million people die annually from ESKD due to lack of treatment access [5, 6].

This chapter addresses three interconnected dimensions: ethical frameworks guiding blood purification provision, economic realities constraining access, and global disparities in availability. We examine strategies to enhance equitable access while maintaining ethical and economic sustainability.

M. Bell (✉)
Karolinska Institutet, Department of Physiology and Pharmacology, Stockholm, Sweden

Perioperative Medicine and Intensive Care, Karolinska University Hospital, Stockholm, Sweden
e-mail: max.bell@regionstockholm.se

S. De Rosa, S. Lassola (eds.), *Next-Gen Blood Purification*,
https://doi.org/10.1007/978-3-032-27033-7_17

17.2 Global Disparities in Access

17.2.1 Chronic Dialysis Access

Dialysis is accessible to more than half of kidney failure patients in only 74% of countries, with dramatic variations: 32% of LICs, 45% of lower-middle-income countries (LMICs), 87% of upper-middle-income countries (UMICs), and 98% of HICs. Regional differences are equally stark—only 14% of South Asian countries and 43% of African nations provide adequate access, compared to universal availability in Eastern Europe, the Middle East, and North/East Asia [7].

In India, 50% of patients stop dialysis due to cost constraints; in Nigeria, financial barriers result in dialysis periods under 1 month [2]. Even with initial access, high attrition rates in resource-limited settings reflect unsustainable financial burden.

17.2.2 Modality-Specific Challenges

Hemodialysis (HD): In-center HD accounts for 78% of RRT globally [8]. Annual costs in LMICs range from $13,510 to $19,263, with public funding covering only 22–30% [2].

Peritoneal Dialysis (PD): Despite advantages for resource-limited settings—lower infrastructure requirements, reduced staffing, home-based capability—PD utilization remains low at 11% globally [9]. Availability ranges from 14% in Africa to 100% in North/East Asia [10]. Barriers include high PD fluid costs, procurement challenges, training deficits, and peritonitis concerns [9].

CRRT: Availability is most constrained in LMICs due to equipment costs, specialized staff requirements, continuous consumables, and lack of laboratory support, forcing reliance on peritoneal dialysis or intermittent hemodialysis [3].

17.2.3 Funding Gaps

Public funding for chronic dialysis in LICs is only 18% and 22% in LMICs, compared to 58% in HICs [2]. Out-of-pocket payments account for 19.7% of ESKD care funding in LMICs [2], creating catastrophic health expenditures affecting 11.1% of patients per HD session in some settings.

The global epidemiology of CKD and AKI and access to treatment options is the context for the ethical discussion below.

17.3 Ethical Frameworks

17.3.1 Core Principles

Four principles guide ethical analysis in blood purification [11]:

- *Autonomy*: Patient right to informed treatment decisions
- *Beneficence*: Obligation to maximize benefit
- *Nonmaleficence*: Minimize harm (clinical and financial)
- *Justice*: Fair allocation of scarce resources

17.3.2 Resource Allocation Ethics

In most LMICs, universal dialysis access is impossible, leading to overt or implicit rationing and exclusion of those unable to pay [12]. This creates profound inequities and imposes emotional burdens on patients, families, and healthcare workers [12].

Priority-setting criteria must be fair, openly communicated, clearly justified, and regularly reviewed [12]. Guidelines should be developed transparently, engaging all stakeholders and considering cost-effectiveness, financial risk protection, and disease burden [12]. Currently, it is practically impossible for LICs to provide universal dialysis, yet the human right to health demands progressive realization of access for all [13].

17.3.3 Special Considerations

End-of-life decisions: Ethical dilemmas arise regarding dialysis futility, treatment risks/benefits, and surrogate decision-making, particularly when families resist or insist on dialysis against clinical judgment [12].

Pandemic allocation: COVID-19 highlighted unique challenges when dialysis centers could serve only some patients in need [14]. Ethical frameworks must balance acute versus maintenance dialysis needs using principles of: (1) maximizing benefits, (2) treating people fairly, (3) prioritizing worst-off individuals, and (4) procedural justice [15].

Vulnerable populations: Special considerations apply to elderly, cognitively impaired, children, and culturally diverse populations, requiring attention to surrogate decision-making and cultural sensitivity [11].

To conclude, healthcare policies in LMICs should focus on allocating resources to improve dialysis access.

17.4 Economic Dimensions

17.4.1 Cost Comparisons

Direct costs vary substantially. In LMICs, annual HD costs range $13,510–$19,263 [2]. Hong Kong data show annual costs: hospital-based HD $400,057 versus PD $118,467 [16]. Malaysia found mean HD cost RM169 per session versus PD RM2,186 per month, with similar annual cost-effectiveness [17].

CRRT costs significantly exceed intermittent modalities due to continuous operation, specialized equipment, intensive nursing, and high consumable use [18].

Indirect costs include transportation, productivity losses, caregiver time, and quality-of-life impacts, with home modalities showing advantages [16].

17.4.2 Cost-Effectiveness Evidence

Multiple studies demonstrate PD's superior cost-effectiveness versus in-center HD. A Canadian analysis found PD dominated HD with lower lifetime costs ($76,915 vs $142,389) and higher quality-adjusted life-years (QALYs: 7.13 vs 6.58) [19]. Swedish, Malaysian, Singaporean, and Brazilian studies consistently confirm PD's cost-effectiveness advantage [20–23].

In summary, PD could be used more in LMICs.

17.5 Continuous Renal Replacement Therapy

17.5.1 CRRT Practice

CRRT is preferred in ICU settings for hemodynamically unstable patients, utilized in 75.2% of RRT sessions [4].

Indications: Volume overload refractory to diuretics, severe electrolyte disturbances, uremia complications, hemodynamic instability, and multiorgan failure.

Timing: KDIGO 2012 recommends emergency RRT for life-threatening changes, but evidence for "early" versus "delayed" initiation beyond absolute indications remains inconclusive. The ELAIN trial showed early start to be beneficial [24], but other trials found no mortality benefit to early initiation of CRRT. Recent large trials found no mortality benefit to early initiation [25, 26]. Very late initiation, as tested in the AKIKI 2 trial, was found to increase mortality [27].

17.5.2 Resource-Limited Settings

CRRT implementation faces multiple barriers in LMICs: specialized equipment, reliable power, purified water, consumable supply chains, trained staff, and prohibitive costs. The ADQI consensus acknowledges these limitations may necessitate alternatives like peritoneal dialysis or intermittent hemodialysis [28].

17.6 Innovations in Blood Purification

17.6.1 Wearable and Implantable Devices

Innovations utilize miniaturization, microfluidics, and nanotechnology toward transportable, wearable, and implantable devices [29].

Wearable Artificial Kidney (WAK): A pilot study of seven ESKD patients demonstrated 24-h treatment was well tolerated with effective solute clearance and electrolyte homeostasis [30]. The device uses sorbent-based dialysate regeneration (zirconium phosphate, hydrous zirconium oxide, activated charcoal), eliminating the need for large dialysate volumes.

Automated WAK (AWAK): Utilizes peritoneal dialysis with sorbent-based regeneration, avoiding vascular access and continuous extracorporeal circulation [29].

Implantable Artificial Kidney (IAK): Combines silicon nanopore membranes with a bioreactor containing renal tubule cells, aiming to replicate both filtration and metabolic functions without immunosuppression [31].

17.7 Strategies to Improve Global Access

17.7.1 Health System Strengthening

Infrastructure: Dialysis centers, water treatment, reliable power, laboratory services, and supply chain management.

Workforce: Training of nephrologists, nurses, and technicians; continuing education; retention strategies; and appropriate task-shifting.

Quality assurance: Standards development, monitoring systems, patient registries, and regular audits.

17.7.2 Financial Protection

Universal Health Coverage (UHC): Progressive public financing expansion through tax-funded systems, social insurance, public-private partnerships, and subsidized care.

Cost containment: Bulk procurement, local production, safe reuse protocols, generic medications, and efficiency improvements without compromising quality.

17.7.3 Appropriate Technology Selection

PD First policies: Given PD's cost-effectiveness and home-based suitability, several countries mandate PD consideration unless contraindicated [19]. This reduces infrastructure requirements, lowers costs, improves autonomy, and preserves vascular access.

CRRT alternatives: In resource-limited ICUs, sustained low-efficiency dialysis (SLED), prolonged intermittent RRT, or acute peritoneal dialysis protocols serve as alternatives.

17.7.4 Prevention and Conservative Management

Prevention: Control diabetes and hypertension; reduce nephrotoxin exposure; ensure clean water/sanitation; implement AKI prevention protocols, including risk assessment and nephrotoxin avoidance.

Disease-modifying therapy: SGLT2 inhibitors and other agents to slow CKD progression.

Conservative Kidney Management (CKM): For patients where dialysis does not align with goals or is unavailable, CKM provides symptom management, dietary modifications, complication management, psychosocial support, and advance care planning. CKM is available in 53% of countries but needs expansion [PMID: 37924060].

17.7.5 Integration and Collaboration

Transplantation: Kidney transplantation offers superior outcomes and cost-effectiveness, requiring living donor programs, deceased donor infrastructure, transplant capacity, and immunosuppression availability.

International cooperation: South-South cooperation sharing successful middle-income country models; North-South partnerships for technology transfer and training; global advocacy through ISN initiatives and World Kidney Day; integration into UHC agendas.

17.8 Policy Recommendations

17.8.1 National Level

1. Develop comprehensive kidney disease strategies integrating prevention through transplantation.
2. Establish national dialysis registries for policy and outcomes tracking.
3. Implement quality standards for all modalities.
4. Ensure sustainable financing through public mechanisms as part of UHC.
5. Invest in workforce development with retention strategies.
6. Promote appropriate technology adoption including PD and home therapies.
7. Establish ethical frameworks for resource allocation.
8. Develop regulatory pathways for innovations.

17.8.2 International Level

1. Support LMIC capacity building through partnerships.
2. Facilitate appropriate technology transfer.
3. Promote research on cost-effective interventions for resource-limited settings.
4. Develop adaptable global standards.
5. Advocate for kidney disease inclusion in global health initiatives.
6. Share best practices through international forums.
7. Support equitable access as a human right.
8. Address catastrophic health expenditures.

17.8.3 Research Priorities

Implementation of science for LMIC dialysis programs; cost-effectiveness analyses in diverse settings; quality-of-life research across modalities; innovation evaluation, including wearables; ethical frameworks for scarcity; prevention trials; workforce optimization studies; and environmental sustainability research.

17.9 Conclusion

Blood purification technologies represent life-sustaining interventions for millions, yet profound access disparities persist. With 2–7 million annual deaths from lack of dialysis access, current global inequity is unacceptable. The disparity between HICs (969 pmp RRT) and LICs (4.4 pmp) demands urgent action.

Economics matter but need not be absolute barriers. Peritoneal dialysis consistently demonstrates superior cost-effectiveness to in-center hemodialysis, yet remains underutilized globally. Innovative financing and appropriate technology selection can expand access within resource constraints.

Ethical frameworks must guide allocation through transparent, accountable, participatory processes. The principles of maximizing benefit, treating people fairly, prioritizing the worst-off, and ensuring procedural justice provide foundations for difficult decisions. Conservative kidney management offers important alternatives where dialysis is unavailable or misaligned with patient goals.

Innovation offers hope. Wearable artificial kidneys, portable devices, novel membranes, and dialysate regeneration may transform blood purification therapy. However, ensuring these innovations reach those most in need requires intentional effort addressing access, affordability, and implementation.

Integration is essential. Effective kidney care requires prevention, early detection, conservative management, dialysis, and transplantation as complementary modalities within broader health systems. Sustainability demands political commitment, adequate financing, workforce development, infrastructure investment, and robust supply chains.

The technologies exist to save millions of lives currently lost to kidney disease. The ethical imperative, and thus the priority actions, are clear. Economic analyses demonstrate feasibility. What remains is political will and global solidarity to ensure birthplace does not determine whether a person with kidney failure receives life-sustaining treatment. This is both a moral obligation and an achievable goal.

References

1. Klomjit N, Kattah AG, Cheungpasitporn W. The cost-effectiveness of peritoneal dialysis is superior to hemodialysis: updated evidence from a more precise model. Kidney Med. 2021;3(1):15–7. https://doi.org/10.1016/j.xkme.2020.12.003.
2. Zafar MN, Rizvi SAH. Providing "free" access to dialysis and transplant to the disfranchised. A sustainable model for low and low middle income countries (LMICs). Transpl Int. 2023;36:11290. https://doi.org/10.3389/ti.2023.11290.
3. Baldwin I, Mottes T. Acute kidney injury and continuous renal replacement therapy: a nursing perspective for my shift today in the intensive care unit. Semin Dial. 2021;34(6):518–29. https://doi.org/10.1111/sdi.12992.
4. Tolwani A. Continuous renal-replacement therapy for acute kidney injury. N Engl J Med. 2012;367(26):2505–14. https://doi.org/10.1056/NEJMct1206045.
5. Kung CW, Chou YH. Acute kidney disease: an overview of the epidemiology, pathophysiology, and management. Kidney Res Clin Pract. 2023;42(6):686–99. https://doi.org/10.23876/j.krcp.23.001.
6. Thurlow JS, Joshi M, Yan G, et al. Global epidemiology of end-stage kidney disease and disparities in kidney replacement therapy. Am J Nephrol. 2021;52(2):98–107. https://doi.org/10.1159/000514550.
7. Zahirian Moghadam T, Powell J, Sharghi A, Zandian H. Economic evaluation of dialysis and comprehensive conservative care for chronic kidney disease using the ICECAP-O and EQ-5D-5L; a comparison of evaluation instruments. Cost Eff Resour Alloc. 2023;21(1):81. https://doi.org/10.1186/s12962-023-00491-3.
8. Farag YMK, El-Sayed E. Global dialysis perspective: Egypt. Kidney360. 2022;3(7):1263–8. https://doi.org/10.34067/KID.0007482021.
9. Okpechi IG, Jha V, Cho Y, et al. The case for increased peritoneal dialysis utilization in low- and lower-middle-income countries. Nephrology (Carlton). 2022;27(5):391–403. https://doi.org/10.1111/nep.14024.
10. Berney T, Bellini MI, Benning L, et al. A year in review. Transpl Int. 2024;2024(37):14243. https://doi.org/10.3389/ti.2024.14243.
11. Davison SN, Holley JL. Ethical issues in the care of vulnerable chronic kidney disease patients: the elderly, cognitively impaired, and those from different cultural backgrounds. Adv Chronic Kidney Dis. 2008;15(2):177–85. https://doi.org/10.1053/j.ackd.2008.01.004.
12. Luyckx VA, Martin DE, Moosa MR, et al. Developing the ethical framework of end-stage kidney disease care: from practice to policy. Kidney Int Suppl. 2020;10(1):e72–7. https://doi.org/10.1016/j.kisu.2019.11.003.
13. Luyckx VA, Moosa MR. Priority setting as an ethical imperative in managing global dialysis access and improving kidney care. Semin Nephrol. 2021;41(3):230–41. https://doi.org/10.1016/j.semnephrol.2021.05.004.
14. Martin DE, Parsons JA, Caskey FJ, Harris DCH, Jha V. Ethics of kidney care in the era of COVID-19. Kidney Int. 2020;98(6):1424–33. https://doi.org/10.1016/j.kint.2020.09.014.

15. Porteny T, Gonzales KM, Aufort KE, et al. Treatment decision making for older kidney patients during COVID-19. Clin J Am Soc Nephrol. 2022;17(7):957–65. https://doi.org/10.2215/CJN.13241021.
16. Wong CKH, Chen J, Fung SKS, et al. Direct and indirect costs of end-stage renal disease patients in the first and second years after initiation of nocturnal home haemodialysis, hospital haemodialysis and peritoneal dialysis. Nephrol Dial Transplant. 2019;34(9):1565–76. https://doi.org/10.1093/ndt/gfy395.
17. Hooi LS, Lim TO, Goh A, et al. Economic evaluation of centre haemodialysis and continuous ambulatory peritoneal dialysis in Ministry of Health hospitals, Malaysia. Nephrology. 2005;10(1):25–32. https://doi.org/10.1111/j.1440-1797.2005.00360.x.
18. Srisawat N, Lawsin L, Uchino S, Bellomo R, Kellum JA, Investigators BK. Cost of acute renal replacement therapy in the intensive care unit: results from the beginning and ending supportive therapy for the kidney (BEST kidney) study. Crit Care. 2010;14(2):R46. https://doi.org/10.1186/cc8933.
19. Wong CKH, Chen J, Fung SKS, et al. Lifetime cost-effectiveness analysis of first-line dialysis modalities for patients with end-stage renal disease under peritoneal dialysis first policy. BMC Nephrol. 2020;21(1):42. https://doi.org/10.1186/s12882-020-1708-0.
20. Sennfalt K, Magnusson M, Carlsson P. Comparison of hemodialysis and peritoneal dialysis--a cost-utility analysis. Perit Dial Int. 2002;22(1):39–47.
21. Surendra NK, Abdul Manaf MR, Hooi LS, et al. Cost utility analysis of end stage renal disease treatment in Ministry of Health dialysis centres, Malaysia: hemodialysis versus continuous ambulatory peritoneal dialysis. PLoS One. 2019;14(10):e0218422. https://doi.org/10.1371/journal.pone.0218422.
22. Yang F, Lau T, Luo N. Cost-effectiveness of haemodialysis and peritoneal dialysis for patients with end-stage renal disease in Singapore. Nephrology (Carlton). 2016;21(8):669–77. https://doi.org/10.1111/nep.12668.
23. de Abreu MM, Walker DR, Sesso RC, Ferraz MB. A cost evaluation of peritoneal dialysis and hemodialysis in the treatment of end-stage renal disease in Sao Paulo, Brazil. Perit Dial Int. 2013;33(3):304–15. https://doi.org/10.3747/pdi.2011.00138.
24. Zarbock A, Kellum JA, Schmidt C, et al. Effect of early vs delayed initiation of renal replacement therapy on mortality in critically ill patients with acute kidney injury: the ELAIN randomized clinical trial. JAMA. 2016;315(20):2190–9. https://doi.org/10.1001/jama.2016.5828.
25. Investigators S-A, Canadian Critical Care Trials G, Australian, et al. Timing of initiation of renal-replacement therapy in acute kidney injury. N Engl J Med. 2020;383(3):240–51. https://doi.org/10.1056/NEJMoa2000741.
26. Barbar SD, Clere-Jehl R, Bourredjem A, et al. Timing of renal-replacement therapy in patients with acute kidney injury and sepsis. N Engl J Med. 2018;379(15):1431–42. https://doi.org/10.1056/NEJMoa1803213.
27. Gaudry S, Hajage D, Martin-Lefevre L, et al. Comparison of two delayed strategies for renal replacement therapy initiation for severe acute kidney injury (AKIKI 2): a multicentre, open-label, randomised, controlled trial. Lancet. 2021;397(10281):1293–300. https://doi.org/10.1016/S0140-6736(21)00350-0.
28. Mehta R, Bagga A, Patibandla R, Chakravarthi R. Detection and management of AKI in the developing world: the 18th acute disease quality initiative (ADQI) international consensus conference. Kidney Int Rep. 2017;2(4):515–8. https://doi.org/10.1016/j.ekir.2017.03.013.
29. Ronco C, Davenport A, Gura V. The future of the artificial kidney: moving towards wearable and miniaturized devices. Nefrologia. 2011;31(1):9–16. https://doi.org/10.3265/Nefrologia.pre2010.Nov.10758.
30. Gura V, Rivara MB, Bieber S, et al. A wearable artificial kidney for patients with end-stage renal disease. JCI Insight. 2016;1(8):e86397. https://doi.org/10.1172/jci.insight.86397.
31. Salani M, Roy S, Fissell WH IV. Innovations in wearable and implantable artificial kidneys. Am J Kidney Dis. 2018;72(5):745–51. https://doi.org/10.1053/j.ajkd.2018.06.005.

Regulatory Challenges and Approval Pathways for Next-Generation Blood Purification Devices

18

Anastasia Maria Anamateros, Agata Sciacca,
Lisa Mathiasen, and Paolo Braganò

18.1 Introduction

Extracorporeal blood purification (EBP) technologies have undergone significant advancements since the introduction of the first artificial kidney device for renal replacement therapy in the early 1940s [1]. Advances in biomaterials, design, and fluid dynamics have progressively expanded the scope of EBP, from life-saving hemodialysis (hemofilters, hemodialyzers, and hemodiafilters) to the introduction of plasma filters, apheresis columns, and adsorbers used across both chronic and acute patient care [2–4].

The goals of innovation have been consistent: improving hemocompatibility and biocompatibility, reducing inflammatory and coagulative responses, enhancing fluid dynamics, and improving molecular retention offset for optimal toxin removal capacity, without compromising essential substances (such as albumin). In terms of removal mechanisms, an EBP device can operate through filtration (diffusion and convection), adsorption, or a combination of both, depending on the materials used and its design. These improvements have widened the clinical spectrum of EBP applications, both in intermittent and continuous modalities [2, 4].

A. M. Anamateros · A. Sciacca · L. Mathiasen
Estor SpA, Pero, Italy
e-mail: anastasia.anamateros@estor.it; agata.sciacca@estor.it; lisa.mathiasen@estor.it

P. Braganò (✉)
Estor SpA, Medical Affairs, Pero, Italy
e-mail: paolo.bragano@estor.it

S. De Rosa, S. Lassola (eds.), *Next-Gen Blood Purification*,
https://doi.org/10.1007/978-3-032-27033-7_18

Meanwhile, the regulatory landscape has become increasingly complex. Pathways for approving medical devices differ substantially from those for pharmaceuticals, and they vary significantly across jurisdictions. The European Medical Device Regulation (EU MDR 2017/745) is often regarded as one of the most stringent frameworks worldwide, influencing classification, conformity assessment, and post-market obligations [5]. At the same time, international discrepancies between the EU, the US (FDA), and Asian-Pacific systems continue to pose a challenge for global manufacturers.

This chapter explores these regulatory challenges, with a particular focus on how next-generation EBP devices are classified, evaluated, and approved across central authorities. By examining both the harmonization efforts and the persisting divergences, this study aims to provide researchers, clinicians, and manufacturers with a comprehensive overview of the approval pathways that will shape the future of advanced EBP technologies.

18.2 General Standard Regulatory Requirements for Medical Devices and Classification

EBP devices are subject to the broader regulatory framework that governs medical devices. Unlike drugs, medical devices are primarily regulated through risk-based classification systems, which determine the level of evidence and conformity assessment required before a device can be used in clinical settings.

Across regions, a common trend is the reliance on risk classes linked to invasiveness, duration of body contact, and intended use. However, each regulatory authority defines these classes differently and applies distinct requirements for clinical evidence, quality systems, and post-market obligations.

The EU has progressively aligned its regulations with international standards, particularly ISO 13485:2021, while introducing stricter obligations for manufacturers under the EU MDR. The regulation emphasizes a life-cycle approach: medical devices must not only demonstrate safety and performance before market entry but also undergo continuous monitoring throughout their clinical use.

In parallel, other regions (such as the US FDA, Japan PMDA, and China NMPA) apply their own frameworks, with varying levels of convergence. For manufacturers of EBP devices—which are often classified in higher-risk categories due to their blood contact and life-supporting role—this creates both opportunities and barriers. A CE-marked device may face additional hurdles before FDA clearance, and vice versa, underscoring the importance of understanding these regulatory systems.

18.3 European Medical Device Regulation (EU MDR 2017/745)

18.3.1 Background and Scope

The main framework for medical device regulation in Europe is the EU Medical Device Regulation (MDR 2017/745) [5], which replaced the earlier Directives 90/385/EEC (Active Implantable Medical Devices) and 93/42/EEC (Medical Devices). Although published in 2017, its enforcement was delayed until 26 May 2021, when it became fully effective.

Unlike the previous directives, which required national transposition and thus led to heterogeneous interpretations, the MDR is a binding regulation, directly applicable in all EU member states. Its purpose is to ensure high standards of safety and performance for medical devices, while harmonizing rules across the EU.

18.3.2 Key Innovations Introduced by the MDR

The MDR imposes more stringent requirements than its predecessors, particularly in terms of transparency, traceability, and post-market surveillance (PMS). Some of its main innovations include:

- *Medical device coordination group (MDCG):* Established in 2017 by the European Commission to support MDR implementation. Although its documents are not legally binding, MDCG guidance plays a crucial role in clarifying requirements for manufacturers, notified bodies, and other stakeholders.
- *Risk-benefit balance:* A continuous demonstration that the benefits of a device outweigh its residual risks throughout its entire life cycle.
- *Expanded obligations for economic operators:* Not only manufacturers, but also importers, authorized representatives, and distributors now carry defined responsibilities under MDR.
- *Quality and safety systems:* Stronger requirements for quality management systems (QMS), post-market surveillance (PMS), vigilance, and risk management, all of which must be documented and continuously updated.
- *Unique device identifier (UDI):* A standardized system for traceability that tracks each device from production to patient use across the entire supply chain.
- *EUDAMED database:* A centralized, publicly accessible, web-based repository that provides transparency and accessibility of device information, including registration, certification, vigilance data, and clinical studies (Fig. 18.1). Some modules are already active, while others are being phased in.
- *Person responsible for regulatory compliance (PRRC):* Each manufacturer and authorized representative must designate a qualified individual to ensure ongoing compliance.

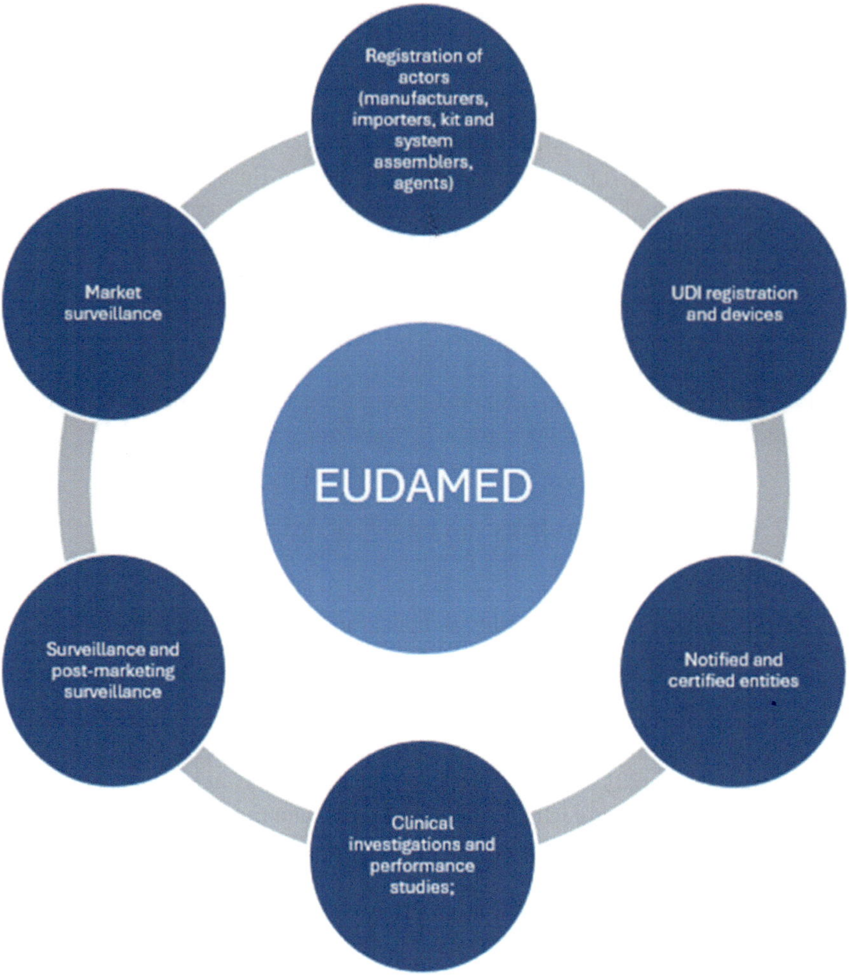

Fig. 18.1 The EUDAMED database structure

18.3.3 Classification of Medical Devices under MDR

The MDR applies a risk-based classification system, codified in Annex VIII, with 22 rules. Classes range from Class I (low risk) to Class III (high risk) (Table 18.1), determined by factors such as invasiveness, duration of contact, systemic vs. local action, and incorporation of medicinal substances and their intended use.

Determining the correct classification is critical, as it defines the regulatory requirements that the medical device needs to comply with. The risk classifications are the same as those present in the previous European Directive. However, the classification criteria are stricter, and with the new EU Regulation, there are more devices in class IIb and in class III.

Table 18.1 Overview of the MDR classification system

Class	Risk level	Examples
Class III	High risk	Long-term, invasive devices, implantable devices, active
Class IIb	Medium-high risk	Long-term, invasive devices active
Class IIa	Medium risk	Short-term invasive devices
Class I	Low risk	Non-invasive or reusable simple devices

Considering specifically EBP devices, most of them fall under Class IIb or Class III (based on critical function and blood contact). This is due to the invasive nature of such medical devices, their blood contact, and their use in life-supporting therapies. The higher the classification of a medical device, the more robust the clinical investigation needs to be.

For extracorporeal blood purification devices, classification typically falls under Class IIb, but they could be compliant with Class III in specific cases due to their invasive nature, blood contact, critical role in sustaining life, presence of drugs, and their intended use.

Hemodialyzers/hemodiafilters (intermittent or continuous): Class IIb or III (Rule 3 or Rule 14)

- Plasma filters (plasma exchange/apheresis): Class IIb or III (Rule 3 or Rule 14)
- Sorbents (hemoadsorption devices): Class IIb or III (Rule 3 or Rule 14)
- Artificial lung membrane: Class IIb

Under the MDR, EBP devices are generally classified as Class IIb due to their significant risk level, unless they meet specific criteria for Class III. For example, devices that directly incorporate a medicinal substance or are intended for modifying blood to a substantial extent, thereby affecting human health, typically fall into Class III.

18.3.4 Conformity Assessment Procedures

The conformity assessment defines how a manufacturer demonstrates compliance with the general safety and performance requirements (GSPRs) in Annex I of MDR.

The risk class of the device dictates which specific procedure, or combination of procedures, must be followed to obtain the CE marking and possible assessment by a Notified Body (NB).

First and foremost, the pathway for conformity assessment for both Class IIb and Class III requires the intervention of a Notified Body (Fig. 18.2).

For IIb medical devices, the regulatory pathway under the MDR (2017/745) intensifies the level of scrutiny by the Notified Body with respect to lower classes.

The manufacturer has two ways to demonstrate conformity to the MDR:

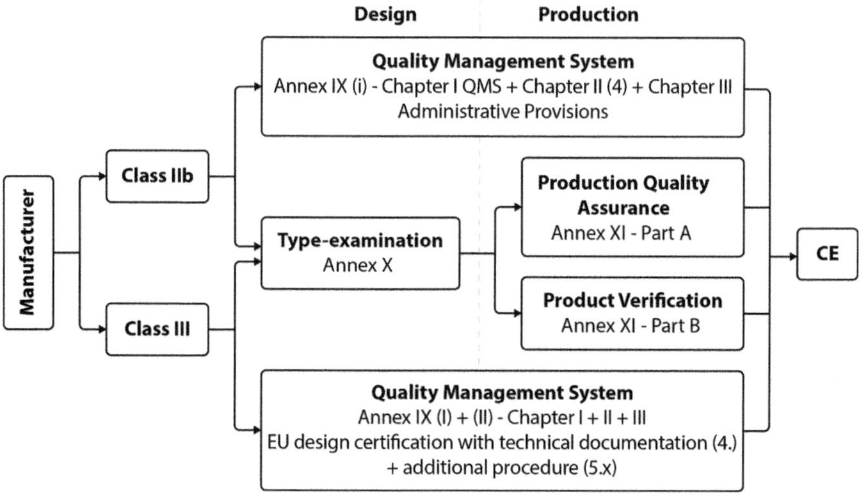

Fig. 18.2 Overview of the regulatory pathways for Class IIb and Class III medical devices under the MDR

- Comprehensive evaluation of the QMS (quality management system) and assessment of the Technical Documentation (Annex IX, Chap. I). The NB must review the technical documentation for at least one representative device per generic device group.
- EU-type examination (Annex X) combined with conformity assessment based on production quality assurance (Annex XI, Part A) or product verification (Annex XI, Part B).

Conformity assessment for Class III devices requires a deep involvement of the Notified Body and rigorous documentation, as well as clinical examination. Also in this case, the manufacturer has two ways to demonstrate conformity to the MDR:

- The most common evaluation for conformity assessment is via Annex IX, which provides for a comprehensive QMS audit, a review of technical documentation, and an in-depth evaluation of the design dossier. The process includes an initial QMS certification followed by a specific design examination for each Class III product. Unlike lower-class devices, where sampling can occur, all Class III device designs are examined individually. This ensures that the manufacturer can demonstrate compliance with all applicable General Safety and Performance Requirements (GSPRs) for that specific product.
- Manufacturers may also pursue a combined Annex IX and Annex X route or use Annex XI (Part A and Part B) for product verification; however, these options are generally reserved for unique production or product configurations.

Regardless of the route chosen, notified bodies perform annual surveillance audits, unannounced inspections, and monitor clinical and PMS data to confirm continued compliance.

For class III devices, the MDR requires:

- A comprehensive clinical evaluation as per Annex XIV. This shall be based on high-quality data, including clinical investigations conducted in accordance with ISO 14155 and MDR Chap. VI. Manufacturers cannot rely solely on equivalence unless they have full access to technical documentation and demonstrate identical device characteristics, biological effects, and clinical use.
- Clinical investigations, which must be designed with statistical justification, defined endpoints, risk-benefit parameters, and follow-up timelines. Data from these studies are used to create the Clinical Assessment Report (CER), a key component of the technical documentation.
- Post-market clinical follow-up (PMCF) must be defined in a PMCF Plan that aligns with the Clinical Evaluation Plan. PMCF may involve observational studies, registry participation, or tracking of long-term outcomes, particularly for implantable or novel devices. The PMCF assessment report shall be updated regularly and submitted together with the periodic safety update report (PSUR).
- Technical documentation, which is extensive and must comply with Annexes II and III of the MDR Regulation. Includes device description and specifications, manufacturing processes, quality and risk management files, performance and safety testing, software validation, and biological compatibility data.
- Summary of Safety and Clinical Performance (SSCP), which shall be reviewed and approved by the notified body. The SSCP is made available to the public through EUDAMED and must be drafted into lay terms for patients and physicians. The SSCP summarizes the intended purpose of the device, indications, contraindications, target populations, clinical outcomes, residual risks, and handling instructions. It is designed to enhance transparency and user understanding, and is subject to ongoing updates.

18.4 From MDD 93/42 to MDR 2017/745: Transition and Key Differences

The Medical Device Directive (MDD 93/42/EEC), in force since 1993, provided the first harmonized framework for medical devices in the EU. However, because directives require national transposition, implementation varied significantly across member states, leading to inconsistencies.

The Medical Device Regulation (MDR 2017/745) was introduced to address these shortcomings. Unlike a directive, the MDR is a directly binding law across the EU, ensuring uniformity. It expands the scope, strengthens classification rules, and imposes stricter requirements for clinical evidence, risk management, and post-market surveillance.

This shift reflects the EU's commitment to a life-cycle approach: medical devices are now monitored not only before market entry but throughout their use, with continuous evaluation of safety and performance. The main similarities and differences between MDD 93/42 and MDR 2017/45 are summarized in Table 18.2, which shows how obligations have evolved regarding clinical evidence requirements, post-market surveillance, traceability, and oversight.

Table 18.2 Main similarities and differences between MDD 93/42 and MDR 2017/745

Aspect	MDD 93/42/EEC	MDR 2017/745
Legal nature	Directive—required transposition into national laws, leading to variations across countries	Regulation—directly applicable in all member states, ensuring uniform implementation
Scope	Medical devices only	Expanded scope: includes certain aesthetic devices, reprocessed single-use devices, and medical software
Purpose	Ensured safety and performance of devices placed on the EU market	Focuses on risk-based approach, safety, transparency, traceability, and stronger post-market requirements
Harmonization	Different national transpositions → inconsistencies between countries	Unified legal framework across the EU; no national deviations allowed
Classification	18 rules; Classes I, IIa, IIb, III	22 rules; stricter criteria → more devices shifted into higher risk classes
Economic operators	Mainly manufacturers and EU representatives	Clearly defined roles for all: manufacturer, authorized representative, importer, distributor
PRRC (person responsible for regulatory compliance)	Not defined	Mandatory designation of a PRRC for manufacturers and authorized representatives
Database/ transparency	Limited; national-level registries only	*EUDAMED* central EU database: registration, vigilance, PMS, clinical investigations; publicly accessible
Traceability	Limited; mostly lot/batch information	*Unique device identifier (UDI):* mandatory system for all devices
Clinical evidence	Often based on equivalence; one-time evaluation	Stricter: robust clinical data required; continuous post-market clinical follow-up (PMCF); risk-benefit analysis integral to CER
Post-market surveillance (PMS)	Less structured; reactive approach (focused on vigilance)	Proactive, continuous PMS required; PMS plan, PMCF plan, and periodic safety update reports (PSURs)
Trend reporting	Not clearly defined	Mandatory reporting of statistically significant increases in incidents
Vigilance	No harmonized definitions for "serious incident" or "adverse event." FSCA reporting fragmented across member states	Harmonized definitions, stricter reporting deadlines, centralized vigilance via EUDAMED; public access to field safety notices
Quality management system (QMS)	Less prescriptive; limited post-market requirements	Stronger requirements aligned with ISO 13485:2021; applies across the entire device life cycle, including PMS and risk management

18.4.1 Comparison of MDD vs MDR

Overall, the MDR represents a fundamental shift from a reactive to a proactive regulatory system. Manufacturers now face stricter documentation, continuous oversight, and greater accountability throughout the device's entire life cycle. While this increases regulatory burden, it also enhances patient safety, transparency, and market confidence. The MDR therefore represents not only a regulatory update but a change of expectations, from premarket verification toward life-cycle accountability and continuous evidence generation.

18.5 MDR and Other Global Regulatory Systems

Although the EU MDR is among the most comprehensive and stringent frameworks worldwide, it is not directly aligned with systems in other regions. Manufacturers seeking global market access must therefore navigate a complex web of regulatory pathways, classifications, and evidence requirements.

While many authorities apply a risk-based classification approach, the specific categories, terminology, and conformity assessments differ. Table 18.3 summarizes the core structural features of the EU, FDA, PMDA, NMPA, and TGA pathways, with emphasis on risk classification tiers, conformity assessment routes, and clinical data expectations.

Table 18.3 Comparison of regulatory systems in the EU, the USA, China, Japan, and Australia

Region/authority	European Union (MDR)	USA (FDA)	China (NMPA)	Japan (PMDA/MHLW)	Australia (TGA/ARTG)
Device classification	Classes I, Ir/Im/Is, IIa, IIb, III (22 rules, risk-based)	Classes I, II, III	Classes I, II, III	Classes I, II, III, IV	Classes I, IIa, IIb, III
System features	Rule-based, invasiveness, contact duration criteria	Risk-based, with "predicate" comparison for new devices	Conservative classification; type testing often mandatory	Risk-based, with common specifications	Risk-based, aligned with the EU system
Conformity assessment and approval	Class I (self-certification if non-sterile/non-measuring). Higher classes → Notified body review.	510(k) for substantial equivalence; De Novo for novel moderate-risk; PMA for high-risk.	Class I → notification. Classes II and III → full registration dossier with NMPA review; local testing may be required.	Class I → notification. Class II/III → certification (if standards exist) or MHLW approval. Class IV → MHLW approval.	ARTG listing required. EU CE or MDSAP evidence often accepted to streamline process.
Clinical evidence requirement	Clinical evaluation required, supported by clinical data; PMCF mandatory.	Varies: 510(k) often literature-based; PMA requires rigorous clinical trials.	Local clinical data often required for Class II/III, though some foreign data may be accepted.	Robust data required for Class III/IV; foreign data sometimes accepted.	Evidence required according to classification; clinical evaluation must demonstrate compliance with essential principles.
Post-market surveillance (PMS)	PMS plan, PSURs (Class IIa+), vigilance reporting to EUDAMED.	Mandatory adverse event reporting, recalls, post-approval studies for PMA.	Annual safety reporting, local vigilance obligations.	MAH responsible for vigilance, annual reports, post-approval studies.	PMS and vigilance reporting required; recalls coordinated via sponsor.
UDI/traceability	Mandatory UDI system (phased rollout).	GUDID (Global UDI Database).	UDI phased in since 2021.	UDI system per PMDA rules.	UDI phased in since 2021.

18.6 Comparison of Regulatory Systems

18.6.1 United States (FDA)

In the US, medical devices are regulated by the Food and Drug Administration (FDA), specifically through the Center for Devices and Radiological Health (CDRH). The FDA's authority covers device marketing, sale, and distribution (not medical practice) [6].

Classification:

- Class I: Low-risk devices, subject to general controls
- Class II: Moderate-risk devices, requiring additional controls
- Class III: High-risk devices, requiring premarket approval (PMA)

Approval Pathways:

- 510(k): Demonstrates substantial equivalence to an existing legally marketed device ("predicate")
- De Novo: For novel, low-to-moderate risk devices lacking a predicate
- PMA: Full scientific and clinical review for high-risk devices

Key Features:

- Devices without a valid predicate are automatically classified as Class III until reclassified.
- PMA requires robust clinical trial data, whereas many 510(k) submissions rely on literature or bench data.
- Post-market obligations include mandatory adverse event reporting, recalls, and (for PMA devices) post-approval studies.

18.6.2 Japan (PMDA/MHLW)

In Japan, medical device oversight is shared between:

- MHLW (Ministry of Health, Labour and Welfare)—policy and final approvals
- PMDA (Pharmaceuticals and Medical Devices Agency)—scientific and technical reviews [7]
- Certification Bodies—designated organizations authorized to approve specific lower-risk devices

Classification:

- Class I (extremely low risk): Notification to PMDA.
- Class II (low risk): Certification if common standards exist; otherwise, MHLW approval.
- Class III (medium risk): Certification (if standards exist) or MHLW approval.
- Class IV (high risk): Always requires MHLW approval.

Approval Categories:

- New medical devices (novel technology)
- Improved medical devices (significant modifications)
- "Me-too" devices (similar to existing approvals)

Key Features:

- High-risk (Class III/IV) devices require rigorous clinical evidence.
- A Designated Marketing Authorization Holder (D-MAH) must be appointed for foreign manufacturers.
- Vigilance responsibilities include annual safety reports and post-approval studies.

18.6.3 China (NMPA)

China's medical devices are regulated by the National Medical Products Administration (NMPA) [8], supported by two specialized entities:

- CMDE (Center for Medical Device Evaluation): Reviews applications and assesses safety and performance
- Center for Medical Device Standards Management: Develops technical standards

Classification:

- Class I (low risk): Notification and registration dossier only
- Class II (medium risk): Full dossier review, including technical and clinical sections
- Class III (high risk): Extensive review of dossier, with mandatory technical and clinical data

Key Features:

- Local type testing in accredited Chinese labs is often required, even if foreign data exists.

- Local clinical studies may be mandatory for Class II/III devices, though biocompatibility studies done abroad may sometimes be accepted.
- Technical standards are published by NMPA (mainly in Chinese) and must be carefully checked before initiating registration.
- Annual safety reporting and local adverse event reporting are compulsory.

18.6.4 Australia (TGA/ARTG)

In Australia, medical devices are regulated by the Therapeutic Goods Administration (TGA) [9]. Devices must be included in the Australian Register of Therapeutic Goods (ARTG) to be marketed.

Classification:

- Class I (including sterile/measuring variants), IIa, IIb, III
- Similar to EU criteria, although with some differences that require careful verification

Conformity Assessment:

- Devices must comply with Essential Principles (EPs) outlined in the Therapeutic Goods (Medical Devices) Regulations 2002.
- There are 15 EPs, covering safety, performance, design, construction, and clinical evidence requirements.
- Manufacturers must complete an Essential Requirements checklist as part of the application.

Key Features:

- The TGA often recognizes EU CE certificates or other MDSAP evidence, which can accelerate market entry.
- Clinical evidence must match the device classification and intended use.
- PMS obligations include incident reporting, recalls, and ongoing compliance oversight by the local sponsor.
- UDI implementation began in 2021 and is being phased in.

In summary, the EU MDR is generally more demanding than the FDA 510(k) pathways, particularly for higher-risk devices. China (NMPA) often requires local type testing and clinical trials, making market entry more time-consuming and costly. Japan (PMDA) applies one of the strictest systems for Class III/IV devices, with detailed clinical and quality requirements. Australia (TGA) is relatively aligned with the EU, often recognizing CE evidence to accelerate approvals.

18.6.5 Regulation in the United Kingdom

The United Kingdom's withdrawal from the EU ("Brexit") on 31 January 2020 had significant consequences for the medical device sector. After the transition period ended on 31 December 2020, the UK established its own regulatory framework.

Currently, medical devices in Great Britain (England, Scotland, Wales) are governed by the UK Medical Devices Regulations 2002 (UK MDR 2002) [10], which originally transposed the EU Directives (MDD, AIMDD, IVDD) into UK law. These regulations have since been amended to reflect Brexit-related changes, including the introduction of the UKCA mark (UK Conformity Assessed).

- Northern Ireland: Under the Northern Ireland Protocol, EU MDR and IVDR remain applicable, with some additional requirements.
- Great Britain: The UKCA mark is gradually replacing CE marking, though CE-marked devices are still accepted during the transition period (currently extended to 2030 depending on device type).
- Future Direction: The UK Medicines and Healthcare products Regulatory Agency (MHRA) is preparing a more stringent framework, closer to the EU MDR. Still, the existing law remains based on the directives.

In summary, the UK operates under a parallel but diverging framework. While closely aligned with EU MDR in intent, manufacturers must address separate requirements, including appointing a UK Responsible Person (UKRP) for market access.

18.6.6 Regulation in Switzerland

Switzerland, although not an EU member, long participated in the single market for medical devices through the Mutual Recognition Agreement (MRA) with the EU. This allowed devices certified under EU rules to circulate freely.

However, with the entry into force of the EU MDR in May 2021, the MRA was not updated, and Switzerland is now treated as a "third country." As a result:

- Swiss authorities introduced the Medical Devices Ordinance (MedDO, 812.213), effective May 26, 2021, which aligns national rules with the EU MDR to maintain comparable safety standards [11].
- Manufacturers outside Switzerland must appoint a Swiss Authorized Representative (CH-REP).
- Despite alignment, Swiss devices no longer enjoy automatic access to the EU market without CE marking, and EU devices must comply with Swiss-specific requirements to enter Switzerland.

Overall, Switzerland's system mirrors the EU MDR in most respects; however, regulatory duplication now applies. Market access requires additional representation and compliance steps, adding complexity for manufacturers operating in both the EU and Switzerland.

18.7 Conclusion

The development of extracorporeal blood purification technologies has progressed considerably since the advent of the artificial kidney, expanding from life-saving renal replacement therapies to a broad array of advanced devices, including plasma filters, apheresis columns, and sorbents, applied across both intermittent and continuous modalities. These innovations have been driven not only by improvements in material science, hemocompatibility, and molecular selectivity, but also by the increasing demand for tailored therapeutic approaches in complex and critically ill patient populations.

In parallel with technological advancements, regulatory frameworks have evolved to provide more stringent oversight, reflecting the increasing importance of device safety, transparency, and performance throughout the entire product life cycle. The EU MDR has emerged as a landmark in this evolution, replacing earlier directives with a binding, risk-based framework that strengthens requirements for clinical evidence, post-market surveillance, and traceability. The MDR's introduction of centralized mechanisms such as EUDAMED, the unique device identifier (UDI) system, and the person responsible for regulatory compliance (PRRC) represents a paradigm shift toward greater accountability and harmonization within the European market.

Nevertheless, significant challenges remain. Regulatory pathways continue to diverge across jurisdictions. While the MDR emphasizes comprehensive clinical evaluation and post-market follow-up, the FDA system relies on predicate-based clearances for moderate-risk devices. In contrast, Asian authorities, such as the NMPA and PMDA, emphasize the importance of comprehensive clinical evaluation and post-market follow-up. The FDA system often requires local testing and clinical data. Even within Europe, the distinct frameworks now operative in the United Kingdom and Switzerland illustrate the persistence of jurisdictional fragmentation despite alignment. For manufacturers of next-generation blood purification devices—most of which fall into higher-risk classes (IIb or III)—these differences translate into increased complexity, prolonged timelines, and substantial resource demands for global market access.

Harmonization initiatives led by international bodies, such as the International Medical Device Regulators Forum (IMDRF) and regional partnerships, remain critical to alleviating these burdens. In the absence of complete harmonization, however, manufacturers must strategically adapt their regulatory strategies to the specificities of each market, ensuring robust quality management systems, comprehensive clinical evidence, and effective post-market surveillance mechanisms.

Ultimately, while regulatory requirements impose significant obligations, they also provide the framework to ensure patient safety, device performance, and public trust. For blood purification technologies—devices inherently invasive, life-supporting, and often used in acute and high-risk clinical settings—such oversight is essential. The future will require a balance between fostering innovation and maintaining rigorous standards, with the long-term aim of ensuring that technological advances in extracorporeal therapies can be translated into safe, effective, and widely accessible clinical solutions worldwide.

References

1. Featherstone PJ, Ball CM. A brief history of haemodialysis and continuous renal replacement therapy. Anaesth Intensive Care. 2019;47(3):220–2.
2. Ronco C, Reis T. Continuous renal replacement therapy and extended indications. Semin Dial. 2021;34(6):550–60.
3. Ronco C, Cruz D. Hemodiafiltration history, technology, and clinical results. Adv Chronic Kidney Dis. 2007;14(3):231–43.
4. Samoni S, et al. Continuous renal replacement therapy in the critically ill patient: from garage technology to artificial intelligence. J Clin Med. 2021;11(1):172.
5. Regulation (EU) 2017/745 of the European Parliament and of the Council of 5 April 2017 on medical devices, amending Directive 2001/83/EC, Regulation (EC) No 178/2002 and Regulation (EC) No 1223/2009 and repealing Council Directives 90/385/EEC and 93/42/EEC (Text with EEA relevance). 2017. p. 1–175.
6. US FDA Medical Device Regulation. Available from: https://www.fda.gov/medical-devices/overview-device-regulation/classify-your-medical-device.
7. Japan PMDA Medical Device Regulation. Available from: https://www.pmda.go.jp/english/.
8. China NMPA Medical Device Regulation. Available from: https://english.nmpa.gov.cn/2024-06/05/c_993242.htm.
9. Australia TGA Medical Device Regulation. Available from: https://www.tga.gov.au.
10. UK MHRA Medical Device Regulation. Available from: https://www.gov.uk/health-and-social-care/medicines-medical-devices-blood-medical-devices-regulation-safety.
11. Switzerland MedDO Medical Device Regulation. Available from: https://www.fedlex.admin.ch/eli/cc/2020/552/en.

Emerging Biotechnologies in Blood Purification

19

Jake Vernon-Elliot, Maxime Schleef, and Emily J. See

19.1 Introduction

Blood purification encompasses extracorporeal therapies that remove metabolic waste products, toxins, excess fluid, and inflammatory mediators from the circulation to support or replace failing organ systems. The core modalities include renal replacement therapy (haemodialysis, hemofiltration, and hemodiafiltration), haemoadsorption, and plasmapheresis.

Renal replacement therapies use diffusion and convection to manage solute clearance and fluid balance in acute kidney injury or end-stage kidney disease. However, currently available devices have notable limitations, including incomplete solute removal, suboptimal selectivity, biocompatibility constraints, and an inability to replicate the kidney's metabolic, endocrine, and immunoregulatory functions [1].

J. Vernon-Elliot
Department of Intensive Care, Royal Melbourne Hospital, Parkville, VIC, Australia
e-mail: jake.vernon-elliot1@wh.org.au

M. Schleef
Department of Nephrology Dialysis and Renal Explorations, Edouard Herriot Hospital, Lyon, France
e-mail: maxime.schleef@chu-lyon.fr

E. J. See (✉)
Department of Intensive Care, Royal Melbourne Hospital, Parkville, VIC, Australia

Department of Nephrology, Royal Melbourne Hospital, Parkville, VIC, Australia

Department of Nephrology, Royal Children's Hospital, Parkville, VIC, Australia

Department of Critical Care, The University of Melbourne, Melbourne, VIC, Australia

Australian and New Zealand Intensive Care Research Centre, Monash University, Melbourne, VIC, Australia
e-mail: emily.see@mh.org.au

S. De Rosa, S. Lassola (eds.), *Next-Gen Blood Purification*,
https://doi.org/10.1007/978-3-032-27033-7_19

They also present practical challenges related to patient quality of life, accessibility, cost, infrastructure, and environmental sustainability [2–4].

Adjunctive blood purification modalities such as haemoadsorption, plasmapheresis, and albumin dialysis expand treatment capabilities by removing larger molecules, protein-bound toxins, and circulating immune factors. They provide additional options for complex metabolic, toxicological, and inflammatory disorders, but lack adequate specificity to deliver consistent, predictable modulation of their target pathways.

The non-selectivity and biological incompatibility of contemporary blood purification technologies represent important gaps in clinical practice, driving the need for innovation in the field. This chapter examines emerging biotechnologies in blood purification that aim to address these limitations of currently available devices. Key areas of innovation include enhancing solute clearance with high-cut-off and medium-cut-off membranes; engineering highly selective, next-generation membranes; maximising circuit biocompatibility through biomimetic surface modifications; leveraging adsorption techniques for targeted removal of cytokines, endotoxins, and pathogenic molecules; and advancing biohybrid and implantable artificial kidney systems to restore broader physiological functions. These emerging biotechnologies arise from multidisciplinary collaboration across materials science, biochemical and tissue engineering, nanotechnology, and translational clinical research. Their successful adoption in clinical practice will depend on overcoming future challenges related to clinical validation, regulatory approval, and manufacturing scalability.

19.2 Advances in Membrane Technology

The semipermeable membrane is the core component of blood purification systems for renal replacement therapy, facilitating the removal of solutes and excess fluid while retaining essential blood components such as proteins, immunoglobulins, and cells [5]. Most membranes are composed of synthetic polymers (e.g., polysulfone, polyacrylonitrile) configured into hollow fibres that maximise surface area within compact dialyzer modules. Membrane efficiency is determined by characteristics such as pore size, uniformity, distribution, and density across the surface of the membrane.

High-flux membranes contain pores of approximately 4 nm radius, permitting the passage of molecules up to ~15–25 kDa [6]. These membranes efficiently clear small water-soluble molecules, but pore size variability leads to suboptimal selectivity and inadequate clearance of middle molecules (500 Da–60 kDa) and protein-bound toxins [5, 7]. Ineffective clearance of these molecules during blood purification holds clinical relevance, especially in the chronic setting, where accumulation is increasingly associated with chronic inflammation and cardiovascular disease [8–10]. Similarly, in critically ill patients, inflammatory mediators implicated in the pathophysiology of multiple organ dysfunction syndrome are not effectively filtered using conventional membranes [11].

19.2.1 High-Cutoff and Medium-Cut Off Membranes

To address the limitations of conventional membranes, advanced membranes with larger pore sizes have been developed (Table 19.1). High-cutoff (HCO) membranes, also referred to as super-flux membranes, incorporate pore sizes substantially larger (~10 nm radius) than those of standard high-flux designs [12]. This expanded permeability enables enhanced removal of larger solutes (25–60 kDa), including free light chains, myoglobin, and cytokines. Established indications for HCO membranes include removal of free light chains in cast nephropathy and severe light chain-mediated acute kidney injury. Their use for myoglobin removal in rhabdomyolysis and for cytokine removal in inflammatory states remains exploratory [6, 13–15]. The principal limitation restricting wider clinical adoption of HCO membranes is the excessive and unintended removal of albumin [16–19].

Medium cut-off membranes (MCO) refine the principles of HCO membrane design by featuring a narrower and more uniform pore size distribution, enabling more selective removal of middle molecules while reducing albumin loss. They are engineered to maximise permeability for solutes up to approximately 45 kDa, with a sharp decline in permeability for larger solutes to minimise albumin passage [5, 20, 21]. Beyond their pore architecture, MCO membranes differ from conventional high-flux membranes in their hydraulic properties, which substantially influence solute clearance. When incorporated into a standard dialysis circuit (as part of "expanded haemodialysis"), the fibre geometry of MCO membranes creates a greater end-to-end pressure gradient within the dialyser [22]. This drives considerable movement from blood to dialysate in the proximal portion of the filter ("internal filtration"), generating convective transport of larger solutes (15–45 kDa). Distally, as the transmembrane pressure reverses, movement from dialysate to blood ("backfiltration") effectively replaces the fluid that was filtered proximally to maintain overall fluid balance [22]. This cycle of internal filtration and backfiltration generates convective clearance comparable to, and for some solutes superior to, high-volume hemodiafiltration.

Clinical investigations have shown that MCO membranes can achieve superior clearance of large middle molecules (e.g., β2-microglobulin, free light chains, specific cytokines, complement factor D) compared with conventional high-flux hemodialysis [23–26]. However, despite increasing clinical uptake, definitive outcome-driven evidence supporting the use of MCO membranes remains limited. In particular, robust data demonstrating improvements in key clinical outcomes, including mortality, cardiovascular events, hospitalisation rates, and patient-reported outcomes, have not been observed [27]. Consequently, the precise role of MCO membranes within the blood purification landscape remains uncertain and will depend on forthcoming long-term outcome data.

Table 19.1 Advanced membranes and biocompatibility strategies

Technology	Key features/mechanism	Application(s)	Evidence	Limitations and challenges
High-cutoff membranes	Pore radius ~ 10 nm; enhanced convective removal of large solutes	Removal of large molecules (e.g., FLCs in cast nephropathy, myoglobin in rhabdomyolysis).	Effective FLC removal Improved IL-6/β2M clearance vs high flux	Significant albumin loss Limited evidence for improved mortality/renal outcomes
Medium-cutoff membranes	Pore radius ~ 5 nm, steep sieving curve above ~45 kDa to minimise albumin loss; internal filtration/backfiltration enhances solute clearance without replacement fluid	Routine chronic HD for enhanced middle molecule clearance	Superior clearance of β2M, FLCs, factor D vs high flux Reduced hospitalisation/ESA use	Lack of RCT data on mortality/CV outcomes vs HF/HDF Long-term cost-effectiveness unclear
Silicon Nanopore membranes	MEMS-fabricated membranes with uniform, engineered nanopores. High permeability and selectivity	Potential for miniaturised wearable/implantable devices	Enhanced diffusive clearance of small molecules in preclinical models Short-term preclinical biocompatibility	Scalability Cost Long-term durability/stability/biocompatibility Stable coatings needed
Other nanomaterials (e.g., MXenes, MOFs, CNTs)	Advanced membranes with high surface area and tunable chemistry. Often provide adsorption-based removal	Potential for enhanced toxin adsorption without need for significant dialysate regeneration	Successful preclinical adsorption of creatinine, uric acid, urea by MXenes	Stability in vivo Biocompatibility Scalable synthesis

Passive membrane modifications (e.g., PEG, heparin)	Modifications often alter hydrophilicity, resist protein/cell adhesion, or provide local anticoagulation (heparin)	Improved biocompatibility of conventional/advanced membranes	Reduced protein adsorption/ platelet adhesion Heparin reduces clotting	Coating stability Potential leaching (i.e., heparin) May not fully eliminate activation
Active membrane modifications (e.g., NO-releasing polymers)	Mimic endothelial function, for example, by actively inhibiting platelet activation/aggregation via NO/cGMP/P-VASP pathway	Achieve high hemocompatibility, potentially without systemic anticoagulation	Reduced thrombus formation, preserved platelets, and reduced monocyte activation in preclinical model without systemic anticoagulation	Long-term NO release kinetics Long-term stability/ durability Clinical translation

β2M Beta-2 Microglobulin, *cGMP* Cyclic Guanosine Monophosphate, *CNTs* Carbon Nanotubes, *Cr* Creatinine, *CV* Cardiovascular, *ESA* Erythropoiesis-Stimulating Agent, *FLCs* Free Light Chains, *HD* Haemodialysis, *HDF* Haemodiafiltration, *HF* Haemofiltration, *IL-6* Interleukin-6, *kDa* Kilodalton, *MEMS* Microelectromechanical Systems, *MOFs* Metal-Organic Frameworks, *MWCO* Molecular Weight Cut-off, *MXenes* Transition Metal Carbides, Nitrides, or Carbonitrides, *NO* Nitric Oxide, *P-VASP* Phosphorylated Vasodilator-Stimulated Phosphoprotein, *PEG* Polyethylene Glycol, *PROs* Patient-Reported Outcomes, *RCT* Randomised Controlled Trial, *SNMs* Silicon Nanopore Membranes

19.2.2 Silicon Nanopore Membranes

Silicon nanopore membranes represent a substantial advancement over conventional synthetic polymer membranes (Table 19.1). Fabricated using microelectromechanical systems adapted from the semiconductor industry, silicon nanopore membranes enable precise nanoscale control over membrane architecture [28, 29]. These membranes typically comprise ultrathin silicon sheets with short diffusion path lengths (~100 μm) perforated by a high density of engineered pores. Unlike the heterogeneous pore structures of polymeric membranes, the pore structure of silicon nanopore membranes is highly uniform in size, shape, and spatial arrangement [28]. This precision in fabrication also enables the design of specific pore geometries, including configurations that mimic biological structures such as the slit-like pores formed by podocyte foot processes, which may optimise hydraulic permeability [28, 30].

The resulting high permeability of silicon nanopore membranes allows for ultrafiltration to be driven by physiological blood pressure alone, potentially eliminating the need for external blood pumps. Concurrently, the uniformity of pore dimensions confers highly selective filtration, permitting effective retention of large proteins while enhancing clearance of middle molecules [28, 30]. Because silicon nanopore membranes achieve high filtration efficiency with minimal membrane surface area (10–50 cm^2) and lower blood flow rates (20–50 mL/min), they support efforts toward device miniaturisation and portability, including the development of wearable kidney replacement technologies [31].

Although silicon nanopore membranes have demonstrated promising performance in ex vivo and preclinical models, they have not yet been evaluated in human studies. A major barrier to clinical translation is the need for scalable, cost-effective fabrication of large-area membranes with consistently uniform, defect-free pores. Long-term biocompatibility also remains uncertain: while short-term hemocompatibility has been favourable, the risks of chronic foreign-body responses, progressive membrane fouling, late-onset thrombosis, and structural degradation of the silicon structure with prolonged blood exposure are not yet characterised and require systematic investigation [28]. Accordingly, silicon nanopore membrane-based hemofiltration systems remain largely in the preclinical phase of development. Although early feasibility studies for implantable artificial kidney applications are ongoing, these technologies have not yet entered human trials. As such, the anticipated advantages of these technologies, including miniaturisation, portability, and pump-free operation, are theoretical at this stage and require validation through rigorous clinical evaluation.

19.2.3 Other Novel Membranes

Bioengineering efforts are also exploring the potential use of alternative nanomaterials, such as MXenes and metal-organic frameworks, for blood purification. These materials provide exceptionally large surface areas and modifiable surface chemistries that enhance adsorption capacity, offering the possibility of more efficient toxin removal [32, 33]. However, significant challenges to the use of such materials remain, including ensuring long-term stability in biologic environments, establishing acceptable biocompatibility, achieving scalable and reproducible synthesis methods, and integrating these materials into safe, functional device architectures.

19.3 Active Biomimetic Membrane Modifications

Beyond solute clearance, enhancing the biocompatibility of extracorporeal circuits remains a major priority in blood purification therapies. Contact between blood and artificial membrane surfaces triggers complement activation, coagulation cascades, and leukocyte recruitment, leading to thrombosis, inflammation, and reduced device performance [34, 35]. As a result, most systems require regional or systemic anticoagulation, which carries a risk of bleeding complications. The pro-inflammatory milieu generated by blood-membrane interactions is also believed to contribute to acute intradialytic symptoms and to chronic inflammation in patients receiving long-term dialysis [36]. Although contemporary membrane modifications have improved biocompatibility relative to earlier membranes, achieving maximally inert surfaces that minimise intradialytic symptoms, improve long-term outcomes, and extend circuit longevity remains an important unmet goal.

Passive surface modifications aimed at reducing membrane reactivity have historically been the primary strategies for improving biocompatibility (Table 19.1). Examples include altering membrane hydrophilicity to influence protein adsorption and complement activation; applying anti-fouling coatings that resist protein deposition and cell adhesion (e.g., polyethylene glycol, vitamin E, fluoropolymers); and covalently binding anticoagulants (e.g., heparin) to membranes to reduce thrombogenicity [37]. Although these methods have improved hemocompatibility compared with earlier membrane technologies, the evolution of the field points toward active biomimetic approaches.

Active biomimetic surface modifications involve engineering membrane interfaces that actively modulate blood responses by mimicking natural endothelial functions (Table 19.1). Examples include synthetic glycocalyx layers that reproduce the protective properties of the endothelial surface, biomimetic polymer brushes designed to reduce thrombosis, and nitric oxide (NO)-releasing polymers that replicate the intrinsic antiplatelet and anticoagulant functions of the vascular endothelium [38]. NO-releasing polymer membranes are of particular interest. These membranes deliver controlled quantities of NO at the blood-material interface, allowing diffusion into adjacent platelets and activation of the cyclic guanosine monophosphate (cGMP) signalling pathway. This leads to phosphorylation of vasodilator-stimulated phosphoprotein and subsequent inhibition of platelet activation, adhesion, and aggregation, thereby preventing thrombus formation.

Proof-of-concept for biomimetic membrane surfaces has been demonstrated in preclinical studies. In a 4-h rabbit model, NO-releasing polymer membranes significantly reduced thrombus formation, preserved platelet counts and function, and demonstrated biochemical evidence of cGMP pathway activation, without the need for systemic anticoagulation [39]. However, these findings are confined to experimental settings. Robust clinical studies evaluating the safety, efficacy, and patient-centred benefits of biomimetic membranes in humans have not been conducted. Therefore, any clinical advantage over existing technologies remains unproven.

19.4 Biohybrid Systems and Bioartificial Kidneys

The development of biohybrid renal replacement systems, such as bioartificial kidneys, represents another emerging biotechnology in blood purification (Table 19.2). These systems integrate living biological components (primarily renal tubular cells) with engineered materials (often advanced membranes and scaffolds) to perform both filtration and metabolic functions [31]. By providing continuous, autonomous renal support, such technologies aim to eliminate the need for scheduled dialysis sessions and address key physiological and patient-centred limitations of current therapies.

The field of biohybrid replacement systems has evolved from extracorporeal bioartificial kidneys, designed for intermittent use in acute care or as bridge therapies, towards fully implantable devices [65, 66]. Notable initiatives include The Kidney Project (UCSF/Vanderbilt), which is developing a coffee cup-sized, pressure-driven biohybrid device combining silicon nanopore membranes with human kidney tubule cells, and the European KIDNEW project, which employs a modular architecture incorporating advanced silicon filters, surface coatings, sensors, and bioreactors with integrated cell monitoring capabilities. Both initiatives have demonstrated significant preclinical progress and secured substantial research funding and early regulatory support. However, clinical trials of implantable bioartificial kidneys in humans have not yet commenced.

19.4.1 Advantages of Biohybrid Systems

Relative to conventional blood purification methods, proposed advantages of biohybrid systems include the potential for continuous, autonomous operation; improved haemodynamic and cardiovascular stability; restoration of renal physiological functions beyond filtration; reduced need for systemic immunosuppression (versus kidney transplantation); and enhanced patient quality of life through greater mobility, autonomy, and the possibility of renal replacement therapy outside of clinical centres [67–70]. Collectively, these benefits may help minimise both disease- and therapy-related complications. Indeed, early clinical studies of extracorporeal bioartificial kidneys have provided proof-of-concept evidence, demonstrating improvements in metabolic control and cardiovascular stability. However, long-term clinical outcomes are yet to be established [71–73].

Table 19.2 Summary of emerging biohybrid systems and bioartificial kidney technologies

Technology	Key features/mechanism	Application(s)	Evidence	Limitations and challenges
Bioartificial kidney	Integrates living biological components (typically renal tubular cells) with artificial components (membranes, scaffolds). Can be extracorporeal or implantable	Treatment of AKI and ESKD	Extracorporeal: Phase I/II trials showed safety for 24 h, metabolic activity (Vit D activation, GSH metabolism), immunomodulatory effects (cytokine reduction), and suggested survival benefit in AKI/MOF patients. Implantable: Preclinical proof-of-concept for bioreactor component using SNMs in pigs demonstrated cell viability/function without immunosuppression for 7 days.	Replicating complex renal physiology Long-term biocompatibility and device durability/failure Vascular access for implants Power source for active components Cost and manufacturing scale-up
Enabling Tech: Cell bioreactor component	Contains cultured renal cells to provide metabolic, endocrine, and transport functions. Cells often cultured on membranes/scaffolds within the device	Physiologic functions not achieved by standard dialysis	Humes RAD trials demonstrated metabolic activity from human cells ex vivo. Kim, 2023 showed >90% viability and function (transporter gene expression, Vit D activation) of human cells in an implanted SNM bioreactor in pigs for 7 days.	Obtaining sufficient functional, stable cells Maintaining long-term viability, phenotype, and sufficient functional cell mass in vivo Achieving proper cell organisation and polarity for effective function

(continued)

Table 19.2 (continued)

Technology	Key features/mechanism	Application(s)	Evidence	Limitations and challenges
Enabling Tech: Membranes (esp. SNMs)	Silicon membranes with uniform, precisely engineered nanopores. High potential hydraulic permeability; potential for pressure-driven filtration (pump-less). Sharp molecular weight cut-offs enable selective filtration and immunoisolation	Haemofiltration and immuno-isolation	High hydraulic permeability demonstrated. Effective immunoisolation shown in vitro (cytokine reduction) and in vivo (7-day human cell survival in pigs without immunosuppression). PEG-coated silicon shows good haemocompatibility (in vitro) and successful short-term implantation in vivo without anticoagulation. Stable performance over 90 h in blood demonstrated.	Long-term in vivo stability and resistance to degradation/failure remains a key challenge Long-term stability of anti-fouling/ biocompatible coatings is critical Scaling up fabrication cost-effectively
Enabling Tech: Dialysate regeneration	Required for portable/wearable/ implantable systems to reuse a small dialysate volume. Sorbent (REDY-based): Uses activated carbon, urease, zirconium phosphate/oxide. Alternatives: Novel adsorbents (MXenes, MIPs), ion concentration - polarisation (ICP)	Enable continuous or prolonged dialysis outside clinical centres with miniaturised devices	Sorbent systems used in early BAK prototypes demonstrate feasibility but technical issues. Electrochemical oxidation/ICP show promise for urea removal in vitro. MXenes show high urea adsorption potential.	Poor urea adsorption (carbon), toxic ammonium production (urease), electrolyte disturbances (zirconium phosphate) Alternative system: Efficiency, selectivity, by-product toxicity, capacity/kinetics, scalability within device constraints

AKI Acute Kidney Injury, *BAK* Bioartificial Kidney, *ESKD* End-Stage Kidney Disease, *GSH* Glutathione, *ICP* Ion Concentration Polarisation, *MIPs* Molecularly Imprinted Polymers, *MOF* Multi-Organ Failure, *MXenes* Transition Metal Carbides, Nitrides, or Carbonitrides, *PEG* Polyethylene Glycol, *RAD* Renal Assist Device, *REDY* Reusable Dialysate System, *SNMs* Silicon Nanopore Membranes, *Vit D* Vitamin D

19.4.2 Challenges of Biohybrid Systems

Successful translation of bioartificial kidney therapies into clinical practice relies on coordinated advances across several core enabling technologies. For example, a miniaturised device incorporating silicon nanopore membranes must also integrate advanced biocompatible surface coatings to mitigate complement activation, inflammatory responses, thrombosis, and membrane fouling [74, 75].

Beyond materials and surface engineering, biological integration presents an equally difficult challenge. Bio-integration and replication of the kidney's complex physiology using a limited cellular component remains a major hurdle for bioartificial kidney development. These systems aim to incorporate functional renal tubular epithelial cells within intracorporeal bioreactors to restore metabolic, endocrine, and transport activities not provided by conventional renal replacement therapy. Key obstacles include sourcing sufficient quantities of viable human renal cells (whether primary, stem cell-derived, or immortalised); maintaining long-term cellular viability and function in vivo; achieving adequate cell mass, sustained polarisations, and phenotypic diversity for clinically meaningful physiological function; and establishing durable immunoisolation to prevent rejection, fibrotic encapsulation, chronic inflammation, and material degradation in the long term [69]. The use of autologous cells, potentially derived from induced pluripotent stem cells, represents one approach to overcome immunological barriers [74].

A further challenge for bioartificial kidney systems is the requirement for efficient dialysate regeneration [76]. Current approaches for dialysate regeneration predominantly rely on sorbent-based technologies derived from the REcirculating DialYsate (REDY) system, which incorporates activated carbon, urease, zirconium phosphate, and hydrous zirconium oxide [66, 76]. However, activated carbon exhibits limited urea adsorption, necessitating enzymatic hydrolysis of urea by urease to ammonium (a potentially neurotoxic intermediate). Subsequent ammonium removal by zirconium phosphate results in sodium release and binding of divalent cations (e.g., calcium and magnesium) with the potential to disturb electrolyte homeostasis [76]. Alternative dialysate regeneration strategies, including ion concentration polarisation (ICP) techniques and molecularly imprinted polymers, are under investigation [68]. Though achieving sufficient adsorption capacity, selectivity, and reaction kinetics within the strict volume constraints of portable or implantable devices remains challenging. In parallel, the development of safe, reliable, durable, and miniaturised power sources for implanted systems requires substantial innovation.

19.5 Haemoadsorption

Haemoadsorption is an emerging blood purification modality that enables targeted removal of pathogenic mediators implicated in the pathogenesis of organ failure during critical illness (Table 19.3) [40]. By selectively removing circulating molecules such as pro-inflammatory cytokines, endotoxin, and bacterial and viral fragments, haemoadsorption seeks to modulate dysregulated inflammatory responses

Table 19.3 Summary of emerging haemoadsorption biotechnologies

Technology	Key features/ mechanism	Application(s)	Evidence	Limitations and challenges
CytoSorb	Porous polymer beads (styrene divinylbenzene)	Remove pro- and anti-inflammatory cytokines + other hydrophobic molecules (bilirubin, myoglobin)	Reduces IL-6/CRP REMOVE trial (IE surgery) showed no benefit in SOFA, mortality, or organ support despite ↓ cytokines	Inconsistent RCT results Non-selective removal (including pharmaceuticals) Cost
oXiris	AN69 membrane, PEI coating, and heparin graft	Bind cytokines and endotoxin	Reduces endotoxin/ cytokines in vitro/ vivo SIRAKI02 trial (cardiac surgery) demonstrates ↓ AKI incidence (mainly milder stages), no difference in mortality/LOS	Limited evidence for improved key clinical outcomes
Jafron HA series (HA-330/ HA-380)	Neutral microporous resins (styrene divinylbenzene)	Binds medium-large molecules like cytokines (e.g., IL-6, IL-10, TNF-α)	Small/retrospective studies suggest ↓inflammation, improved organ function in sepsis/ COVID/cardiac surgery Additional trials ongoing	Limited high-quality RCT evidence Potential antibiotic adsorption
Polymyxin B	Affinity adsorption of endotoxin via lipid A binding to polymyxin B immobilised on polystyrene fibres	Endotoxin removal	EUPHRATES trial (sepsis, EAA $\geq$ 0.60): No overall ↓28 d mortality. Post-hoc analysis demonstrated potential benefit in EAA 0.6–0.89 subgroup TIGRIS trial ongoing	Limited evidence for improved key clinical outcomes Optimal patient selection (EAA range) unclear Cost

AKI Acute Kidney Injury, *AN69* Acrylonitrile and sodium methallyl sulphonate copolymer, *COVID* Coronavirus Disease, *CRP* C-Reactive Protein, *EAA* Endotoxin Activity Assay, *HA* Haemoadsorption, *IE* Infective Endocarditis, *IL-6* Interleukin-6, *IL-10* Interleukin-10, *kDa* Kilodalton, *LOS* Length of Stay, *LPS* Lipopolysaccharide, *PEI* Polyethylenimine, *RCT* Randomised Controlled Trial, *SOFA* Sequential Organ Failure Assessment, *TNF-α* Tumour Necrosis Factor-alpha observed in conditions such as sepsis and during major cardiac surgery requiring cardiopulmonary bypass. The therapeutic goal is not indiscriminate detoxification, but rather partial restoration of immune homeostasis. From a biological standpoint, it is plausible that removal of mediators central to vasodilation, capillary leak, and organ dysfunction may translate into improved physiological stability and patient-centred outcomes [40].

Several haemoadsorption technologies are already available for clinical use [40]. The CytoSorb device employs porous polymer beads to remove circulating cytokines. Although in vivo and early clinical studies suggested potential benefit [41, 42], a systematic review of 34 studies (including 12 randomised controlled trials) found no difference in IL-6 concentration, serum lactate, length of stay, or mortality with CytoSorb compared with standard care in patients with sepsis and other inflammatory conditions.

The oXiris device utilises a surface-modified AN69 membrane with high affinity for cytokines and endotoxin. In a systematic review of 14 studies (including 4 randomised controlled trials), oXiris use was associated with lower IL-6 concentration, reduced noradrenaline requirements, lower Sequential Organ Failure Assessment (SOFA) scores, and improvements in length of stay and mortality. Furthermore, the SIRAKI02 trial demonstrated a reduction in the incidence of acute kidney injury during cardiac surgery with oXiris. This was largely driven by a decrease in stage 1 acute kidney injury and did not translate into improved long-term outcomes [43].

Resin-based devices, including the Jafron HA series (HA-330, HA-380), have also been employed clinically, particularly in Asia. These devices utilise neutral microporous resins to adsorb medium-to-large molecular weight solutes, including cytokines. Evidence supporting their efficacy in sepsis remains limited to case reports and small observational studies. [44–48] Ongoing randomised clinical trials evaluating HA-380 in septic shock (e.g., NCT04997421 and NCT04306419) are expected to provide more robust evidence to inform their use [49].

Polymyxin B haemoadsorption (PMX) employs cartridges containing immobilised polymyxin B to selectively bind circulating endotoxin [50, 51]. The concurrent development of the endotoxin activity assay (EAA) allows identification of patients with high endotoxin levels (EAA ≥ 0.60) who may derive the greatest benefit from PMX [52]. The EUPHAS trial reported improvements in vasopressor requirements, SOFA scores, and mortality in patients with septic shock treated with PMX compared with usual care. However, these findings were not replicated in the larger ABDOMIX and EUPHRATES trials. [53] *Post hoc* analysis of EUPHRATES suggested a potential benefit in patients with moderate endotoxin activity (EAA 0.6–0.9), a hypothesis that will be prospectively tested in the ongoing TIGRIS trial (NCT03901807) [54].

19.5.1 Further Applications of Haemoadsorption

Beyond their primary investigation in sepsis, cardiac surgery, and related inflammatory states, the principles and technologies underlying selective adsorption hold broader potential across a range of critical illnesses [55]. In acute respiratory distress syndrome, where dysregulated inflammation plays a central pathophysiological role, both preclinical and early clinical studies suggest that cytokine adsorption may attenuate lung injury [56]. In acute and acute-on-chronic liver failure, extracorporeal circuits incorporating haemoadsorption devices like CytoSorb or resin-based cartridges can facilitate removal of accumulated toxins, including bilirubin and ammonia [57]. In the field of organ transplantation, ex situ machine perfusion platforms combined with haemoadsorption have emerged as a potential strategy to improve organ preservation and, potentially, to recondition marginal donor organs prior to implantation [58]. Additional applications include the management of selected drug intoxications and acute autoimmune disease. Collectively, these diverse indications highlight the versatility of blood purification platforms beyond renal replacement therapy and the treatment of sepsis-associated inflammation.

19.5.2 Limitations in Haemoadsorption

Despite strong pathophysiological rationale and ongoing technological refinement, haemoadsorption faces significant barriers to widespread clinical adoption. Foremost among these is the absence of robust evidence from large, adequately powered randomised controlled trials demonstrating meaningful improvements in patient-centred outcomes, particularly mortality. This limitation is closely linked to challenges in identifying appropriate patient subgroups within heterogeneous critical illness syndromes, uncertainty regarding optimal timing and duration of therapy, unwanted removal of substances (e.g., antibiotics), and the frequently observed disconnect between successful target molecule removal and downstream clinical outcomes. In addition, the cost and operational complexity of haemoadsorption therapies within resource-intensive critical care environments necessitate clear demonstration of both clinical efficacy, safety, and cost-effectiveness before broader implementation can be justified.

19.5.3 Frontiers in Haemoadsorption

Ongoing research efforts are focussed on the development of highly selective sorbents to enable precision blood purification. Two principal strategies currently dominate this field: molecularly imprinted polymers (MIPs) and affinity ligand-based systems [59–61]. MIPs are synthetic polymers created using a template molecule, resulting in nanocavities that are structurally and chemically complementary to the target and capable of selective rebinding. Proof-of-concept prototypes have demonstrated effective binding of targets such as hemoglobin [60]. In principle, libraries of MIPs could be engineered to selectively capture a wide range of uremic toxins, cytokines, endotoxins, and drugs, offering broad potential applicability across diverse clinical contexts.

Affinity ligand-based systems utilise a complementary strategy, whereby ligands with high binding specificity for a target molecule are immobilised onto a sorbent matrix [61]. An established clinical example includes protein A columns for IgG removal in autoimmune disease. More recent developments encompass affinity ligands derived from monoclonal antibodies, synthetic peptides, and nucleic acid aptamers, enabling selective capture of targets ranging from endotoxin to specific inflammatory mediators or autoantibodies [61–63]. Although these systems offer high specificity by mimicking biological binding interactions, their clinical translation is constrained by limited ligand capacity and the cost and complexity of manufacturing biological ligands such as recombinant proteins. Moreover, even when biochemical target removal is achieved, this does not necessarily translate into improved clinical outcomes in complex conditions like sepsis [64].

19.6 Translational Outlook and Future Directions

While emerging biotechnologies hold substantial promise for overcoming the limitations of existing blood purification modalities, significant translational challenges must be overcome before widespread clinical integration can be achieved. Rigorous clinical validation through adequately powered randomised controlled trials focusing on patient-centred outcomes remains essential, alongside robust demonstration of cost-effectiveness to justify adoption within resource-constrained healthcare systems.

Key technological barriers also persist. These include the development of durable and highly biocompatible materials and membranes, the achievement of reliable long-term function and immunocompatibility for implantable or biohybrid devices, and the optimisation of efficient, scalable dialysate regeneration systems. In parallel, consideration of the environmental footprint of blood purification, the integration of sustainable manufacturing and disposal practices, and the promotion of equitable global access to these potentially transformative technologies represent important ethical and societal considerations [3, 77, 78].

Addressing these challenges will require sustained multidisciplinary collaboration across materials science, biochemical and tissue engineering, nanotechnology, and translational clinical research. Such coordinated efforts are essential to translate innovation into safe, effective, and accessible next-generation blood purification therapies.

19.7 Conclusion

Although current blood purification modalities are life-sustaining, they inadequately address the full spectrum of physiological disturbances that occur with severe renal dysfunction and critical illness, underscoring the need for continued innovation. Emerging strategies offer considerable promise: advanced membrane technologies (e.g., MCO, HCO, and silicon nanopore membranes) aim to optimise solute removal profiles; active surface modifications seek to enhance biocompatibility and reduce reliance on anticoagulation; bioartificial kidneys pursue the ambitious goal of restoring comprehensive renal function; and haemoadsorption therapies provide mechanisms for targeted removal of pathogenic mediators in critical illness. Together, the emergence of these technologies highlights the shift toward precision, biologically informed blood purification.

Despite this progress, translation into widespread clinical practice remains challenging and dependent on robust outcome data, regulatory approval, and scalability. MCO membranes, while demonstrating improved middle molecule clearance, require definitive long-term outcome data to establish their clinical value. Bioartificial kidney systems remain largely in preclinical or early clinical development, facing complex challenges related to cell sourcing, long-term viability, immunoisolation, device integration, and dialysate regeneration. Haemoadsorption therapies, although effective in reducing circulating inflammatory mediators, have not consistently improved clinical endpoints, highlighting the importance of appropriate patient selection and therapeutic timing.

Future progress hinges on continued advances in materials science; a deeper mechanistic understanding of uremic and inflammatory pathophysiology to inform targeted interventions; rigorous clinical evaluation prioritising patient-centred outcomes and health economic impact; and proactive consideration of sustainability, equitable access, and ethical implementation. While the potential to transform care is considerable, overcoming these scientific, clinical, and translational barriers will be essential to realise the full promise of next-generation blood purification technologies.

Bibliography

1. National KF. KDOQI clinical practice guideline for hemodialysis adequacy: 2015 update. Am J Kidney Dis. 2015;66(5):884–930.
2. Liyanage T, Ninomiya T, Jha V, Neal B, Patrice HM, Okpechi I, et al. Worldwide access to treatment for end-stage kidney disease: a systematic review. Lancet. 2015;385(9981):1975–82.
3. Yeo SC, Ooi XY, Tan TSM. Sustainable kidney care delivery and climate change –a call to action. Glob Health. 2022;18(1):75.
4. Raoofi S, Pashazadeh Kan F, Rafiei S, Hoseinipalangi Z, Rezaei S, Ahmadi S, et al. Hemodialysis and peritoneal dialysis-health-related quality of life: systematic review plus meta-analysis. BMJ Support Palliat Care. 2023;13(4):365–73.
5. Ronco C, Clark WR. Hemodialysis membranes. Nat Rev Nephrol. 2018;14(6):394–410.
6. Reis T, Anwar S, Neves F, Ronco C. Disruptive technologies for hemodialysis: medium and high cutoff membranes. Is the future now? J Bras Nefrol. 2021;43(3):410–6.
7. Rosner MH, Reis T, Husain-Syed F, Vanholder R, Hutchison C, Stenvinkel P, et al. Classification of uremic toxins and their role in kidney failure. Clin J Am Soc Nephrol. 2021;16(12):1918–28.
8. Lekawanvijit S, Kompa AR, Wang BH, Kelly DJ, Krum H. Cardiorenal syndrome: the emerging role of protein-bound uremic toxins. Circ Res. 2012;111(11):1470–83.
9. Ito S, Yoshida M. Protein-bound uremic toxins: new culprits of cardiovascular events in chronic kidney disease patients. Toxins (Basel). 2014;6(2):665–78.
10. Wolley M, Jardine M, Hutchison CA. Exploring the clinical relevance of providing increased removal of large middle molecules. Clin J Am Soc Nephrol. 2018;13(5):805–14.

11. Bottari G, Ranieri VM, Ince C, Pesenti A, Aucella F, Scandroglio AM, et al. Use of extracorporeal blood purification therapies in sepsis: the current paradigm, available evidence, and future perspectives. Crit Care. 2024;28(1):432.
12. Boschetti-de-Fierro A, Voigt M, Storr M, Krause B. Extended characterization of a new class of membranes for blood purification: the high cut-off membranes. Int J Artif Organs. 2013;36(7):455–63.
13. Weidhase L, de Fallois J, Haussig E, Kaiser T, Mende M, Petros S. Myoglobin clearance with continuous veno-venous hemodialysis using high cutoff dialyzer versus continuous veno-venous hemodiafiltration using high-flux dialyzer: a prospective randomized controlled trial. Crit Care. 2020;24(1):644.
14. Hutchison CA, Heyne N, Airia P, Schindler R, Zickler D, Cook M, et al. Immunoglobulin free light chain levels and recovery from myeloma kidney on treatment with chemotherapy and high cut-off hemodialysis. Nephrol Dial Transplant. 2012;27(10):3823–8.
15. Hutchison CA, Harding S, Mead G, Goehl H, Storr M, Bradwell A, et al. Serum free-light chain removal by high cutoff hemodialysis: optimizing removal and supportive care. Artif Organs. 2008;32(12):910–7.
16. Atan R, Peck L, Visvanathan K, Skinner N, Eastwood G, Bellomo R, et al. High cut-off hemofiltration versus standard hemofiltration: effect on plasma cytokines. Int J Artif Organs. 2016;39(9):479–86.
17. Chelazzi C, Villa G, D'Alfonso MG, Mancinelli P, Consales G, Berardi M, et al. Hemodialysis with high cut-off hemodialyzers in patients with multi-drug resistant gram-negative sepsis and acute kidney injury: a retrospective. Case-Control Study Blood Purif. 2016;42(3):186–93.
18. Villa G, Chelazzi C, Morettini E, Zamidei L, Valente S, Caldini AL, et al. Organ dysfunction during continuous veno-venous high cut-off hemodialysis in patients with septic acute kidney injury: a prospective observational study. PLoS One. 2017;12(2):e0172039.
19. Atan R, Peck L, Prowle J, Licari E, Eastwood GM, Storr M, et al. A double-blind randomized controlled trial of high cutoff versus standard hemofiltration in critically ill patients with acute kidney injury. Crit Care Med. 2018;46(10):e988–e94.
20. Boschetti-de-Fierro A, Voigt M, Storr M, Krause B. MCO membranes: enhanced selectivity in high-flux class. Sci Rep. 2015;5:18448.
21. Ronco C. The rise of expanded hemodialysis. Blood Purif. 2017;44(2):I–VIII.
22. Zhang Z, Yang T, Li Y, Li J, Yang Q, Wang L, et al. Effects of expanded hemodialysis with medium cut-off membranes on maintenance hemodialysis patients: a review. Membranes (Basel). 2022;12(3):253.
23. Cho NJ, Park S, Islam MI, Song HY, Lee EY, Gil HW. Long-term effect of medium cut-off dialyzer on middle uremic toxins and cell-free hemoglobin. PLoS One. 2019;14(7):e0220448.
24. Weiner DE, Falzon L, Skoufos L, Bernardo A, Beck W, Xiao M, et al. Efficacy and safety of expanded hemodialysis with the Theranova 400 dialyzer: a randomized controlled trial. Clin J Am Soc Nephrol. 2020;15(9):1310–9.
25. Kirsch AH, Lyko R, Nilsson LG, Beck W, Amdahl M, Lechner P, et al. Performance of hemodialysis with novel medium cut-off dialyzers. Nephrol Dial Transplant. 2017;32(1):165–72.
26. Sevinc M, Hasbal NB, Yilmaz V, Basturk T, Ahbap E, Sakaci T, et al. Comparison of circulating levels of uremic toxins in hemodialysis patients treated with medium cut-off membranes and high-flux membranes: Theranova in Sisli Hamidiye Etfal (THE SHE) randomized control study. Blood Purif. 2020;49(6):733–42.
27. Fiorentino M, La Fergola F, De Rosa S. Medium cut-off dialyzer for middle molecular uremic toxins in AKI and chronic dialysis. J Nephrol. 2024;37(1):23–37.
28. Kim S, Feinberg B, Kant R, Chui B, Goldman K, Park J, et al. Diffusive silicon nanopore membranes for hemodialysis applications. PLoS One. 2016;11(7):e0159526.
29. Kensinger C, Karp S, Kant R, Chui BW, Goldman K, Yeager T, et al. First implantation of silicon nanopore membrane hemofilters. ASAIO J. 2016;62(4):491–5.
30. Fissell WH, Dubnisheva A, Eldridge AN, Fleischman AJ, Zydney AL, Roy S. High-performance silicon nanopore hemofiltration membranes. J Memb Sci. 2009;326(1):58–63.

31. Tang YS, Tsai YC, Chen TW, Li SY. Artificial kidney engineering: the development of dialysis membranes for blood purification. Membranes (Basel). 2022;12(2):177.
32. Javaherchi P, Zarepour A, Khosravi A, Heydari P, Iravani S, Zarrabi A. Innovative applications of MXenes in dialysis: enhancing filtration efficiency. Nanoscale. 2025;17(8):4301–27.
33. Deng L-E, Guo M, Deng Y, Pan Y, Wang X, Maduraiveeran G, et al. MOF-based platform for kidney diseases: advances, challenges, and prospects. Pharmaceutics. 2024;16(6):793.
34. Hakim RM. Clinical implications of hemodialysis membrane biocompatibility. Kidney Int. 1993;44(3):484–94.
35. Clark WR, Hamburger RJ, Lysaght MJ. Effect of membrane composition and structure on solute removal and biocompatibility in hemodialysis. Kidney Int. 1999;56(6):2005–15.
36. Kohlová M, Amorim CG, Araújo A, Santos-Silva A, Solich P, Montenegro MCBSM. The biocompatibility and bioactivity of hemodialysis membranes: their impact in end-stage renal disease. J Artif Organs. 2019;22(1):14–28.
37. Nazari S, Abdelrasoul A. Impact of membrane modification and surface immobilization techniques on the Hemocompatibility of hemodialysis membranes: a critical review. Membranes. 2022;12(11):1063.
38. Frost MC, Reynolds MM, Meyerhoff ME. Polymers incorporating nitric oxide releasing/generating substances for improved biocompatibility of blood-contacting medical devices. Biomaterials. 2005;26(14):1685–93.
39. Major TC, Handa H, Annich GM, Bartlett RH. Development and hemocompatibility testing of nitric oxide releasing polymers using a rabbit model of thrombogenicity. J Biomater Appl. 2014;29(4):479–501.
40. Bellomo R, Ankawi G, Bagshaw SM, Baldwin I, Basu R, Bottari G, et al. Hemoadsorption: consensus report of the 30th acute disease quality initiative workgroup. Nephrol Dial Transplant. 2024;39(12):1945–64.
41. Diab M, Lehmann T, Bothe W, Akhyari P, Platzer S, Wendt D, et al. Cytokine hemoadsorption during cardiac surgery versus standard surgical care for infective endocarditis (REMOVE): results from a multicenter randomized controlled trial. Circulation. 2022;145(13):959–68.
42. Steindl D, Schroeder T, Krannich A, Nee J. Hemoadsorption in the management of septic shock: a systematic review and meta-analysis. J Clin Med. 2025;14(7):2285.
43. Pérez-Fernández X, Ulsamer A, Cámara-Rosell M, Sbraga F, Boza-Hernández E, Moret-Ruíz E, et al. Extracorporeal blood purification and acute kidney injury in cardiac surgery: the SIRAKI02 randomized clinical trial. JAMA. 2024;332(17):1446–54.
44. Kurniawan A, Partiningrum DL, Olivera I, Sanjaya S, Djunarko J, Yusri NH, et al. Effect of hemoperfusion in critically ill COVID-19 patients: a case series from a single-center hospital in Indonesia. J Infect Dev Ctries. 2024;18(12.1):S206–S13.
45. Chen L, Zhou S, Wang C, Qie G, Tai Z, Wang F, et al. Efficacy of HA380 hemoperfusion in the treatment of septic shock. J Transl Crit Care Med. 2024;6(3):e24–00008.
46. Ryazanova D, Tobylbayeva Z, Mironova O, Kakenov E, Sazonov V. Comparison of CytoSorb and Jafron HA330 hemoadsorption devices in pediatric oncological patients with sepsis: retrospective observational study. J Clin Med. 2024;13(24):7694.
47. Nurmykhametova Z, Lesbekov T, Kaliyev R, Bekishev B, Jabayeva N, Novikova S, et al. Preliminary report of extracorporeal blood purification therapy in patients receiving LVAD: Cytosorb or Jafron HA330. J Extra Corpor Technol. 2024;56(1):10–5.
48. Lesbekov T, Nurmykhametova Z, Kaliyev R, Kuanyshbek A, Faizov L, Bekishev B, et al. Hemoadsorption in patients requiring V-A ECMO support: comparison of Cytosorb versus Jafron HA330. Artif Organs. 2023;47(4):721–30.
49. Li Y, Han M, Yang M, Su B. Hemoperfusion with the HA330/HA380 cartridge in intensive care settings: a state-of-the-art review. Blood Purif. 2024;54(2):122–37.
50. Roncoa PPC. Polymyxin-B hemoperfusion and endotoxin removal: lessons from a review of the literature. Contrib Nephrol. 2010;167:77–82.
51. Cruz DN, Bellomo R, Ronco C. Clinical effects of polymyxin B-immobilized fiber column in septic patients. Contrib Nephrol. 2007;156:444–51.

52. Pinciroli R, Checchi S, Bottiroli M, Monti G, Casella G, Fumagalli R. Endotoxin activity assay for the detection of whole blood Endotoxemia in critically ill patients. J Vis Exp. 2019;148
53. Dellinger RP, Bagshaw SM, Antonelli M, Foster DM, Klein DJ, Marshall JC, et al. Effect of targeted Polymyxin B Hemoperfusion on 28-day mortality in patients with septic shock and elevated endotoxin level: the EUPHRATES randomized clinical trial. JAMA. 2018;320(14):1455–63.
54. Klein DJ, Foster D, Walker PM, Bagshaw SM, Mekonnen H, Antonelli M. Polymyxin B hemoperfusion in endotoxemic septic shock patients without extreme endotoxemia: a post hoc analysis of the EUPHRATES trial. Intensive Care Med. 2018;44(12):2205–12.
55. Becker S, Lang H, Vollmer Barbosa C, Tian Z, Melk A, Schmidt BMW. Efficacy of CytoSorb®: a systematic review and meta-analysis. Crit Care. 2023;27(1):215.
56. Szigetváry CE, Turan C, Kovács EH, Kói T, Engh MA, Hegyi P, et al. Hemoadsorption as adjuvant therapy in acute respiratory distress syndrome (ARDS): a systematic review and meta-analysis. Biomedicine. 2023;11(11):3068.
57. Turan C, Szigetváry CE, Kói T, Engh MA, Atakan I, Zubek L, et al. Hemoadsorption therapy for critically ill patients with acute liver dysfunction: a meta-analysis and systematic review. Biomedicine. 2023;12(1):67.
58. Jiao C, Sun K, Shamugarajah K, Zhang M, Wehrle CJ, Panconesi R, et al. From critical care to organ preservation: the potential role of hemoadsorption in transplantation—a narrative review. Hepatobiliary Surg Nutr. 2025;4(4):608–29.
59. Vasapollo G, Sole RD, Mergola L, Lazzoi MR, Scardino A, Scorrano S, et al. Molecularly imprinted polymers: present and future prospective. Int J Mol Sci. 2011;12(9):5908–45.
60. Ergun C, Eskizengin H. Recent updates on blood purification: use of smart polymer materials. J Biomed Mater Res A. 2025;113(3):e37883.
61. Xue A, Fan S. Matrices and affinity ligands for antibody purification and corresponding applications in radiotherapy. Biomolecules. 2022;12(6):830.
62. Zhao W-W, Liu F-F, Shi Q-H, Dong X-Y, Sun Y. Biomimetic design of affinity peptide ligands for human IgG based on protein A-IgG complex. Biochem Eng J. 2014;88:1–11.
63. Arora S, Saxena V, Ayyar BV. Affinity chromatography: a versatile technique for antibody purification. Methods. 2017;116:84–94.
64. Lipcsey M, Tenhunen J, Pischke SE, Kuitunen A, Flaatten H, De Geer L, et al. Endotoxin removal in septic shock with the Alteco LPS Adsorber was safe but showed no benefit compared to placebo in the double-blind randomized controlled trial-the asset study. Shock. 2020;54(2):224–31.
65. Nalesso F, Garzotto F, Cattarin L, Bettin E, Cacciapuoti M, Silvestre C, et al. The future for end-stage kidney disease treatment: implantable bioartificial kidney challenge. Appl Sci. 2024;14(2):491.
66. Ramada DL, de Vries J, Vollenbroek J, Noor N, Ter Beek O, Mihaila SM, et al. Portable, wearable and implantable artificial kidney systems: needs, opportunities and challenges. Nat Rev Nephrol. 2023;19(8):481–90.
67. Song S, Faleo G, Yeung R, Kant R, Posselt AM, Desai TA, et al. Silicon nanopore membrane (SNM) for islet encapsulation and immunoisolation under convective transport. Sci Rep. 2016;6:23679.
68. Kim W, Hong S, Kim K, Lee S, Shin DA, Yang SH, et al. Scalable ion concentration polarization dialyzer for peritoneal dialysate regeneration. J Nanobiotechnol. 2025;23(1):255.
69. Tasnim F, Deng R, Hu M, Liour S, Li Y, Ni M, et al. Achievements and challenges in bioartificial kidney development. Fibrogenesis Tissue Repair. 2010;3:14.
70. Pino CJ, Yevzlin AS, Tumlin J, Humes HD. Cell-based strategies for the treatment of kidney dysfunction: a review. Blood Purif. 2012;34(2):117–23.
71. Humes HD, Buffington DA, Lou L, Abrishami S, Wang M, Xia J, et al. Cell therapy with a tissue-engineered kidney reduces the multiple-organ consequences of septic shock. Crit Care Med. 2003;31(10):2421–8.

72. Humes HD, Sobota JT, Ding F, Song JH. A selective cytopheretic inhibitory device to treat the immunological dysregulation of acute and chronic renal failure. Blood Purif. 2010;29(2):183–90.
73. Humes HD, Weitzel WF, Bartlett RH, Swaniker FC, Paganini EP, Luderer JR, et al. Initial clinical results of the bioartificial kidney containing human cells in ICU patients with acute renal failure. Kidney Int. 2004;66(4):1578–88.
74. Kim EJ, Chen C, Gologorsky R, Santandreu A, Torres A, Wright N, et al. Feasibility of an implantable bioreactor for renal cell therapy using silicon nanopore membranes. Nat Commun. 2023;14(1):4890.
75. Muthusubramaniam L, Lowe R, Fissell WH, Li L, Marchant RE, Desai TA, et al. Hemocompatibility of silicon-based substrates for biomedical implant applications. Ann Biomed Eng. 2011;39(4):1296–305.
76. van Gelder MK, Jong JAW, Folkertsma L, Guo Y, Blüchel C, Verhaar MC, et al. Urea removal strategies for dialysate regeneration in a wearable artificial kidney. Biomaterials. 2020;234:119735.
77. Vanholder R. Future directions for dialysis. Kidney Dial. 2022;2(2):153–62.
78. Jimenez MDA, Audije-Gil J, Martinez R, Martin Vaquero N, Gomez M, Portillo J, et al. How to improve the environmental impact in hemodialysis: small actions, big changes. Clin Kidney J. 2025;18(2):sfae407.

Case-Based Applications: Real-World Scenarios in Extracorporeal Therapies

20

Alexandre Klopp and Kevin Roedl

20.1 Introduction

Extracorporeal therapies have evolved from single-organ support systems into adaptable, modular platforms that can manage complex multiorgan dysfunction in critically ill patients. The transition from conventional single-organ replacement therapies to multimodal circuits capable of providing simultaneous renal, hepatic, and pulmonary support opens up new therapeutic possibilities but also presents new challenges in terms of patient selection, appropriate timing, and tailored integration.

This chapter presents three clinical scenarios to demonstrate the application of next-generation blood purification techniques: (1) sepsis-associated acute kidney injury (AKI) with hyperinflammation, (2) acute-on-chronic liver failure (ACLF) with hepatorenal syndrome-AKI (HRS-AKI), and (3) refractory hypercapnic respiratory failure. Each case outlines the decision-making process, therapy integration, and clinical outcomes and concludes with key take-home points and future perspectives.

Each scenario is followed by a focused discussion that contextualizes the individual case within the current evidence base, highlighting both clinical rationale and existing limitations.

A. Klopp
III. Department of Medicine, University Medical Center Hamburg-Eppendorf, Hamburg, Germany

Hamburg Center for Kidney Health (HCKH), University Medical Center Hamburg-Eppendorf, Hamburg, Germany
e-mail: a.klopp@uke.de

K. Roedl (✉)
Department of Intensive Care Medicine, University Medical Centre Hamburg-Eppendorf, Hamburg, Germany
e-mail: k.roedl@uke.de

S. De Rosa, S. Lassola (eds.), *Next-Gen Blood Purification*,
https://doi.org/10.1007/978-3-032-27033-7_20

20.2 Case 1—Sepsis-Induced Acute Kidney Injury with Hyperinflammation: Continuous Renal Replacement Therapy Combined with Hemadsorption

A 58-year-old man was admitted to the emergency department (ED) with a 48-h history of fever, productive cough, and progressive dyspnea. His past medical history included arterial hypertension, treated with candesartan and amlodipine, and hyperlipidemia on statin therapy. He was a former smoker with a total of 30 pack-years. No prior kidney disease was known.

On presentation in the ED, the patient was hypotensive (mean arterial pressure 58 mmHg), tachycardic (up to 130/min), febrile (39.4 °C), and hypoxic with an SpO_2 of 86% while receiving 10 L/min oxygen via face mask. Laboratory testing revealed markedly elevated C-reactive protein (310 mg/L), leukocytosis (23 × 10^9/L), and hyperlactatemia (4.8 mmol/L). Thoracic computed tomography demonstrated bilateral consolidation of the right and left lower lobes, consistent with community-acquired pneumonia (CAP).

Given the severely reduced clinical condition with sepsis due to severe CAP, the patient was admitted to the intensive care unit (ICU). Guideline-based (Surviving Sepsis Campaign 2021 [1]) initial sepsis management included crystalloid fluid resuscitation, broad-spectrum antibiotic therapy with meropenem initiated within 1 h, adjunctive intravenous hydrocortisone [2], and vasopressor support with norepinephrine via central venous catheter for blood pressure stabilization. Due to the severe hypoxemia, high-flow nasal cannula therapy was initiated (FiO_2 0.8, flow 50 L/min) in alternation with non-invasive ventilation. However, non-invasive oxygenation strategies failed, with further worsening of hypoxemia and hypercapnia, necessitating endotracheal intubation on the day of admission. After blood cultures confirmed *Streptococcus pneumoniae*, antibiotic therapy was de-escalated to intravenous penicillin.

Within 24 h of ICU admission, further clinical deterioration occurred. Despite norepinephrine at 0.6 μg/kg/min, the target mean arterial pressure (MAP) of 65 mmHg was barely achieved. Therefore, vasopressin was added as a second-line vasopressor to improve hemodynamic support. Urine output declined to <50 mL/h over the preceding 12 h, serum creatinine increased from a baseline of 1.0 mg/dL to 3.5 mg/dL, and metabolic acidosis progressed (pH 7.18, bicarbonate 12 mmol/L). Lactate rose to 6.8 mmol/L. Extended laboratory diagnostics revealed an IL-6 concentration exceeding 10,000 pg/mL, indicating a pronounced hyperinflammatory state.

With acute kidney injury at KDIGO stage 3, refractory metabolic acidosis, hyperkalemia (K^+ 6.0 mmol/L), oliguria with progressive hypervolemia, and ongoing hemodynamic instability, continuous renal replacement therapy (CRRT) delivered as continuous veno-venous hemodialysis (CVVHD) was initiated. Given the degree of cytokine release and persistent vasoplegia, the addition of a hemadsorption device to the CRRT circuit was considered as a rescue option.

The decision to initiate hemadsorption was based primarily on:

- Pathophysiological rationale—high circulating concentrations of proinflammatory mediators are believed to contribute to vasoplegia and multiorgan failure in septic shock [3].
- Risk–benefit assessment—although high-quality evidence for a survival benefit remains limited, in this critically unstable patient, the potential for rapid hemodynamic stabilization and attenuation of hyperinflammation was considered more relevant than the uncertainty regarding long-term outcomes.

The extracorporeal circuit was configured with the hemadsorber in a pre-filter position. CRRT was prescribed at 35 mL/kg/h using regional citrate anticoagulation. Blood flow was maintained at 100–150 mL/min. Hemadsorption was performed for a total of 72 h, with adsorber exchanges every 24 h. Monitoring included continuous assessment of hemodynamics, filter pressures, and circuit integrity, as well as daily measurement of IL-6 and CRP, and close evaluation of lactate clearance.

During the first 36 h, norepinephrine requirements decreased by approximately 50%, lactate levels began to decline, and IL-6 fell from >10,000 pg/mL to 3800 pg/mL by day 3. Urine output gradually improved, and by day 7, a dialysis-free trial was initiated, which was successful. Renal function continued to recover over the following 2 weeks, with serum creatinine at 1.3 mg/dL at hospital discharge.

20.3 Discussion and Key Learning Points

While the observed clinical improvement in this patient was temporally associated with the initiation of cytokine adsorption, interpretation of such findings requires careful consideration of the existing evidence. This case illustrates how the combination of CRRT and hemadsorption can be considered in patients with refractory septic shock, severe AKI, and hyperinflammation. Large randomized controlled trials have not demonstrated improvements in mortality or organ dysfunction scores with hemadsorption [4, 5]. In contrast, smaller prospective studies have reported short-term benefits, including improved hemodynamic stability and reductions in inflammatory markers, particularly in highly unstable patients [6]. However, these therapies carry important limitations and risks. The immune system relies on a delicate balance of pro- and anti-inflammatory cytokines, and indiscriminate removal of both may disrupt normal host defense, hinder infection control, or impair tissue repair. Potential adverse effects, therefore, include sustained immune dysregulation, cellular dysfunction, and organ injury if cytokine clearance is not precisely controlled [7]. Additional concerns include the potential removal of antibiotics, additional costs, the requirement for technical expertise, and—most importantly—the lack of strong guideline recommendations and robust evidence for improved long-term outcomes. Consequently, hemadsorption should not be used routinely; its application should be limited to carefully selected cases or within randomized controlled trials. Further research is essential to clarify optimal timing, patient selection, and biomarker thresholds for initiating such therapies.

20.4 Case 2: Acute-on-Chronic Liver Failure with Hepatorenal Syndrome Treated with ADVOS as Bridge-to-Transplant

A 65-year-old man with a history of alcoholic cirrhosis (Child–Pugh B) was admitted with progressive abdominal distension, fatigue, and confusion for approximately 1 week. He reported abstinence from alcohol for 7 months, though several prior admissions for decompensated cirrhosis had occurred. Baseline creatinine was 1.1 mg/dL, and he had never required RRT.

On arrival at the emergency department, he was febrile (38.6 °C), hypotensive (MAP 55 mmHg), tachycardic (110 bpm), and markedly confused, consistent with hepatic encephalopathy grade II (West Haven). Physical examination revealed tense ascites, scleral icterus, and asterixis. Laboratory results showed leukocytosis (17×10^9/L), total bilirubin 16 mg/dL, INR 3.5, creatinine 2.6 mg/dL, sodium 128 mmol/L, and lactate 3.4 mmol/L. Diagnostic paracentesis confirmed spontaneous bacterial peritonitis (SBP) with >250 neutrophils/μL. The patient was admitted to the ICU, and treatment was initiated with intravenous ceftriaxone and metronidazole, albumin infusion (1.5 g/kg), and norepinephrine infusion targeting a MAP ≥65 mmHg. A trial of terlipressin for suspected HRS-AKI was also initiated but discontinued after 48 h due to lack of hemodynamic and renal response, as well as its known unfavorable side-effect profile, including ischemic complications such as bowel ischemia and pulmonary complications [8].

Despite these measures, clinical deterioration occurred within 72 h. Renal function worsened (creatinine 4.0 mg/dL, urine output <100 mL/day), encephalopathy progressed to grade III, and a severe mixed metabolic and respiratory acidosis developed (pH 7.12, bicarbonate 13 mmol/L, $PaCO_2$ 62 mmHg). Taken together, these findings were consistent with ACLF with HRS-AKI and progressive multiorgan failure. At this stage, escalation from conventional supportive therapy to extracorporeal multiorgan support was considered. Especially, given the present liver and kidney dysfunction with incipient respiratory failure, the multidisciplinary team initiated ADVanced Organ Support (ADVOS) therapy. ADVOS is an integrated extracorporeal multiorgan support system capable of simultaneously supporting liver, kidney, and acid-base homeostasis. It efficiently removes water-soluble and protein-bound toxins, corrects metabolic and respiratory acidosis, and can facilitate fluid management through ultrafiltration. The rationale of using ADVOS included:

- The ability to integrate multiorgan support in a single device.
- Efficient detoxification with removal of both water-soluble and protein-bound toxins at levels comparable to state-of-the-art therapies such as RRT [9] or molecular adsorbent recirculating system (MARS) [10].
- Correction of metabolic and respiratory acidosis via liquid-based direct removal of acids and CO_2 [11].

Six 24-h ADVOS sessions with regional citrate anticoagulation were performed. Optimization of arterial pCO2 and pH was achieved by adjusting the parameters to the patient's actual needs (e.g., dialysate pH 8.5, blood flow of 200 mL/min, and alkaline concentrate with reduced bicarbonate). Continuous ultrafiltration was applied to improve fluid balance and respiratory mechanics. Within the first 24 h, the combined respiratory and metabolic acidosis improved significantly (pH 7.25 vs. 7.12 at baseline). Vasopressor requirements declined (norepinephrine 0.1 μg/kg/min vs. 0.35 μg/kg/min at initiation). Total bilirubin decreased from 16 to 13 mg/dL, neurological status improved, and creatinine stabilized at 3.1 mg/dL with mildly increased urine output (0.5 mL/kg/h).

ADVOS was discontinued on day 6 due to clinical improvement. However, persistent renal impairment necessitated ongoing RRT. With a peak MELD score of 36 and a stabilized clinical condition, the patient was considered eligible for urgent liver transplantation. A suitable graft became available on day 12. Following transplantation, renal function gradually recovered, with creatinine improving to 1.5 mg/dL by postoperative day 10, without further extracorporeal support. The patient was discharged from the ICU on day 26 and from the hospital 3 weeks later, with good graft function and near-normal cognitive performance.

20.5 Discussion and Key Points

In this patient, ADVOS functioned primarily as a bridge-to-transplant strategy rather than as definitive therapy, highlighting the distinction between short-term stabilization and long-term outcome. Although this case illustrates the potential role of ADVOS as a bridging therapy in patients with acute-on-chronic liver failure complicated by HRS-AKI, it is important to acknowledge that almost all currently available data originate from small, uncontrolled clinical studies and observational cohorts [9–13]. Previous extracorporeal liver support systems, such as MARS and Prometheus, have been tested in randomized controlled trials but failed to demonstrate significant improvements in survival or long-term outcomes, highlighting the experimental nature of these therapies [14]. While initial results with ADVOS are promising, adequately powered randomized controlled trials are still lacking, and thus, the true clinical impact of ADVOS remains uncertain. Future research should aim to define clear surrogate markers and patient populations most likely to benefit, for example, individuals like in this case with acute-on-chronic liver failure and concomitant renal dysfunction. Beyond liver failure, ADVOS has also shown encouraging results in patients with ARDS and multiorgan failure [15, 16], particularly through its ability to support acid–base homeostasis and facilitate CO_2 removal. Ongoing and planned clinical studies, such as ADVOVENT (DRKS00015874), are exploring additional indications for ADVOS, including the facilitation of ultraprotective ventilation strategies by enabling extracorporeal CO_2 removal and thereby potentially reducing the need for invasive mechanical ventilation. The establishment of robust evidence will be crucial if ADVOS is to achieve wider acceptance within the international intensive care and liver transplant community.

20.6 Case 3—Severe ARDS Refractory to Conventional Therapy: Escalation from multiECCO$_2$R to vv-ECMO with Fatal Outcome

A 54-year-old woman with obesity class II (BMI 37 kg/m^2), COPD, arterial hypertension, and type 2 diabetes mellitus presented to the emergency department after 5 days of progressive dyspnea, fever, and productive cough. On admission, she was tachypneic (respiratory rate 38/min), tachycardic (HR 125/min), hypoxemic (SpO_2 78% on 12 L/min oxygen via face mask), and hemodynamically unstable (MAP 62 mmHg, norepinephrine 0.2 μg/kg/min).

Chest CT revealed bilateral diffuse ground-glass opacities and consolidations, consistent with severe pneumonia-related ARDS (PaO_2/FiO_2 68 mmHg). Endotracheal intubation was performed on the day of admission, with an initial attempt at lung-protective ventilation (tidal volume < 6 mL/kg predicted body weight, PEEP 14 cmH_2O). Despite progressive escalation of ventilatory pressures into the non-protective range, inhaled nitric oxide (NO) and prolonged prone positioning (>16 h/day), the patient developed worsening hypercapnia with severe respiratory acidosis ($PaCO_2$ > 95 mmHg, pH 7.10).

Given refractory hypercapnia and worsening renal function, a CRRT with an extracorporeal carbon dioxide removal ("multiECCO$_2$R gas exchanger") was initiated to facilitate CO_2 removal. Shortly after initiation, $PaCO_2$ decreased from 95 to 75 mmHg and pH improved transiently to 7.22. However, oxygenation remained critically impaired, and over the next 24 h, the patient developed progressive hypoxemia (PaO_2/FiO_2 < 60 mmHg) and worsening hemodynamic instability despite escalating vasopressor support (norepinephrine 0.45 μg/kg/min).

At this point, the patient fulfilled EOLIA criteria for veno-venous ECMO (vv-ECMO) initiation (PaO_2/FiO_2 < 80 mmHg for >6 h and pH < 7.25 with $PaCO_2$ > 60 mmHg >6 h) [17]. A vv-ECMO was therefore implanted (femoro-jugular cannulation, initial flow >2.4 L/min, continuous heparin anticoagulation, aPTT target 40–50 s). ECMO provided improvement in oxygenation (PaO_2/FiO_2 ~ 120 mmHg), allowing reduction of ventilatory pressures (plateau <28 cmH_2O). Prone positioning was continued under ECMO support.

Over the following days, the patient developed multiple severe complications. Thrombocytopenia (25 × 10^9/L) and recurrent bleeding at cannulation sites required temporary interruption of anticoagulation. Despite broad anti-infective therapy with meropenem and vancomycin, inflammatory markers remained elevated. Persistent renal dysfunction with oliguria necessitated continuation of CRRT. Vasoplegia persisted with rising lactate levels (>8 mmol/L) despite vv-ECMO flow adjustments and maximal vasopressor therapy.

Despite optimized vv-ECMO management and full intensive care support, oxygenation deteriorated once more (PaO_2/FiO_2 < 100 mmHg), hypercapnia remained uncontrolled, and the patient's hemodynamic instability worsened. On day 10 of ICU admission, the patient developed refractory septic shock with irreversible cardiovascular collapse and cardiac arrest, unresponsive to resuscitation efforts. This unfavorable outcome underscores the need to distinguish between technological feasibility and meaningful clinical benefit when escalating extracorporeal support.

20.7 Discussion and Learning Points

In this case, multiECCO$_2$R was initiated as an intermediate step to control refractory hypercapnia. Besides facilitating extracorporeal CO_2 removal, such systems may offer additional benefits through their integration with RRT platforms, enabling simultaneous correction of acidosis, fluid balance, and electrolyte disturbances. However, multiECCO$_2$R remains an experimental therapy with very limited clinical evidence and should therefore be restricted to highly selected patients or ideally applied within randomized controlled trials. These devices are further limited by their reliance on the patient's own cardiac output and are largely ineffective in correcting severe hypoxemia. While multiECCO$_2$R may serve as a bridge in patients with predominant hypercapnic failure (e.g., COPD exacerbations), its role in fulminant ARDS with life-threatening hypoxemia is limited. In such settings, vv-ECMO is generally considered the preferred rescue strategy. Vv-ECMO is in fact an established treatment option for severe, refractory ARDS and has been shown to improve survival, with reported survival rates between 50% and 70% in experienced centers [17, 18]. However, it is a highly invasive treatment with substantial risks, requiring strict patient selection, clear indications, and expert management. Complications such as bleeding, thrombocytopenia, and infection remain common and can significantly impact outcome. Guidelines recommend that vv-ECMO therapy should only be performed in high-volume centers (>20 cases/year) with specialized expertise [19, 20].

This case illustrates that vv-ECMO is not a guarantee of recovery, but rather a bridge therapy in selected patients. Even with timely escalation and technically correct management, ECMO-related complications and poor outcomes remain part of the clinical reality in intensive care. Careful patient selection, early initiation, and continuous reassessment of therapy goals are crucial to optimize outcomes while acknowledging the inherent limitations of extracorporeal support.

20.8 Conclusion

The three cases presented in this chapter illustrate the broad spectrum of extracorporeal therapies in critical care—from CRRT combined with hemadsorption in septic shock, to advanced organ support in acute-on-chronic liver failure, and the escalation from extracorporeal carbon dioxide removal devices (ECCO$_2$R) to vv-ECMO in severe ARDS. These examples highlight both the potential and the limitations of extracorporeal support.

While in some patients, extracorporeal techniques can provide life-saving stabilization or bridge to transplantation, in others, even optimal application may not alter the fatal trajectory of critical illness. Therefore, strict patient selection, individualized timing of initiation, and careful monitoring remain key. Together, these cases demonstrate how extracorporeal therapies may serve as rescue, bridge, or supportive strategies depending on disease trajectory and patient selection.

The current evidence base is still limited: most modalities are supported by small clinical trials, registries, or observational data rather than large randomized controlled studies. Nevertheless, emerging data, ongoing trials, and technological improvements suggest a growing role of extracorporeal therapies in the future.

Ultimately, extracorporeal support should be understood as part of a multimodal, interdisciplinary intensive care strategy, not as a stand-alone solution. Collaboration between nephrology, hepatology, cardiology, and critical care teams, along with structured training and concentration of experience in specialized centers, will be crucial to maximize patient benefit and ensure safe application of these complex technologies.

References

1. Evans L, Rhodes A, Alhazzani W, Antonelli M, Coopersmith CM, French C, et al. Surviving sepsis campaign: international guidelines for management of sepsis and septic shock 2021. Crit Care Med. 2021;49(11):e1063–e143.
2. Dequin P-F, Meziani F, Quenot J-P, Kamel T, Ricard J-D, Badie J, et al. Hydrocortisone in severe community-acquired pneumonia. N Engl J Med. 2023;388(21):1931–41.
3. Burgdorff A-M, Bucher M, Schumann J. Vasoplegia in patients with sepsis and septic shock: pathways and mechanisms. J Int Med Res. 2018;46(4):1303–10.
4. Schädler D, Pausch C, Heise D, Meier-Hellmann A, Brederlau J, Weiler N, et al. The effect of a novel extracorporeal cytokine hemoadsorption device on IL-6 elimination in septic patients: a randomized controlled trial. PLoS One. 2017;12(10):e0187015.
5. Diab M, Lehmann T, Bothe W, Akhyari P, Platzer S, Wendt D, et al. Cytokine hemoadsorption during cardiac surgery versus standard surgical care for infective endocarditis (REMOVE): results from a multicenter randomized controlled trial. Circulation. 2022;145(13):959–68.
6. Friesecke S, Stecher S-S, Gross S, Felix SB, Nierhaus A. Extracorporeal cytokine elimination as rescue therapy in refractory septic shock: a prospective single-center study. J Artif Organs. 2017;20(3):252–9.
7. Graf H, Gräfe C, Bruegel M, Happich FL, Wustrow V, Wegener A, et al. Extracorporeal elimination of pro-and anti-inflammatory modulators by the cytokine adsorber CytoSorb® in patients with hyperinflammation: a prospective study. Infect Dis Ther. 2024;13(9):2089–101.
8. Sagi SV, Mittal S, Kasturi KS, Sood GK. Terlipressin therapy for reversal of type 1 hepatorenal syndrome: a meta-analysis of randomized controlled trials. J Gastroenterol Hepatol. 2010;25(5):880–5.
9. Kaps L, Ahlbrand C, Gadban R, Nagel M, Labenz C, Klimpke P, et al. Applicability and safety of discontinuous ADVanced organ support (ADVOS) in the treatment of patients with acute-on-chronic liver failure (ACLF) outside of intensive care. PLoS One. 2021;16(4):e0249342.
10. Falkensteiner C, Kortgen A, Leonhardt J, Bauer M, Sponholz C. Comparison of albumin dialysis devices molecular adsorbent recirculating system and ADVanced organ support system in critically ill patients with liver failure—a retrospective analysis. Ther Apher Dial. 2021;25(2):225–36.
11. Fuhrmann V, Weber T, Roedl K, Motaabbed J, Tariparast A, Jarczak D, et al. Advanced organ support (ADVOS) in the critically ill: first clinical experience in patients with multiple organ failure. Ann Intensive Care. 2020;10(1):96.

12. Huber W, Henschel B, Schmid R, Al-Chalabi A. First clinical experience in 14 patients treated with ADVOS: a study on feasibility, safety and efficacy of a new type of albumin dialysis. BMC Gastroenterol. 2017;17(1):32.
13. Fuhrmann V, de Garibay APR, Faltlhauser A, Tyczynski B, Jarczak D, Lutz J, et al. Registry on extracorporeal multiple organ support with the advanced organ support (ADVOS) system: 2-year interim analysis. Medicine. 2021;100(7):e24653.
14. García Martínez JJ, Bendjelid K. Artificial liver support systems: what is new over the last decade? Ann Intensive Care. 2018;8(1):109.
15. Allescher J, Rasch S, Wiessner JR, Ruiz P, de Garibay A, Huberle C, Hesse F, et al. Extracorporeal carbon dioxide removal with the advanced organ support system in critically ill COVID-19 patients. Artif Organs. 2021;45(12):1522–32.
16. Huber W, Lorenz G, Heilmaier M, Böttcher K, Sahm P, Middelhoff M, et al. Extracorporeal multiorgan support including CO2-removal with the ADVanced organ support (ADVOS) system for COVID-19: a case report. Int J Artif Organs. 2021;44(4):288–94.
17. Combes A, Peek GJ, Hajage D, Hardy P, Abrams D, Schmidt M, et al. ECMO for severe ARDS: systematic review and individual patient data meta-analysis. Intensive Care Med. 2020;46(11):2048–57.
18. Munshi L, Walkey A, Goligher E, Pham T, Uleryk EM, Fan E. Venovenous extracorporeal membrane oxygenation for acute respiratory distress syndrome: a systematic review and meta-analysis. Lancet Respir Med. 2019;7(2):163–72.
19. Combes A, Brodie D, Bartlett R, Brochard L, Brower R, Conrad S, et al. Position paper for the organization of extracorporeal membrane oxygenation programs for acute respiratory failure in adult patients. Am J Respir Crit Care Med. 2014;190(5):488–96.
20. Tonna JE, Abrams D, Brodie D, Greenwood JC, Mateo-Sidron JAR, Usman A, et al. Management of adult patients supported with venovenous extracorporeal membrane oxygenation (VV ECMO): guideline from the extracorporeal life support organization (ELSO). ASAIO J. 2021;67(6):601–10.

21 The Future of Blood Purification: What's Next?

Silvia De Rosa and Sergio Lassola

21.1 Introduction

Blood purification has a long and fascinating history, stretching from ancient bloodletting to the highly engineered extracorporeal systems we know today. Early medicine saw blood removal as a universal cure, based on humoral theory rather than physiology [1]. The twentieth century marked the first true paradigm shift, with Willem Kolff's pioneering rotating drum kidney in the 1940s proving that extracorporeal removal of toxins could sustain life. From there, progress accelerated [2]. Regenerated cellulose membranes dominated the early decades, offering basic small-solute clearance but limited biocompatibility. The introduction of synthetic polymers in the 1970s–1980s (polysulfone, polyethersulfone, polyacrylonitrile) revolutionized dialysis [3], allowing higher fluxes, better middle-molecule clearance, and improved hemocompatibility. Parallel to this, sorbent technologies emerged: coated charcoal and ion-exchange resins extended extracorporeal therapy

Supplementary Information The online version contains supplementary material available at https://doi.org/10.1007/978-3-032-27033-7_21.

S. De Rosa (✉)
Centre for Medical Sciences, University of Trento, Trento, Italy

Anesthesia and Intensive Care, Santa Chiara Hospital, Trento, Italy
e-mail: silvia.derosa@unitn.it

S. Lassola
Anesthesia and Intensive Care, Santa Chiara Hospital, Trento, Italy
e-mail: sergio.lassola@apss.tn.it

S. De Rosa, S. Lassola (eds.), *Next-Gen Blood Purification*,
https://doi.org/10.1007/978-3-032-27033-7_21

to toxin removal, inflammatory modulation, and multi-organ support [4]. Hybrid systems integrating membranes and sorbents expanded capabilities, enabling simultaneous diffusive, convective, and adsorptive clearance. This evolution mirrored a philosophical change: dialysis and blood purification were no longer seen solely as "survival therapy" for end-stage kidney disease, but as tools to improve quality of life, preserve residual function, and even intervene early in acute illness [5]. This chapter outlines the anticipated trajectory of blood purification technologies, highlighting near-term innovations expected by 2035 and longer-term breakthroughs that could redefine the boundaries of extracorporeal therapy in the decades ahead.

21.2 The Current Landscape of Blood Purification

Today, blood purification encompasses a spectrum of membrane and sorbent-based technologies tailored to diverse clinical needs. High-flux membranes dominate modern hemodialysis, providing superior removal of middle molecules such as β_2-microglobulin [5]. High cut-off (HCO) membranes, with even larger pores, are used for specific scenarios like removing myeloma light chains, albeit with the trade-off of potential albumin loss [6]. Medium cut-off (MCO) membranes offer a balanced approach, delivering strong middle-molecule clearance with minimal protein leakage, increasingly becoming the standard for both chronic and acute settings. Sorbent integration has gained renewed interest, particularly in sepsis, liver failure, and intoxication [7]. Devices such as hemoperfusion cartridges and hemoadsorption columns can be used alone or in series with dialyzers, targeting protein-bound and hydrophobic toxins beyond the reach of membranes alone. Multifunctional systems now combine high-performance membranes with dedicated sorbent modules, offering comprehensive clearance profiles in a single circuit [8]. Wearable and home-based blood purification technologies are emerging, aiming to provide continuous, low-intensity therapy that aligns with patients' daily lives. Miniaturized dialyzers, portable sorbent-based detox units, and low-power pump systems are being tested in both chronic kidney disease and high-risk acute care populations. These solutions promise to reduce hospital dependency, expand treatment access, and shift the paradigm toward patient-centered, lifestyle-compatible care [9]. In sum, modern blood purification is no longer a one-size-fits-all intervention. It is a modular, multimodal, and increasingly personalized field, shaped by advances in materials science, bioengineering, and clinical insight and poised for further transformation in the era of digital health and precision medicine.

21.3 Achievements and Unresolved Challenges

Over the past decades, blood purification technologies have transformed survival prospects for patients with kidney failure, severe intoxications, and critical illnesses. Modern high-flux membranes, sorbents, and hybrid systems have improved small and middle molecule clearance, reduced treatment times, and expanded the scope of extracorporeal therapies beyond nephrology to sepsis [10], liver failure, and autoimmune disorders. These advances have not only extended life expectancy but also improved patient-reported outcomes such as fatigue, functional status, and quality of life. Biocompatibility has seen remarkable progress. Early cellulose membranes often triggered inflammation and clotting, whereas today's synthetic, surface-modified materials reduce complement activation, platelet adhesion, and cytokine release. Yet, the risk of chronic microinflammation, vascular access complications, and albumin loss persists, particularly in high cut-off or sorbent-based systems [11]. Accessibility remains a central challenge. While advanced dialyzers and multifunctional cartridges are available in high-income settings, their cost, infrastructure demands, and maintenance requirements limit adoption in low- and middle-income countries [12]. Portable and home-based systems hold promise for decentralizing care, but affordability, training, and technical support must be addressed to prevent widening global disparities. Economic considerations intersect with clinical decision-making. Health systems must balance investment in cutting-edge technology with long-term sustainability, reimbursement policies, and equitable access [13]. Regulatory frameworks, especially those governing water purity, dialysate quality, and device safety, have tightened in response to high-profile contamination events, raising the standard for manufacturing and clinical operation. Nevertheless, disparities in enforcement remain across regions, leaving some patients at greater risk. The field now faces a dual mission: consolidate the achievements of the past half-century while tackling persistent shortcomings. The goal is not simply to remove toxins more efficiently, but to integrate these technologies into care pathways that are patient-centered, cost-effective, and globally accessible.

Table 21.1 summarizes the evolution of blood purification from its historical roots to current capabilities and future ambitions, highlighting technological, clinical, and collaborative shifts that underpin the field's transformation.

Table 21.1 From past to future: key themes in the evolution of blood purification

Theme	Past	Present	Future
Technology	Cellulose membranes, basic diffusion	Synthetic high-flux and MCO membranes, hybrid sorbent systems	Biohybrid, implantable, AI-driven devices
Clinical scope	End-stage kidney disease survival therapy	Chronic and acute kidney care, liver failure, sepsis	Multi-organ support platforms
Treatment model	Hospital-based, intermittent	Mixed hospital and home therapies	Fully portable, continuous, home-integrated
Goals	Life-saving	Improved quality of life and function	Continuous, personalized, preventive therapy
Collaboration	Isolated expertise	Multidisciplinary clinical–engineering links	Global, open-access innovation networks

Notes: *MCO* Medium Cut-Off membrane, *AI* Artificial Intelligence

21.4 The Innovation Pipeline

The next generation of blood purification technologies is being shaped by a convergence of engineering, materials science, and digital health. Nanotechnology now allows unprecedented precision in pore geometry, enabling membranes that can selectively target uremic toxins while sparing essential proteins. Surface functionalization, through molecular coatings or embedded bioactive agents, adds new capabilities, such as reducing clot formation or neutralizing inflammatory mediators directly on the membrane [14]. Artificial intelligence and biosensors are beginning to transform how therapies are delivered. Real-time monitoring of solute levels, hemodynamic parameters, and patient biomarkers can enable adaptive treatment, where device settings adjust automatically to changing physiological conditions. This approach promises not only greater efficiency but also personalization of therapy to individual patient needs. Miniaturization is another frontier. Wearable artificial kidneys (WAKs), compact portable devices, and even fully implantable systems are moving from prototype to early clinical testing. These devices aim to free patients from fixed treatment schedules, offering continuous purification that more closely mimics natural kidney function. However, challenges remain in power supply, clot prevention, and ensuring safety outside specialized centers [15]. Biohybrid approaches are also on the horizon, integrating living cells into synthetic scaffolds to create regenerative filtration units. These could eventually combine mechanical clearance with metabolic and endocrine functions, representing a true leap toward artificial organ replacement [16]. A schematic overview of the expected evolution of blood purification technologies over the next two decades is shown in Fig. 21.1.

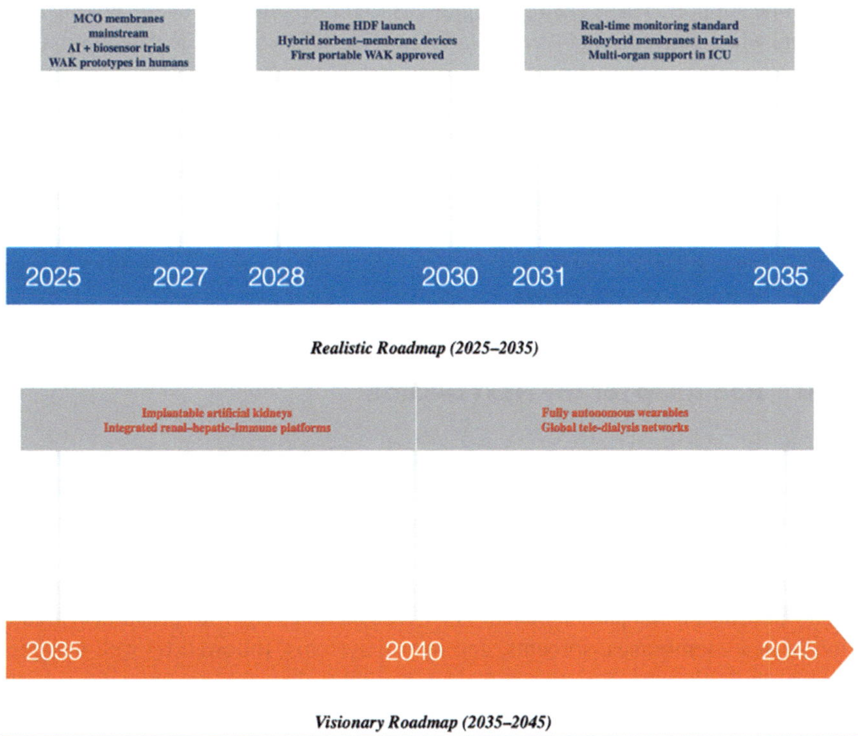

Fig. 21.1 Roadmap for the next two decades in blood purification technologies. This timeline outlines realistic milestones expected between 2025 and 2035, including the adoption of MCO membranes, AI integration, and wearable dialysis devices, as well as visionary goals for 2035–2045 such as implantable artificial kidneys and global tele-dialysis networks. The roadmap distinguishes near-term developments based on current R&D from long-term innovations requiring major breakthroughs. It serves as a guide for clinicians, engineers, and policymakers to align strategies and investments. *Notes*: *MCO*, Medium Cut-Off Membrane, *AI* Artificial Intelligence, *HDF* Hemodiafiltration, *WAK* Wearable Artificial Kidney, *ICU* Intensive Care Unit

21.5 Looking Beyond the Kidney

Blood purification has traditionally been synonymous with renal replacement, but its scope is expanding into multi-organ support. Advanced platforms can now integrate renal, hepatic, and immunomodulatory functions in a single circuit, opening possibilities for patients with complex, multi-system failure. In sepsis, where a dysregulated immune response drives organ damage, extracorporeal devices equipped with sorbents or immunoactive membranes can selectively remove cytokines, endotoxins, and other inflammatory mediators. Such "immune rebalancing" strategies are being tested as adjuncts to standard care, with the aim of reducing mortality and preventing long-term disability [17]. For hepatic failure, albumin dialysis systems and bioartificial livers combine filtration, adsorption, and metabolic support. These can bridge patients to transplant or recovery, buying critical time when conventional therapy falls short [18]. Beyond acute care, detoxification systems are being explored for rare metabolic disorders, oncology-related toxin removal, and even enhancing recovery from major surgery. This broadening of indications requires careful tailoring of membrane and sorbent properties, along with integration into existing care pathways [18]. The future is likely to see "all-in-one" extracorporeal platforms capable of supporting multiple organs, guided by continuous data streams and AI-driven decision support. In this vision, blood purification becomes less a stand-alone therapy and more a core component of personalized, multi-system critical care.

21.6 Roadmap for the Next Decade

The coming decade will define how blood purification technologies move from promising prototypes to routine, life-changing interventions. Success will depend on coordinated progress across science, engineering, clinical practice, and health policy.

Translational research priorities should focus on closing the gap between laboratory innovation and patient benefit [19]. This includes rigorous preclinical validation of new membranes, sorbents, and hybrid systems, followed by well-designed clinical trials that measure not just clearance rates, but also patient-centered outcomes such as functional recovery, quality of life, and long-term survival. Special emphasis should be placed on devices that enable continuous, physiologically aligned therapy, whether in the ICU, outpatient setting, or at home.

Collaborative networks will be the engine of progress. Bringing together clinicians, biomedical engineers, material scientists, and industry partners in structured consortia can shorten development cycles and ensure that design decisions are clinically relevant from the outset [20]. Such networks should also engage regulatory bodies early, aligning safety standards and trial endpoints with emerging technologies. International registries and open-access data sharing can accelerate learning and avoid duplication of effort.

Policy and reimbursement frameworks will be critical in determining how quickly patients can access next-generation devices. Payers and policymakers must recognize the long-term economic and societal benefits of therapies that reduce hospitalizations [21], improve productivity, and enhance quality of life. Bundled payment models and value-based reimbursement can incentivize adoption while ensuring sustainability for healthcare systems. Public–private partnerships could play a pivotal role in de-risking investment in novel but costly technologies, such as wearable artificial kidneys or biohybrid devices.

Education and patient empowerment must evolve alongside technology. Clinicians will need updated training on device selection, troubleshooting, and integration into care pathways. Patients and caregivers should receive accessible, personalized education that enables them to confidently manage home-based therapies. Digital tools, such as smartphone-linked biosensors and virtual coaching platforms, can enhance engagement and adherence [22].

Finally, the roadmap must remain *flexible and adaptive,* incorporating feedback from early adopters and adjusting to unexpected challenges—whether these are technical failures, safety concerns, or shifts in healthcare delivery models. The ultimate goal is a blood purification ecosystem that is more patient-centric, seamlessly integrated into multi-organ support, and capable of delivering individualized therapy anywhere, anytime. If achieved, this vision will not only improve survival but also redefine what it means to live well with kidney disease, liver failure, sepsis, or other conditions where extracorporeal support plays a role. The next decade offers a rare opportunity to align scientific ambition with real-world impact, and the time to act is now.

21.7 Conclusions

Over the past century, blood purification has evolved from a last-resort survival intervention to a cornerstone of modern critical and chronic care. Advances in membrane engineering, sorbent technology, and hybrid systems have broadened its clinical scope, improved patient outcomes, and laid the groundwork for a new era of personalized, continuous therapy. The next decade presents an opportunity to translate promising prototypes—such as wearable artificial kidneys, AI-guided treatment platforms, and biohybrid devices—into everyday clinical practice.

Success will require a coordinated effort that bridges scientific innovation and real-world adoption. Clinicians, engineers, regulators, and industry must work together in structured, data-driven networks, ensuring that emerging technologies are safe, effective, and aligned with patient needs. Policies and reimbursement strategies must recognize the long-term value of reducing hospitalizations, improving quality of life, and enabling home-based care, while equitable access must remain a guiding principle.

Ultimately, the vision is for blood purification to become seamlessly integrated into daily life, continuous, adaptive, and multi-organ in scope—offering not just survival but a fuller, healthier life for patients with kidney disease, liver failure, sepsis, or other complex conditions. Achieving this will require flexibility, global collaboration, and an unwavering focus on the patient experience. If realized, the transformation will redefine the boundaries of extracorporeal medicine for decades to come.

References

1. Ronco C. Continuous renal replacement therapy: forty-year anniversary. Int J Artif Organs. 2017;40:257–64.
2. Sharma N, Khav E, Elahmadi A, Ong J, Parag S. Dr. Willem Kolff: the father of the artificial kidney. Cureus. 2024;16:e69098.
3. Wang S, Lu A, Zhang L. Recent advances in regenerated cellulose materials. Prog Polym Sci. 2016;53:169–206.

4. Clark WR, Ferrari F, La Manna G, Ronco C. Extracorporeal sorbent technologies: basic concepts and clinical application. In: La Manna G, Ronco C, editors. Contributions to nephrology. Basel: S. Karger AG; 2017. p. 43–57.
5. Vega-Vega O, Ronco C, Martínez-Rueda AJ. Pushing the boundaries of hemodialysis: innovations in membranes and sorbents. Rev Investig Clin. 2023;75:274–88.
6. Gondouin B, Hutchison CA. High cut-off dialysis membranes: current uses and future potential. Adv Chronic Kidney Dis. 2011;18:180–7.
7. Zweigart C, Boschetti-de-Fierro A, Hulko M, Nilsson L-G, Beck W, Storr M, Krause B. Medium cut-off membranes – closer to the natural kidney removal function. Int J Artif Organs. 2017;40:328–34.
8. Damianaki A, Stambolliu E, Alexakou Z, Petras D. Expanding the potential therapeutic options of hemoperfusion in the era of improved sorbent biocompatibility. Kidney Res Clin Pract. 2023;42:298–311.
9. Armignacco P, Lorenzin A, Neri M, Nalesso F, Garzotto F, Ronco C. Wearable devices for blood purification: principles, miniaturization, and technical challenges. Semin Dial. 2015;28:125–30.
10. De Rosa S, Marengo M, Fiorentino M, et al. Extracorporeal blood purification therapies for sepsis-associated acute kidney injury in critically ill patients: expert opinion from the SIAARTI-SIN joint commission. J Nephrol. 2023;36:1731–42.
11. Bonomini M, Piscitani L, Di Liberato L, Sirolli V. Biocompatibility of surface-modified membranes for chronic hemodialysis therapy. Biomedicine. 2022;10:844.
12. Haroon S, Davenport A. Choosing a dialyzer: what clinicians need to know. Hemodial Int. 2018;22(S2):S65–74. https://doi.org/10.1111/hdi.12702.
13. Sapkota S, Dhakal A, Rushton S, Van Teijlingen E, Marahatta SB, Balen J, Lee AC. The impact of decentralisation on health systems: a systematic review of reviews. BMJ Glob Health. 2023;8:e013317.
14. Wieszczycka K, Staszak K, Woźniak-Budych MJ, Litowczenko J, Maciejewska BM, Jurga S. Surface functionalization—the way for advanced applications of smart materials. Coord Chem Rev. 2021;436:213846.
15. Jin X, Liu C, Xu T, Su L, Zhang X. Artificial intelligence biosensors: challenges and prospects. Biosens Bioelectron. 2020;165:112412.
16. Wang C, Zhang Z, Wang J, Wang Q, Shang L. Biohybrid materials: structure design and biomedical applications. Mater Today Bio. 2022;16:100352.
17. Mehta Y, Paul R, Ansari AS, et al. Extracorporeal blood purification strategies in sepsis and septic shock: an insight into recent advancements. World J Crit Care Med. 2023;12:71–88.
18. Tsipotis E, Shuja A, Jaber BL. Albumin dialysis for liver failure: a systematic review. Adv Chronic Kidney Dis. 2015;22:382–90.
19. Mahalmani V, Sinha S, Prakash A, Medhi B. Translational research: bridging the gap between preclinical and clinical research. Indian J Pharmacol. 2022;54:393–6.
20. Sankaran RR, Ameling JM, Cohn AEM, Grum CM, Meddings J. A practical guide for building collaborations between clinical researchers and engineers: lessons learned from a multidisciplinary patient safety project. J Patient Saf. 2021;17:e1420–7.
21. Wagenschieber E, Blunck D. Impact of reimbursement systems on patient care—a systematic review of systematic reviews. Health Econ Rev. 2024;14:22.
22. Nguyen AM, Rivera AM, Gualtieri L. A new health care paradigm: the power of digital health and E-patients. Mayo Clin Proc Digit Health. 2023;1:203–9.

Index

S. De Rosa, S. Lassola (eds.), *Next-Gen Blood Purification*,
https://doi.org/10.1007/978-3-032-27033-7